New developments in quantitative coronary arteriography

DEVELOPMENTS IN CARDIOVASCULAR MEDICINE

Recent volumes

Hanrath P, Bleifeld W, Souquet, J. eds: Cardiovascular diagnosis by ultrasound. Transesophageal, computerized, contrast, Doppler echocardiography. 1982. ISBN 90-247-2692-1.

Roelandt J, ed: The practice of M-mode and two-dimensional echocardiography. 1983. ISBN 90-247-2745-6.

Meyer J, Schweizer P, Erbel R, eds: Advances in noninvasive cardiology. 1983. ISBN 0-89838-576-8.

Morganroth J, Moore EN, eds: Sudden cardiac death and congestive heart failure: Diagnosis and treatment. 1983. ISBN 0-89838-580-6.

Perry HM, ed: Lifelong management of hypertension. 1983. ISBN 0-89838-582-2.

Jaffe EA, ed: Biology of endothelial cells. 1984. ISBN 0-89838-587-3.

Surawicz B, Reddy CP, Prystowsky EN, eds: Tachycardias. 1984. ISBN 0-89838-588-1.

Spencer MP, ed: Cardiac Doppler diagnosis. 1983. ISBN 0-89838-591-1.

Villarreal H, Sambhi MP, eds: Topics in pathophysiology of hypertension. 1984. ISBN 0-89838-595-4.

Messerli FH, ed: Cardiovascular disease in the elderly. 1984. ISBN 0-89838-596-2.

Simoons ML, Reiber JHC, eds: Nuclear imaging in clinical cardiology. 1984. ISBN 0-89838-599-7.

Ter Keurs HEDJ, Schipperheyn JJ, eds: Cardiac left ventricular hypertrophy. 1983. ISBN 0-89838-612-8.

Sperelakis N, ed: Physiology and pathophysiology of the heart. 1984. ISBN 0-89838-615-2.

Messerli FH, ed: Kidney in essential hypertension. 1984. ISBN 0-89838-616-0.

Sambhi MP, ed: Fundamental fault in hypertension. 1984. ISBN 0-89838-638-1.

Marchesi C, ed: Ambulatory monitoring: Cardiovascular system and allied applications. 1984. ISBN 0-89838-642-X.

Kupper W, MacAlpin RN, Bleifeld W, eds: Coronary tone in ischemic heart disease. 1984. ISBN 0-89838-646-2.

Sperelakis N, Caulfield JB, eds: Calcium antagonists: Mechanisms of action on cardiac muscle and vascular smooth muscle. 1984. ISBN 0-89838-655-1.

Godfraind T, Herman AS, Wellens D, eds: Calcium entry blockers in cardiovascular and cerebral dysfunctions. 1984. ISBN 0-89838-658-6.

Morganroth J, Moore EN, eds: Interventions in the acute phase of myocardial infarction. 1984. ISBN 0-89838-659-4.

Abel FL, Newman WH, eds: Functional aspects of the normal, hypertrophied, and failing heart. 1984. ISBN 0-89838-665-9.

Sideman S, Beyar R, eds: Simulation and imaging of the cardiac system. 1985. ISBN 0-89838-687-X.

Van der Wall E, Lie KI, eds: Recent views on hypertrophic cardiomyopathy. 1985. ISBN 0-89838-694-2.

Beamish RE, Singal PK, Dhalla NS, eds: Stress and heart disease. 1985. ISBN 0-89838-709-4.

Beamish RE, Panagio V, Dhalla NS, eds: Pathogenesis of stress-induced heart disease. 1985. ISBN 0-89838-710-8.

Morganroth J, Moore EN, eds: Cardiac arrhythmias. 1985. ISBN 0-89838-716-7.

Mathes E, ed: Secondary prevention is coronary artery disease and myocardial infarction. 1985. ISBN 0-89838-736-1.

Lowell Stone H, Weglicki WB, eds: Pathology of cardiovascular injury. 1985. ISBN 0-89838-743-4.

Meyer J, Erbel R, Rupprecht HJ, eds: Improvement of myocardial perfusion. 1985. ISBN 0-89838-748-5.

Reiber JHC, Serruys PW, Slager CJ: Quantitative coronary and left ventricular cineangiography. 1986. ISBN 0-89838-760-4.

Fagard RH, Bekaert IE, eds: Sports cardiology. 1986. ISBN 0-89838-782-5.

Reiber JHC, Serruys PW, eds: State of the art in quantitative coronary arteriography. 1986. ISBN 0-89838-804-X.

Roelandt J, ed: Color Doppler Flow Imaging. 1986. ISBN 0-89838-806-6.

Van der Wall EE, ed: Noninvasive imaging of cardiac metabolism. 1986. ISBN 0-89838-812-0.

Liebman J, Plonsey R, Rudy Y, eds: Pediatric and fundamental electrocardiography. 1986. ISBN 0-89838-815-5.

Hilger HH, Hombach V, Rashkind WJ, eds: Invasive cardiovascular therapy. 1987. ISBN 0-89838-818-X.

Serruys PW, Meester GT, eds: Coronary angioplasty: a controlled model for ischemia. 1986. ISBN 0-89838-819-8.

Tooke JE, Smaje LH: Clinical investigation of the microcirculation. 1986. ISBN 0-89838-833-3.

Van Dam RTh, Van Oosterom A, eds: Electrocardiographic body surface mapping. 1986. ISBN 0-89838-834-1.

Spencer MP, ed: Ultrasonic diagnosis of cerebrovascular disease. 1987. ISBN 0-89838-836-8.

Legato MJ, ed: The stressed heart. 1987. ISBN 0-89838-849-X.

Roelandt J, ed: Digital techniques in echocardiography. 1987. ISBN 0-89838-861-9.

Sideman S, Beyar R, eds: Activation, metabolism and perfusion of the heart. 1987. ISBN 0-89838-871-6.

Safar ME et al., eds: Arterial and venous systems in essential hypertension. 1987. ISBN 0-89838-857-0.

Ter Keurs HEDJ, Tyberg JV, eds: Mechanics of the circulation. 1987. ISBN 0-89838-870-8.

Aliot E, Lazzara R, eds: Ventricular tachycardias. 1987. ISBN 0-89838-881-3.

Schneeweiss A, Schettler G, eds: Cardiovascular drug therapy in the elderly. 1987. ISBN 0-89838-883-X.

Chapman JV, Sgalambro A, eds: Basic concepts in Doppler echocardiography. 1987. ISBN 0-89838-888-0.

Chien S, Dormandy J, Ernst E, Matrai A, eds: Clinical hemorheology. 1987. ISBN 0-89838-807-4.

Morganroth J, Moore EN, eds: Congestive heart failure. 1986. ISBN 0-89838-955-0.

Messerli FH, ed: Cardiovascular disease in the elderly, 2nd ed. 1987. ISBN 0-89838-962-3.

Heintzen PH, Bursch JH, eds: Progress in digital angiocardiography. 1987. ISBN 0-89838-965-8.

Scheinman M, ed: Catheter ablation of cardiac arrhythmias. 1987. ISBN 0-89838-967-4.

Spaan JAE, Bruschke AVG, Gittenberger AC, eds: Coronary circulation. 1987. ISBN 0-89838-978-X.

Visser C et al., eds: Echocardiography in coronary artery disease. 1987. ISBN 0-89838-979-8.

Bayes de Luna A, ed: Therapeutics in cardiology. 1987. ISBN 0-89838-981-X.

Mirvis DM, ed: Body surface electrocardiographic mapping. 1987. ISBN 0-89838-983-6.

Konstam MA, Isner JM, eds: The right verticle. 1987. ISBN 0-89838-987-9.

Kappagoda CT, Greenwood PV, eds: Long-term management of patients after myocardial infarction. 1988. ISBN 0-89838-352-8.

Gaasch WH, Levine HJ, eds: Chronic aortic regurgitation. 1988. ISBN 0-89838-364-1.

Singal PK, ed: Oxygen radicals in the pathophysiology of heart disease. 1988. ISBN 0-89838-375-7.

Reiber JHC, Serruys PW, eds: New developments in quantitative coronary arteriography. 1988. ISBN 0-89838-377-3.

NEW DEVELOPMENTS IN QUANTITATIVE CORONARY ARTERIOGRAPHY

edited by

JOHAN H. C. REIBER PhD and
PATRICK W. SERRUYS MD FACC
*Institute of Cardiology, Thoraxcenter, Erasmus University,
Rotterdam and University Hospital Dijkzigt, Rotterdam, The Netherlands*

Kluwer Academic Publishers
DORDRECHT / BOSTON / LONDON

Library of Congress Cataloging in Publication Data

New developments in quantitative coronary arteriography / edited by
  Johan H.C. Reiber and Patrick W. Serruys.
      p.   cm. -- (Developments in cardiovascular medicine)
   Based on a symposium held in Rotterdam in June 1987.
   Includes index.
   ISBN-13:978-94-010-7082-9   e-ISBN-13:978-94-009-1309-7
   DOI: 10.1007/978-94-009-1309-7

   1. Angiocardiography--Digital techniques--Congresses. 2. Coronary
 arteries--Imaging--Congresses. 3. Coronary heart disease-
 -Diagnosis--Congresses.   I. Reiber, J. H. C. (Johan H. C.)
 II. Serruys, P. W. III. Series.
   [DNLM: 1. Angiography--methods--congresses. 2. Coronary Vessels-
 -radiography--congresses.   W1 DE997VME / WG 300 N5315 1987]
 RC683.5.A5N48 1988
 616.1'207572--dc19
 DNLM/DLC
 for Library of Congress   88-8982
                                                    CIP

ISBN-13:978-94-010-7082-9

Published by Kluwer Academic Publishers,
P.O. Box 17, 3300 AA Dordrecht, The Netherlands

Kluwer Academic Publishers incorporates
the publishing programmes of
D. Reidel, Martinus Nijhoff, Dr W. Junk and MTP Press.

Sold and distributed in the U.S.A. and Canada
by Kluwer Academic Publishers,
101 Philip Drive, Norwell, MA 02061, U.S.A.

In all other countries, sold and distributed
by Kluwer Academic Publishers Group,
P.O. Box 322, 3300 AH Dordrecht, The Netherlands.

Contents

THE STENT, A BREAKTHROUGH?

List of contributors

BEATT KJ, MD
Catheterization Laboratory, Thoraxcenter, Erasmus University and University Hospital Dijkzigt, P.O. Box 1738, 3000 DR Rotterdam, The Netherlands

BONZEL T, MD
Medical Clinic, Department of Cardiology, University of Freiburg, Hugstetter Strasse 55, 7800 Freiburg i.Br., Germany

BOUNHOURE JP, MD
Service de Cardiologie, CHU Rangueil, Chemin du Vallon, 31054 Toulouse, France

BRAND M vd, MD
Catheterization Laboratory Thoraxcenter, Erasmus University and University Hospital Dijkzigt, P.O. Box 1738, 3000 DR Rotterdam, The Netherlands

BRENNECKE R, PhD
2. Medical Clinic, Johannes Gutenberg-University, Langenbeckstrasse 1, 6500 Mainz, Germany

BÜRSCII JII, MD
Department of Pediatric Cardiology and Biomedical Engineering, University of Kiel, Schwanenweg 20, 2300 Kiel 1, Germany

CAPUTO, GR
Department of Cardiology, LDS Hospital, University of Utah, Salt Lake City, Utah 84143, USA

COURTAULT A, MD
Service de Cardiologie, CHU Rangueil, Chemin du Vallon, 31054 Toulouse, France

DORIOT P-A, PhD
Centre de Cardiologie, Hôpital Cantonal Universitaire, CH-1211 Geneva 4, Switzerland

ECKEL L
Center of Surgery, Department of Cardiovascular and Thoracic Surgery, Klinikum der Universität, Theodor Stern Kai 7, 6000 Frankfurt 70, Germany

EIGLER NE, MD
Division of Cardiology, Cedars-Sinai Medical Center, Box 48750, Los Angeles, CA 90048-0750, USA

FEYTER PJ de, MD
Catheterization Laboratory, Thoraxcenter, Erasmus University and University Hospital Dijkzigt, P.O. Box 1738, 3000 DR Rotterdam, The Netherlands

FORRESTER JS, MD
Division of Cardiology, Cedars-Sinai Medical Center, Box 48750, Los Angeles, CA 90048-0750, USA

GALINIER M, MD
Service de Cardiologie, CHU Rangueil, Chemin du Vallon, 31054 Toulouse, France

GLICK D, MD
Cedars-Sinai Medical Center, Box 48750, Los Angeles, CA 90048-0750, USA

GOLF S, MD
Departement de Cardiologie, Centre Hospitalier Universitaire Vaudois, CH-1011, Lausanne, Switzerland

GRUNDFEST WS, MD
Laser Research Center, Cedars-Sinai Medical Center, Box 48750, Los Angeles, CA 90048-0750, USA

HADDAH J, MD
Service de Cardiologie, CHU Rangueil, Chemin du Vallon, 31054 Toulouse, France

HANGIANDREOU N, MSc
University of Wisconsin Hospital, Madison, WI, USA

HERRINGTON DM, MD
Department of Medicine, Harvey 502, Divisions of Internal Medicine and Cardiology, Johns Hopkins Hospital, 601 N. Wolfe St., Baltimore, MD 21205, USA

HICKEY A, MD
Cedars-Sinai Medical Center, Box 48750, Los Angeles, CA 90048-0750, USA

HIRATZKA LF, MD
Department of Internal Medicine, Cardiovascular Center, University of Iowa Hospital, Iowa City, IA 52242, USA

JOFFRE F, MD
Service de Cardiologie, CHU Rangueil, Chemin du Vallon, 31054 Toulouse, France

JUILLIÈRE Y, MD
Centre Hospitalier Régional et Universitaire de Nancy, Hôpitaux de Brabois, Rue du Morvan, 54511 Vandoeuvre Cedex, France

JUST H, MD
Medical Clinic, Department of Cardiology, University of Freiburg, Hugstetter Strasse 55, 7800 Freiburg i.Br., Germany

KALTENBACH M, MD
Center of Internal Medicine, Department of Cardiology, Klinikum der Universität, Theodor Stern Kai 7, 6000 Frankfurt 70, Germany

KAPPENBERGER L, MD
Departement de Cardiologie, Centre Hospitalier Universitaire Vaudois, CH-1011, Lausanne, Switzerland

KAUFMANN U, MD
Departement de Cardiologie, Centre Hospitalier Universitaire Vaudois, CH-1011 Lausanne, Switzerland

KERBER RE, MD
Department of Internal Medicine, Cardiovascular Center, University of Iowa Hospital, Iowa City, IA 52242, USA

KIESO RA, MSc
Department of Internal Medicine, Cardiovascular Center, University of Iowa Hospital, Iowa City, IA 52242, USA

KOBER G, MD
Center of Internal Medicine, Department of Cardiology, Klinikum der Universität, Theodor Stern Kai 7, 6000 Frankfurt 70, Germany

KRAUSE E
Center of Surgery, Department of Cardiovascular and Thoracic Surgery, Klinikum der Universität, Theodor Stern Kai 7, 6000 Frankfurt 70, Germany

LEE P,
Medical Clinic, Department of Cardiology, University of Freiburg, Hugstetter Strasse 55, 7800 Freiburg i.Br., Germany

LITVACK F, MD
Laser Research Center, Cedars-Sinai Medical Center, Box 48750, Los Angeles, CA 90048-0750, USA

LUIJTEN HE, MD
Catheterization Laboratory, Thoraxcenter, Erasmus University and University Hospital Dijkzigt, P.O. Box 1738, 3000 DR Rotterdam, The Netherlands

MANCINI GBJ, MD
Division of Cardiology, Veterans Administration Medical Center, 2215 Fuller Road, Ann Arbor, MI 48103, USA

MARCUS ML, MD
Department of Internal Medicine, Cardiovascular Center, University of Iowa Hospital, Iowa City, IA 52242, USA

MARSHALL HW
Department of Cardiology, LDS Hospital, University of Utah, Salt Lake City, Utah 84143, USA

McPHERSON DD, MD
Department of Internal Medicine, Cardiovascular Center, University of Iowa Hospital, Iowa City, IA 52242, USA

MISTRETTA C, PhD
Department of Radiology, University of Wisconsin Hospital, Madison, WI, USA

MOHR F, MD
Cedars-Sinai Medical Center, Box 48750, Los Angeles, CA 90048-0750, USA

MÜLLER T
Center of Internal Medicine, Department of Cardiology, Klinikum der Universität, Theodor Stern Kai 7, 6000 Frankfurt 70, Germany

PARKER DL, PhD
Department of Medical Informatics, LDS Hospital, University of Utah, Salt Lake City, Utah 84143, USA

PEARSON TA, MD
Division of Cardiology, Harvey 502, Johns Hopkins Hospital, 601 N Wolfe St., Baltimore, MD 21205, USA

PEPPLER W, PhD
University of Wisconsin Hospital, Madison, WI, USA

PFAFF JM, PhD
Division of Cardiology, Cedars-Sinai Medical Center & UCLA School of Medicine, Box 48750, Los Angeles, CA 90048-0750, USA

POPE DL
Department of Medical Informatics, LDS Hospital, University of Utah, Salt Lake City, Utah 84143, USA

PUEL J, MD
Service de Cardiologie, CHU Rangueil, Chemin du Vallon, 31054 Toulouse, France

RADÜNZ N
Center of Internal Medicine, Department of Cardiology, Klinikum der Universität, Theodor Stern Kai 7, 6000 Frankfurt 70, Germany

REIBER JHC, PhD
Laboratory for Clinical and Experimental Image Processing, Thoraxcenter, Erasmus University and University Hospital Dijkzigt, P.O. Box 1738, 3000 DR Rotterdam, The Netherlands

ROUSSEAU H, MD
Service de Cardiologie, CHU Rangueil, Chemin du Vallon, 31054 Toulouse, France

RUTISHAUSER W, MD
Centre de Cardiologie, Hôpital Cantonal Universitaire, CH-1211 Geneva 4, Switzerland

SANZ M, MD
Division of Cardiology, Veterans Administration Medical Center, 2215 Fuller Road, Ann Arbor, MI 48103, USA

SARAI K
Center of Surgery, Department of Cardiovascular and Thoracic Surgery, Klinikum der Universität, Theodor Stern Kai 7, 6000 Frankfurt 70, Germany

SATTER P
Center of Surgery, Department of Cardiovascular and Thoracic Surgery, Klinikum der Universität, Theodor Stern Kai 7, 6000 Frankfurt 70, Germany

SCHRÄDER R
Center of Internal Medicine, Department of Cardiology, Klinikum der Universität, Theodor Stern Kai 7, 6000 Frankfurt 70, Germany

SEGALOWITZ J, MD
Cedars-Sinai Medical Center, Box 48750, Los Angeles, CA 90048-0750, USA

SERRUYS PW, MD
Catheterization Laboratory, Thoraxcenter, Erasmus University and University Hospital Dijkzigt, P.O. Box 1738, 3000 DR Rotterdam, The Netherlands

SIEVERT H
Center of Internal Medicine, Department of Cardiology, Klinikum der Universität, Theodor Stern Kai 7, 6000 Frankfurt 70, Germany

SIGWART U, MD
Departement de Cardiologie, Centre Hospitalier Universitaire Vaudois, CH-1011 Lausanne, Switzerland

SIRNA SJ, MD
Department of Internal Medicine, Cardiovascular Center, University of Iowa Hospital, Iowa City, IA 52242, USA

SOLZBACH U
Medical Clinic, Department of Cardiology, University of Freiburg, Hugstetter Strasse 55, 7800 Freiburg i.Br., Germany

SURYAPRANATA H, MD
Catheterization Laboratory, Thoraxcenter, Erasmus University and University Hospital Dijkzigt, P.O. Box 1738, 3000 DR Rotterdam, The Netherlands

TOGGART EJ, MD
University of Wisconsin Hospital, Madison, WI, USA

VALLBRACHT C
Center of Internal Medicine, Department of Cardiology, Klinikum der Universität, Theodor Stern Kai 7, 6000 Frankfurt 70, Germany

VAN BREE, R
Department of Medical Informatics, LDS Hospital, University of Utah, Salt Lake City, Utah 84143, USA

VOGEL RA, MD
Division of Cardiology, University of Maryland Hospital, 22 S. Greene St., Baltimore, MA 21201, USA

WALFORD GA, MD
Divisions of Cardiology, Harvey 502, Johns Hopkins Hospital, 601 N. Wolfe St., Baltimore, MD 21205, USA

WENDT Th, MD
Center of Internal Medicine, Department of Cardiology, Klinikum der Universität, Theodor Stern Kai 7, 6000 Frankfurt 70, Germany

WHITING JS, PhD
Division of Cardiology, Cedars-Sinai Medical Center, Box 48750, Los Angeles, CA 90048-0750, USA

WOLLSCHLÄGER H, MD
Medical Clinic, Department of Cardiology, University of Freiburg, Hugstetter Strasse 55, 7800 Freiburg i.Br., Germany

WU J
Department of Medical Informatics, LDS Hospital, University of Utah, Salt Lake City, Utah 84143, USA

ZEIHER AM
Medical Clinic, Department of Cardiology, University of Freiburg, Hugstetter Strasse 55, 7800 Freiburg i.Br., Germany

ZIJLSTRA F, MD
Catheterization Laboratory, Thoraxcenter, Erasmus University and University Hospital Dijkzigt, P.O. Box 1738, 3000 DR Rotterdam, The Netherlands

Introduction

There are few techniques that have influenced therapeutic strategies in modern cardiology to a similar extent as coronary arteriography. Bypass surgery as well as transluminal coronary angioplasty would not have been possible without coronary angiography serving as a 'midwife' in their evolution. Despite the widespread and long-standing use in clinical practice, however, the interpretation of coronary angiograms has not changed very much since the early days. Most angiograms are still reviewed in a visual and semi-quantitative and thus often very subjective way. In the face of an almost exploding field for interventional catheterization including thrombolysis, balloon dilatation, and other rapidly evolving techniques for transluminal revascularization or recanalization, a more detailed and quantitative analysis of coronary arteriograms is urgently required. In addition to the delineation of coronary morphology, we need dynamic and functional information about flow and perfusion to understand the physiological significance of anatomic abnormalities. Coronary arteriography contains and can provide most of this information. With the application of appropriate techniques, it can be made available in the catheterization laboratory even during the patient's investigation, thus facilitating and improving clinical decision making. Objective and reproducible analysis will furthermore enhance our understanding about the pathophysiology of coronary disease.

After a first symposium in 1985, leading experts within the field of quantitative and digital coronary arteriography gathered again in Rotterdam in June, 1987, to discuss the present and future aspects of digital techniques for the quantitative analysis of coronary function and morphology from angiocardiography. This book has been based on a coherent selection of important contributions characterising the state of the art in quantitative coronary arteriography, including new complementary methods such as high frequency echocardiography or coronary angioscopy.

We hope that this book may stimulate those active in the field and that it may help in the development of better diagnostic and investigational tools,

J. C. Reiber & P. W. Serruys (eds.), New Developments in Quantitative Coronary Arteriography,
xvii—xviii.

since many examples have shown that the scientific work and method of today may well be the clinical routine of tomorrow.

RÜDIGER W. R. SIMON
Working Group 'Coronary
Blood Flow and Angina pectoris'
European Society of Cardiology.

1. Digital imaging systems for coronary angiography

RÜDIGER BRENNECKE

SUMMARY. The optimization of digital imaging systems requires the matching of the image quality parameters in the digital and in the analog parts of the system. Therefore, a brief overview on image generation, including the analog components (generator, X-ray tube, image intensifier, video camera) and the digital components (ADC, memory devices, DAC) is given. Next, the differences between the architecture of a standard general-purpose computer and the architectures of image processors are demonstrated. Future developments such as high capacity archival systems and new system architectures are discussed as well. Future systems should be able to handle not only image data, but also physiological data (such as ECG and pressure signals) and general patient information by presenting all of this information in a generalized database environment to the user.

1. Introduction

A general interest in digital imaging was created by the demonstration of the feasibility of digital video subtraction for image enhancement in clinical studies. However, additional features that became available with digital storage and processing of angiocardiograms, such as real-time image retrieval and quantitative image analysis, are equally important. The development of digital imaging systems with this degree of flexibility is still in progress. As a further development, functional imaging was introduced to improve the analysis of myocardial perfusion. Presently, we see not only progress in diagnostic power through the application of digital techniques, but also improvements in matters relevant to clinical image management, such as the rapid availability of image data during PTCA and the archiving of image data.

This chapter reviews the system parameters which are responsible for the quality of image storage and processing. Physical and technical parameters must be seen in a common context. An example of this relationship is the dependency of image quality on the quality of an analog device, the image intensifier, and on the matrix size of the digital system. Since digitization is

J. C. Reiber & P. W. Serruys (eds.), New Developments in Quantitative Coronary Arteriography,
1–12.

performed at the end of a chain consisting of X-ray generator, X-ray tube, patient, image intensifier and electronic camera, the spatial and temporal resolution of the digitization process must be seen in relation to the image quality of this chain. While in earlier studies the geometric resolution of imaging systems (measured, for instance, in line-pairs per mm) was considered to be of primary importance, we shall stress here the aspect of contrast resolution that became important in subtraction imaging. We shall also show that quite general differences exist in system optimization between the analog parts of the system and the digital parts.

Although image quality considerations have governed the discussion of the 'ideal system' for a long time, it will before long be more or less standardized in digital systems. At that time, image management considerations will be essential in any system comparison, including topics such as fast interactive image processing, the design of the image data base provided and the design of the human-computer interface.

2. Analog and digital components

2.1. The components of the imaging chain

2.1.1. Analog imaging components
The first element in the imaging chain is the X-ray tube. The tube load and therefore the density of radiation energy are limited [1]. Thus, integration of energy is always necessary at the receiver end (film or video camera) of the chain. Some elegant schemes for scatter reduction using moving slits for collimating the radiation, or similar devices [2], are probably ruled out, at least for angiocardiographic applications, since temporal resolution is decreased by the need to integrate each linear image segment for a period of time comparable to a frame pulse (1 to 5 msec).

The total radiation dose applied is primarily limited by the patient exposure that we are willing to accept, and it depends also to some extent on the amount of contrast material administered. The rule that is applicable in these cases is very general. It says that for each diagnostic question, we must minimize both the X-ray dose and the amount of contrast material, as long as the certainty of the diagnostic decision does not decrease. In digital subtraction imaging, the radiation dose and the amount of contrast material are strongly interdependent [3]. Thus, a reduction in the amount of contrast material by a factor of 2 must be compensated for by an increase in X-ray dose by a factor of 4 to keep image contrast (noise contrast) constant.

Another critical point is the detection quantum efficiency (DQE, percentage of converted X-ray photons) of the X-ray intensifier. A high DQE means a high signal-to-noise ratio (SNR) at a given dose of radiation and amount of contrast material. For a typical X-ray spectrum (ICRU), this number varies between 35 and more than 70 percent [4]. A high DQE and a high spatial resolution (measured, as is usually done, using a high contrast phantom) are presently conflicting requirements. In digital angiography, the trend is to stress the importance of a high DQE more than of a high spatial resolution, since the perceptibility of low contrast details depends on the noise structure and this is, at a fixed patient dose, a function of the DQE.

The video camera is the first component in the imaging chain that can be considered to be an electronic device. The video camera is usually coupled to the output screen of the image intensifier by a lens system. The optical system produces an inhomogeneity in the geometric resolution at larger openings of the iris. A direct coupling of the output screen of the intensifier and the TV-camera by fiber optics would reduce this error while producing veiling glare, and therefore introducing errors in digital densitometry.

The principal role of the iris (f-stop) must be emphasized, since its setting determines the SNR of the digital image. A well exposed X-ray image will always map a value of, for example, 1000 gray scale steps to the total range of brightness provided by the output screen of the image intensifier. Since the maximum brightness, however, will correspond to 100 times more photons at an input dose of 10 μR per frame as compared to a typical fluoroscopic dose of 0.1 μR, the noise is smaller by a factor of 10 in the first case, although the brightness of the electronic image is the same. Therefore, after subtraction smaller amounts of contrast material can be detected. Digital video techniques coupled with a pulsed fluoroscopy mode of the X-ray generator allows for the first time to use a wide spectrum of X-ray dose rates.

The video camera assumes two roles in digitization. Its first function is to freeze the X-ray image by integrating, at each pixel location, the brightness over time due to the pulsed radiation. Its second function is to convert the resulting two-dimensional charge distribution into a serial video signal. Therefore, together with the analog-to-digital converter, the technical parameters of the video camera determine the spatial resolution or matrix size of the imaging chain [5]. There are, however, other important factors determining spatial resolution. The distance between the object and the entrance screen of the image intensifier, the zooming factor or field-of-view and the focal spot size of the X-ray tube all contribute to the usable resolution of the total system. In a new design, a further improvement in resolution is obtained by scanning only a rectangular region of the circular output window of the image intensifier. Even if all the other factors have been optimized, the digital matrix size of 512 by 512 pixels in use today can degrade the usable spatial resolution. Model computations lead to matrix size requirements of about 1024 $\times$ 1024 pixels to match under all circumstances the resolution provided by a modern image intensifier (4 line-pairs per mm) at a field-of-view of 25 cm. However, we doubt that model calculations based on objects with a high contrast (such as a lead test pattern) can describe adequately the performance of the imaging chain under the low contrast conditions typical for imaging contrast material distributions in the heart, the great vessels and especially in the coronary arteries. Preliminary results indicate that a resolution between 512×512 and 1024×1024 pixels should be adequate for all of these applications including coronary angiography. The change from the interlaced to the progressive mode of scanning the video image [5] has greatly improved video imaging.

There are two principal aspects that play a role in the discussion of the resolution of a digital system. The increase in spatial (and temporal) resolution also increases the data rate and the data capacity to be handled. However, we can only obtain more information from this increased amount of data if we increase, at the same time, the X-ray dose or the amount of contrast material (or both) applied to the patient. Otherwise, an increase in noise variance due to the smaller pixel size will interfere. Considering this relationship between cost (dose) and gain (usable resolution) of the imaging process, it becomes important to clarify further the question of what resolution is necessary for a given decision, be it the decision to perform a coronary angioplasty or the operative correction of a congenital malformation of the heart.

If we were only to match the performance of the digital image acquisition components to the technical specifications of the analog components of the system, we might end up with a large amount of overhead in our data and might find that we have to increase the load to the patient (contrast and X-ray dose). Therefore, a bottleneck for some of the parameters just mentioned may be advantageous at the interface between analog and digital systems. Of course, careful design is necessary to transform, for instance, an overhead in resolution provided by the image intensifier into an increase in the signal-to-noise ratio of the total system.

2.1.2. Digital imaging components
The interface between the analog and the digital world is the analog-to-digital converter (ADC). After this conversion, image quality can be kept arbitrarily high, depending only on the cost we are willing to pay. Techniques such as spatial multiplexing can be used to match physically slower digital devices to the primary data rate provided by the ADC. In spatial multiplexing, the primary data stream is distributed into several parallel streams, the rate of each stream being a fraction of the original rate. An example is the use of parallel disk magnetic drives. Although each single disk is too slow for image storage at the data rate provided by the ADC, the real-time distribution of ADC data to four or eight of these devices operating in parallel (at a rate of only 1/4 or 1/8 of the original rate) solves the

problem of real-time image sequence storage. For display, the data streams from the group of parallel disks are, of course, merged again. It must be noted, however, that depending on the details of the multiplexing techniques applied, random access to selected images can be much slower in a system of multiplexed disk drives than in a system based on a large semiconductor memory. Image processing can also be speeded up by the implementation of parallel processors, as will be discussed in the next paragraph. Here again, the efficient coupling of the processors is far from trivial.

Besides data multiplexing, data reduction is an approach to decreasing the data rate and data capacity requirements of the digital system. By statistical analysis of image data, it is possible to detect which part of the image data can be derived from data already transferred. These data are 'redundant'. On the basis of this analysis, it is possible to transfer only new or 'nonredundant' data. These require a lower data rate and a smaller storage capacity. Of course, we can reconstruct the original data from the nonredundant data without error (reversible coding). Under real-time conditions, the statistical analysis is limited to relatively simple algorithms. Nevertheless, 'compression factors' of 2 : 1 to 3 : 1 are achievable in typical imagery. Most digital storage systems for angiocardiography that are based on magnetic disks rely on schemes of data reduction.

As a consequence, the limiting step in digital imaging is not the high data rate required but, in the first place, the archival storage of the large amount of data acquired from each patient. The storage of 60 s of angiograms at 25 frame/s and at a matrix size of $512 \times 512 \times 8$ bits requires about 400 MBytes of storage capacity. With 1200 patients per year, we end up with about 500 GBytes per year. Conventional magnetic tape and magnetic disk technology were not able to solve the problem of storage of such a large amount of data involved in angiocardiographic examinations. In some digital systems, a photographic (matrix) camera system was provided with a cine-camera to record the original and processed images on film again. The advent of optical disk technology using a laser beam to store up to 2 gigabytes per disk has changed this situation to some degree [6]. Digital magnetic tape technology is also making progress and we expect within 2 years that digital tape recorders with a capacity of 5 to 15 gigabytes per tape with a form factor similar to the VHS-standard as it is used in home video equipment will become available. A transfer rate of only a few minutes per patient's data is necessary, requiring data transfer rates of several MBytes per second.

A critical point about magnetic media is the stability of storage. There is, of course, no experience yet on the durability of these media in terms of 15 or 30 years of storage time, a question of utmost concern in image archiving. Probably, one must rerecord the data every 5 to 10 years by an automatic archival system. This also increases storage cost.

Therefore, the archival problem must not be considered as a long term bottleneck in digital angiocardiography. The flexibility provided by digital systems will help to reduce the amount of data by irrelevancy reduction and redundancy reduction. Irrelevancy reduction will, at the same time, help to reduce the X-ray dose applied to the patient (and the personnel) during the examination.

2.1.3. Digital processing architectures

In a digital imaging system for angiocardiography, the video camera signal is digitized in real time (Fig. 1). The digital data stream is then usually stored in a digital semiconductor memory at a high transfer rate. Systems developed recently, also allow for the real-time acquisition of larger amounts of data on magnetic media such as Winchester disks. These data are re-transferred to a semiconductor memory for digital processing. Archival storage requires another device, as will be discussed later. The entire system is controlled by a general-purpose computer. Image processing functions, such as the videometric evaluation of stored images, are also increasingly performed by this general-purpose computer.

There are, in general, two principal levels of architecture in any digital computer system:

(a) *Hardwired functions.* They can provide high speed. However, the resources such as memories and processors included into a hardwired function can be used in only a relatively narrow range of problems.

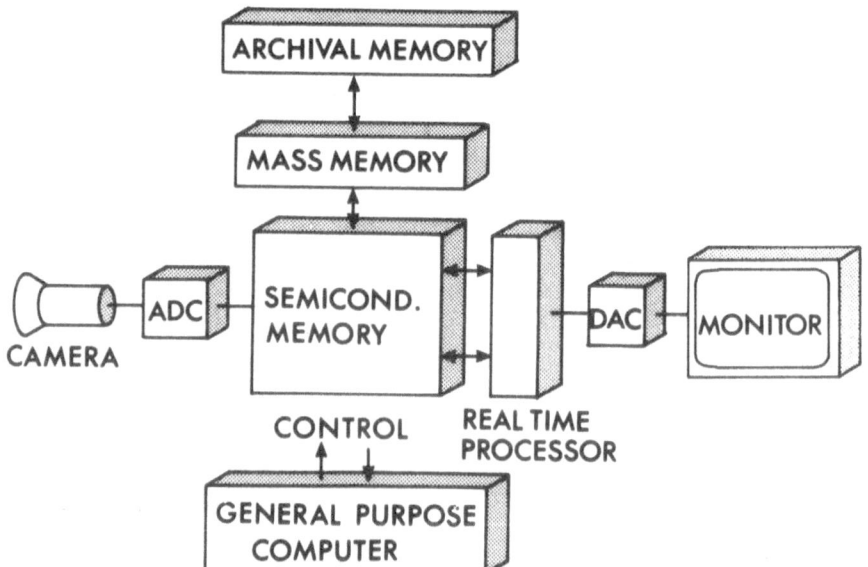

Figure 1. Components of a digital imaging system for angiocardiography.

(b) *Programmable functions.* A well-designed system of this kind can be very flexible. This means also that the system's resources can be put to work in many different contexts. However, programmable architectures perform generally much more slowly than hardwired functions. The primary reason for this state of design is that the vast majority of programmable computers are based on the classical von Neumann computer model. This describes a sequential machine performing essentially one operation at a time.

Because of these speed limitations, the first and the second generation of digital hardware for angiocardiography depended to a great extent on hardwired functions. The programmable general-purpose computer included was used for control purposes only. These configurations were directly derived from the most basic and most common algorithm applied: image subtraction. Background images can be stored and integrated (for random noise reduction) in a semiconductor memory. Dye images are stored or processed in another memory. The stored images can be combined using a subtraction circuit (real-time processor). A look-up table (LUT) allows selective contrast enhancement. Finally, a digital-to-analog converter performs the generation of video signals compatible with analog video monitors.

The general-purpose computer included in the configuration performs the dialogue between the operator and the system and controls all system functions. Second-generation designs added an array processor to the general-purpose computer. Programs and data are loaded down to the array processor which in turn provides processed data and status information. Array processors are optimized for the fast execution of a relatively broad range of operations from matrix subtraction to fast Fourier transforms. Thus, their position is in-between hardwired and totally programmable systems. However, the passage of the large amount of image data needed in image sequence analysis from mass memory via the bus system (and possibly also main memory) of the host to the array processor can produce a severe bottleneck.

Flexible systems will, therefore, apply a much closer coupling between the main (semiconductor) memory of the image processor and advanced functional units optimized for functions, such as buffering of the input and output data streams, subtraction and parameter extraction.

As is shown in Fig. 2, future systems with an enhanced structure will be structured around two levels of internal communication called 'interface levels'. The first level handles primarily image data transfer, while the second level handles control information and the transfer of data requiring lower transfer rates, such as derived data (e.g. densograms), context data (e.g. physiological signals) and control information. Standardization of these levels of communication for the functional units has two advantages:

8

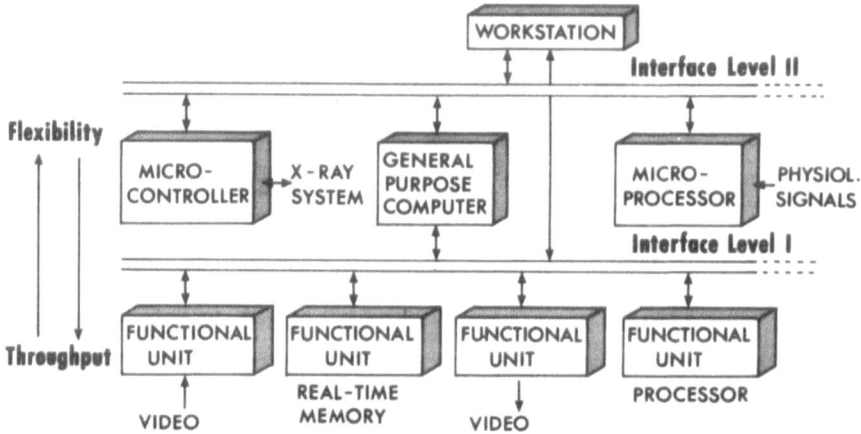

Figure 2. Interconnection of system components in a modular digital imaging system for angiocardiography. Two levels of interfaces are shown. Level I handles image data at a high throughput rate, while level II handles control information at a lower speed, but with a much more flexible communication protocol.

(a) If the transfer rate (bandwidth) of these communication channels is chosen adequately, parallel operation of many functional units can be implemented with a resulting increase in throughput of the system.

(b) The standardized interface levels simplify a modular expandability and upgrading of the system.

A hardware approach to the implementation of the second interface level is the Ethernet standard that, in addition, standardizes several levels of a communication protocol. The remaining levels of this protocol must be implemented by the manufacturers of the equipment to be interconnected. One example is DEC-net (Digital Equipment) now available for micro- and minicomputers from Digital Equipment and for personal computers from IBM. At this interface level in particular, the link between heart catheterization systems providing physiological data and the image processing systems could be realized with this standard.

Standardization of the first interface level (fast image data transfer) is much less likely. More important than this standardization aspect of a communication 'bus' is that it can provide a system 'backbone' for flexible parallel processing. A time-multiplexed scheme [7] will probably show decisive advantages over the spatially multiplexed systems typical of present equipment. A more detailed review of the architectures of digital imaging systems has been given elsewhere [7]. In commercially available systems, the general trend is towards the replacement of hardwired 'subtraction' processors by array processors with large memories, while flexible, truly parallel processors (Fig. 2) have not yet been implemented.

3. Software considerations

3.1. The development of algorithms

Generally, the algorithms implemented in digital systems for angiocardiography perform the following types of operations:

1. Digital image storage
2. Contrast enhancement
   — Subtraction [8, 9]
   — Temporal filtering [8, 10]
3. Parameter extraction [11, 12]
4. Image restoration [13, 14]
5. Image analysis [15, 16, 17].

The groups of techniques listed imply increasing complexity and, therefore, decreasing speed of operation. With present technology, groups 1 and 2 can be performed in real time. Some of the known simple techniques of parameter extraction could be the next candidates for real-time performance, but today these algorithms require several minutes. Image restoration and analysis such as compensation for veiling glare and flow measurement are still not standard in digital imaging systems. Geometric analysis (e.g. stenosis measurement) is usually performed interactively. For this kind of problem, real-time hardware is not available and may be entirely unnecessary. Often, however, attempts are made to complement the geometric analysis of the degree of stenosis with a densitometric approach.

A final general consideration in system design is the expandibility of the system. A modular design [18] is important in obviating early obsolescence.

3.2. Human-computer interface

The user must have access not only to images but also to a large amount of related data. These items differ with regard to the data capacity required and their structural complexity:

(a) Image sequences
   — Raw data
   — Processed data
(b) Regions of interest
   — in the time domain (gating)
   — in the spatial domain (windows)
   — in the density domain (gray level windows)

(c) Signals
  — derived from images
    — densograms
    — line profiles
  — related non-image signals
    — ECG
    — pressure curves
    — Doppler flow catheter
(d) Parameters
  — Percent stenosis
  — End-diastolic/end-systolic volumes
  — Regional wall motion
(e) Patient data
  — patient history
  — patient management data

The integration of these data into a single framework and the development of well-designed user interfaces for accessing these data and certain functionally related subgroups is of crucial importance to progress in routine applications of digital angiocardiography. There does not exist as yet much experience with user interfaces for complex systems like these. We shall probably have to wait for a gradual change in the general attitude towards computers, until convincing human-computer interfaces for complex image sequence processors can be designed. Without doubt, the advent of the personal computer will result in substantial progress in this direction.

To make it rapidly adaptable to different groups of users and to new trends in human-computer interfaces, we have designed our image processing software in such a way that the computing portions of the programs are systematically separated from the interactive portions (input of control from the user and output of status information). A special shell program handles the interactive tasks. We expect that this shell program can be easily changed if, for instance, all users or a certain group of users should prefer a command-driven interaction approach over a menu-driven interaction or vice versa. It cannot, however, be overlooked that these shell programs tend to become extremely complex.

4. Future developments

The main development in imaging hardware will be in the increase in spatial resolution of the video camera. Semiconductor (CD) cameras could be used in order to remove the time-lag typical of vacuum tube cameras.

The trends in hardware design, stated in the previous paragraph, can be summarized as a development towards programmable parallel computers. This trend would also mean a radical change in software development. Data-driven computer architectures [7] are among the concepts that may in the future provide the necessary hardware and software for the design of flexible, modular and fast image processing systems for digital angiocardiography.

Another future trend will be the development of a database approach to the integration of all types of information relevant in the context of angiocardiographic image display, archival storage and analysis. The primary prerequisite for this is the development of archival media capable of storing the large amounts of data involved. Without data compression, up to one gigabyte of data per examination is to be expected. Optical disk technology and magnetic tape technology are candidates for future archival devices.

Finally, data acquired in the catheterization laboratory will not be separated from other diagnostic information. Digital communication networks will provide for the access to image data by means of viewing stations positioned in the cardiology department and with the cardiac surgeon.

References

1. Leeuw P de: Quality considerations on ciné-imaging and PTCA-fluoroscopy anticipating a digital future. In: Reiber JHC, Serruys PW (eds): State of the art in quantitative coronary arteriography. Martinus Nijhoff, Dordrecht, Boston, 1986, pp 3—16.
2. Shaw C-G, Plewes DB: Quantitative digital subtraction angiography: two scanning techniques for correction of scattered radiation and veiling glare. Radiology 157: 247—253, 1985.
3. Balter S, Ergun D, Tscholl E, Buchmann F, Verhoeven L: Digital subtraction angiography: fundamental noise characteristics. Radiology 152: 195—198, 1984.
4. Hoffmann FW: Image intensifiers. In: Just H, Heintzen PH (eds): Angiocardiography. Springer-Verlag, Berlin, Heidelberg, New York, 1986, pp 15—20.
5. Seibert JA: Improved fluoroscopic and ciné-radiographic display with pulsed exposures and progressive TV scanning. Radiology 159: 277—278, 1986.
6. James AE, Carroll F, Pickens III DR, Chapman JC, Robinson RR, Pendergrass HP, Zaner R: Medical Image Management. Radiology 160: 847—851, 1986.
7. Brennecke R: Image processors for digital angiography. In: Kereiakes JG, Thomas SR, Orton CG (eds): Digital radiology. Plenum, New York, 1986, pp 13—33.
8. Heintzen PH, Brennecke R: Digital imaging in cardiovascular radiology. Thieme, Stuttgart, New York, 1983.
9. Kruger RA, Mistretta CA, Houk TL, Riederer SJ, Shaw CG, Goodsitt MM, Crummy AB, Zwiebel W, Lancaster JC, Rowe GG, Flemming D: Computerized fluoroscopy in real time for noninvasive visualization of the cardiovascular system. Radiology 130: 49—57, 1979.
10. Kruger RA: A method for time domain filtering using computerized fluoroscopy. Med Phys 8: 466—470, 1981.
11. Bürsch JH, Hahne HJ, Brennecke R, Grönemeier D, Heintzen PH: Assessment of arterial blood flow measurements by digital angiography. Radiology 141: 39—47, 1981.
12. Vogel RA: Digital assessment of coronary flow reserve. In: Buda AJ, Delp EJ (eds): Digital Cardiac Imaging. Martinus Nijhoff, Boston, 1985, pp 106—115.

13. Brennecke R, Hahne HJ, Bürsch JH, Heintzen PH: Digital videodensitometry: some approaches to radiographic image restoration and analysis. In: Heuck FHW (ed): Radiological functional analysis, Springer, New York, 1983, pp 79—88.

14. Shaw C-G, Ergun DL, Myerowitz PD, Van Lysel MS, Mistretta CA, Zarnstorff WC, Crummy AB: A technique for scatter and glare correction for videodensitometric studies in digital subtraction videoangiography. Radiology 142: 209—213, 1982.

15. Heintzen PH, Bürsch JH: Roentgen-video-techniques. Thieme, Stuttgart, New York, 1978.

16. Sigwart U, Heintzen PH: Ventricular wall motion. Thieme, Stuttgart, New York, 1984.

17. Reiber JHC, Serruys PW: State of the art in quantitative coronary arteriography. Martinus Nijhoff Publishers, Dordrecht, Boston, Lancaster, 1986.

18. Brennecke R, Jung D, Clas W, Erbel R, Meyer J: TALISMAN: An interpreter language for image sequence management in digital angiography and echocardiography. Comput Cardiol: 363—366, 1985.

2. Optimal biplane imaging of coronary segments with computed triple orthogonal projections

HELMUT WOLLSCHLÄGER, A. M. ZEIHER, P. LEE, U. SOLZBACH, T. BONZEL, and H. JUST

SUMMARY. A new method for improved imaging of coronary segments with exact triple orthogonal projections was developed. By means of this method, the two X-ray gantries of a biplane mutidirectional unit can be readjusted perpendicular to the long axis of an object of interest and perpendicular to each other using the results of spatial computations from a surveying view. The method was verified with phantom studies and applied in the clinical setting.

Introduction

One of the basic prerequisites for quantitative measurements from coronary angiograms is an optimal visualization of the coronary segment of interest, i.e. the portraying X-ray beams must be oriented perpendicular to the long axis of the segment. This is especially important, if reliable densitometric measurements of coronary arteries are to be performed, where orthogonal visualization is a necessity. In addition — following one of the most basic rules in radiology — at least two views, perpendicular to each other should be applied [1].

Therefore, most useful information can be derived from an angiographic study if this concept of triple orthogonality is applied: two projections perpendicular to the long axis of a coronary segment *and* perpendicular to each other.

In the practice of coronary angiography, this seemingly trivial requirement is difficult to meet: since the exact spatial orientation of an individual coronary segment is not known, currently repeated trials are sometimes necessary to approximate orthogonal projections empirically.

However, modern biplane multidirectional X-ray equipment with known geometric properties offer a solution by the fact that three-dimensional information can be obtained from two simultaneous two-dimensional images [2, 3, 4].

J. C. Reiber & P. W. Serruys (eds.), New Developments in Quantitative Coronary Arteriography,
13–21.

Using these mathematical prerequisites, we have developed a new method for:

1. the exact determination of the spatial orientation of any coronary segment in the fields of view of the two X-ray systems,
2. the calculation of the angles of projection of this coronary segment, and
3. computed readjustment of the X-ray gantries following the concept of triple orthogonality.

Method

Rationale

The basis for this method is the definition of a patient oriented 'global' three-dimensional coordinate system with the axes x, y, and z around the isocenter of the biplane unit. Knowing the geometrical properties of the X-ray system in use, the spatial positions of the centers of the image intensifier entrance fields and of the X-ray foci can be calculated for any projection from the rotational parameters (angles of angulation) and from the distances between the image intensifiers and the isocenter.

For the derivation of three-dimensional information from the two-dimensional images, 'local' two-dimensional coordinate systems with the axes k and l (Fig. 1) are defined on the surfaces of the image intensifier entrance fields.

The spatial orientation of a coronary segment is determined from optional surveying simultaneous biplane views, e.g. the standard RAO- or LAO-projections. The directions of the central X-ray beams of these projections are calculated as vectors in the global coordinate system (FA-0, FB-0 in Fig. 1).

For the computations, corresponding projections of the coronary segment of interest have to be identified by selecting simultaneous frames from planes A and B. Then, tangential lines have to be constructed to the projections of the vessel segment in both planes. This is performed:

1. by interactive marking of the projections of a well definable point in both planes (CA and CB in Fig. 2 — e.g. the center of a coronary stenosis or a branching point of the coronary tree), and
2. by interactive alignment of straight lines which are oriented tangentially to the vessel segment nearby CA and CB, respectively.

Next, the zero-crossings of these tangential lines with the corresponding axes of the local 2-dimensional coordinate systems are calculated (SA, TA, and SB, TB, respectively). Since the angles of rotation and the focus—image

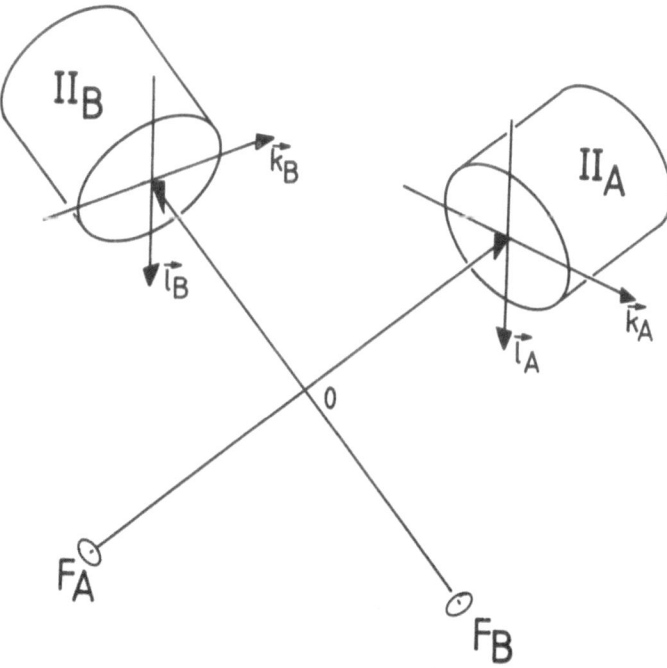

Figure 1. Schematic representation of the local two-dimensional coordinate systems (axes k and l) on the image-intensifier-entrance-fields (II). F = X-ray focus, 0 = isocenter of the system (all abbreviations indexed for systems A and B).

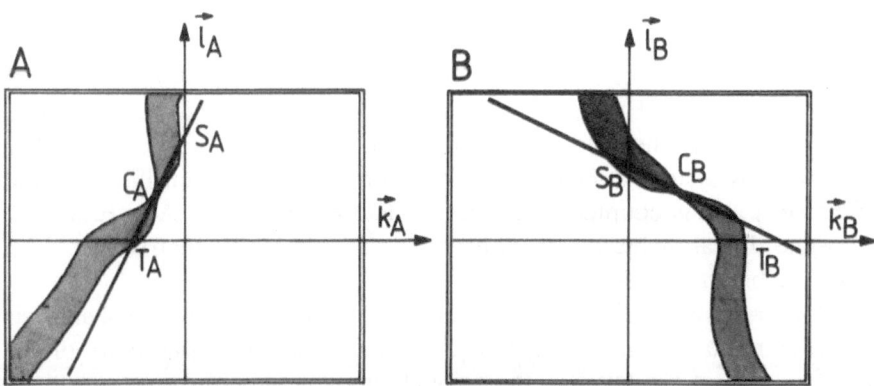

Figure 2. Construction of tangential lines at well definable points (C) in a schematic representation of a coronary artery segment in simultaneous biplane views (A and B). k and l: axes of local coordinate systems. The tangential lines are constructed interactively and are mathematically determined by the zero-crossings (S and T) with the horizontal axes of the local coordinate systems.

intensifier distances of these distinct projections are known for both planes, the exact spatial positions of these points SA, TA, and SB, TB can be determined in the 3-dimensional 'global' coordinate system. Thereafter, two subsidiary planes (actually triangles) are constructed which include the spatial positions of the corresponding X-ray focus and the zero-crossings on the image intensifier entrance field, i.e. plane FA-SA-TA, and plane FB-SB-ST.

The computed line of intersection of these two planes represents the spatial orientation of the axis of the vessel segment, and is expressed as a vector **v** in the global coordinate system.

The actual angle of projection of this surveying view of the coronary segment can be calculated from the orientation of the vector v and the direction of the portraying X-ray beam (dot product) for both planes.

Then — knowing the spatial orientation of the axis v — exact triple orthogonal projections can be calculated:

1. one of the X-ray systems is positioned perpendicular to v using an algorithm developed previously [5], and
2. the second X-ray gantry is adjusted perpendicular to v and perpendicular to the first one by calculation of the vector product (vector of the central X-ray beam of the first system and vector v).

The calculated orthogonal projections are valid only for the central X-ray beams. Therefore, the vessel segment of interest including the well-defined point C, must be shifted into the isocenter of the biplane unit by adjustment of the position of the craddle.

Imaging system

The mathematical algorithms have been solved for the biplane BICOR system (Siemens AG, Erlangen) with two C-arm gantries, which are mounted on the ceiling and at the head side of the supine patient.

The BICOR system is equipped with dual mode image intensifiers (5″ and 7″ diameter) and is coupled to the DIGITRON 3 (Siemens AG, Erlangen) for on-line digital image acquisition (512 × 512 × 10 bit matrix size, 12.5 images/s in biplane mode).

The programmable DIGITRON has been used for the geometrical analysis and the computation of orthogonal projections: the surveying views of the coronary segment are taken with optional simultaneous biplane projections (including hemiaxial views) and stored in the image memory for further processing. The technician selects two corresponding images at the same phase in the cardiac cycle (e.g. at end diastole). Next, the coronary segment is identified in both images by marking a well definable point (e.g. the center of a stenosis) using a graphic pad. After constructing the tangential lines in both planes, the spatial orientation of the segment is computed using the angles of rotation of the X-ray gantries and the distances between the X-ray foci and the image intensifiers.

From these data triple orthogonal projections are calculated. The operator then shifts the coronary segment into the isocenter of the BICOR unit and the gantries are readjusted using the computed angles of angulation. The coronary segment is visualized again, now under optimal geometrical conditions.

In case of overlapping with other anatomical details such as coronary branches, or in case of impending collision of the gantries with the patient or with each other, another pair of triple orthogonal projections must be selected from the (in theory) infinite number of possible solutions.

Verification

To verify the method we have performed phantom measurements with a small disc affixed perpendicular to a little metal rod which served as a model of a short straight coronary segment.

In all views different from 90° the projection of the disc appears with an elliptical shape. Only in a view perpendicular to the orientation of the rod, the projection of the disc appears as a straight line. The phantom was positioned in the fields of view of the BICOR system and digital images were obtained from randomly chosen simultaneous biplane projections. As can be seen in Fig. 3 (top), the projection of the disc has an elliptical shape, indicating oblique directions of the X-ray beams.

From these biplane views the spatial orientation of the rod was assessed, triple orthogonal projections were calculated, and the phantom was filmed again after shifting it into the isocenter and readjusting the gantries using the computed results. The projections of the disc are now straight lines, indicating orthogonal views.

Clinical application

We have applied this method in the clinical setting to short stenotic segments of coronary arteries. Figure 4 depicts the digital images of a clinical example, a stenotic segment of the proximal LAD. The two images at the top show the surveying views with the standard RAO and LAO projections. The axes of the local coordinate systems and the tangential lines to the vessel segment are outlined. The calculated angles of projection were 73° for the RAO view, and 23° for the LAO view.

The two images at the bottom of Fig. 4 demonstrate the result after

18

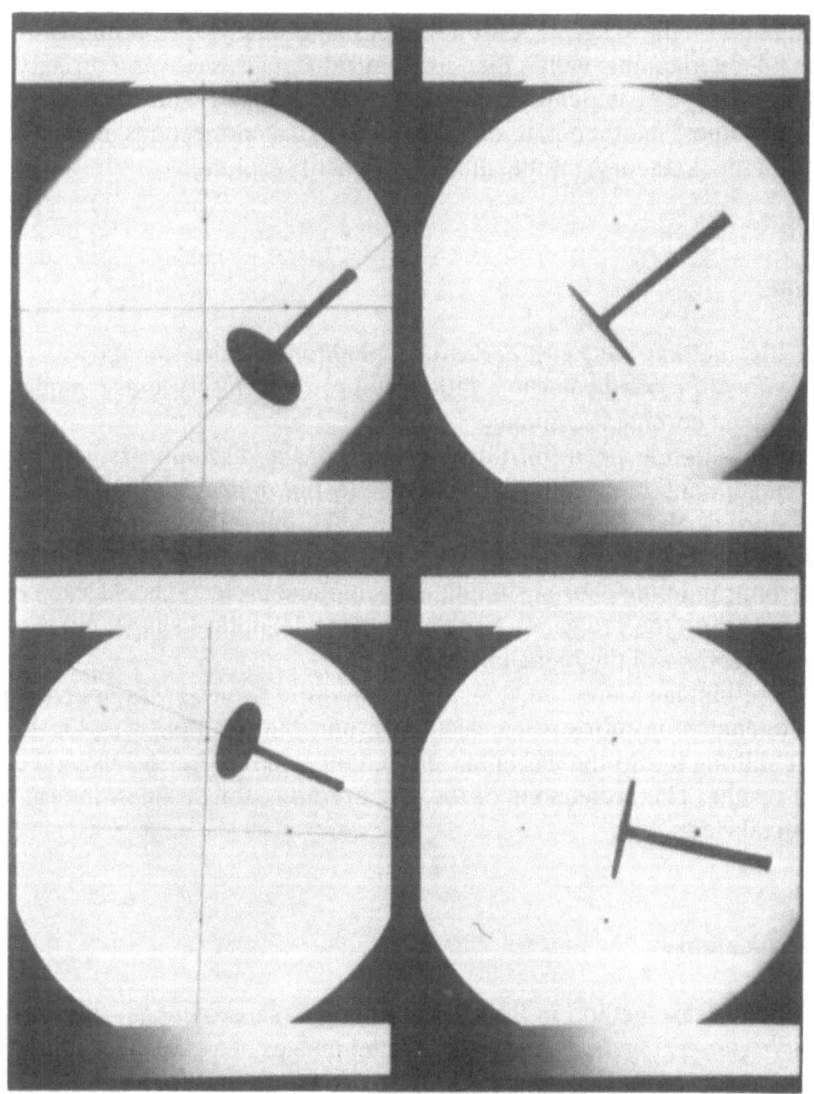

Figure 3. Simultaneous biplane views of the phantom. TOP: Surveying views with randomly chosen angles of angulation: the projection of the disc has an elliptical shape. BOTTOM: Same phantom with triple orthogonal projections after readjustment of the gantries: the projections of the disc are now straight lines indicating orthogonal projections.

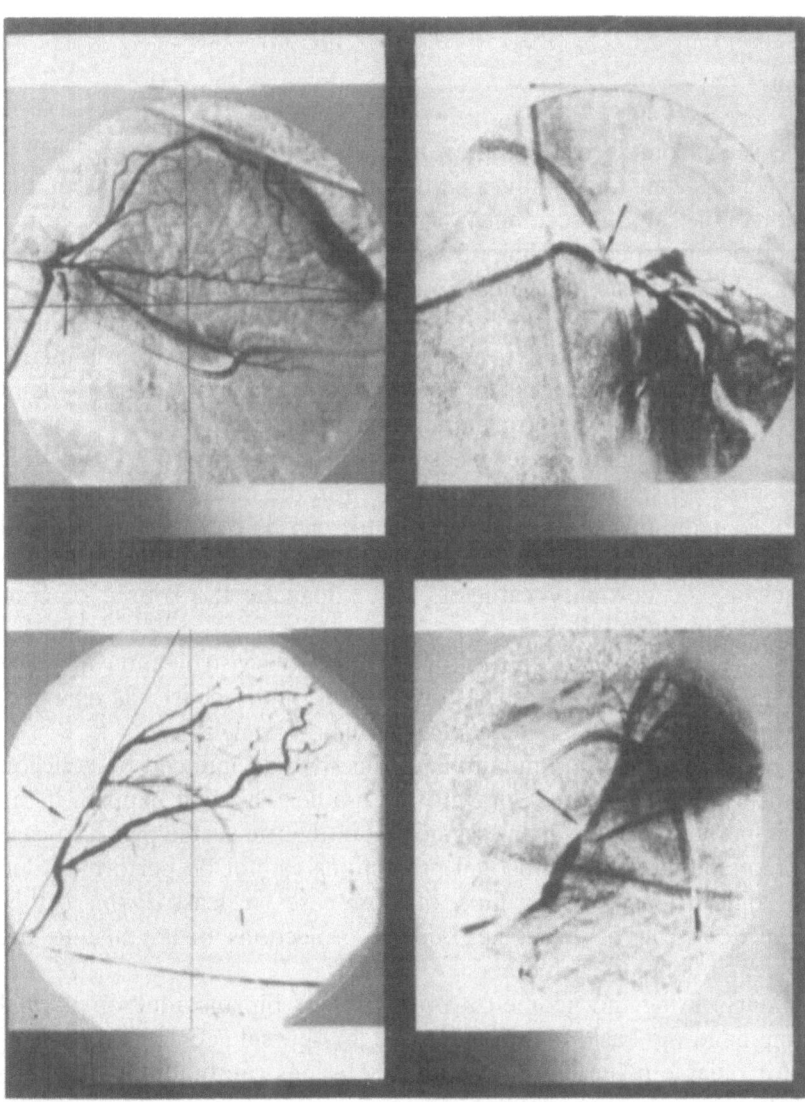

Figure 4. Simultaneous biplane views of a stenosis in the proximal LAD (indicated by arrows). TOP: Surveying views (the axes of the local coordinate systems and the tangential lines are outlined). BOTTOM: Same stenosis after computed readjustment of the X-ray systems.

computed readjustment of the gantries: two orthogonal projections with significantly improved geometrical visualization of the stenosis.

The time necessary for the entire procedure is about 4 to 6 minutes and will be reduced by directly interfacing the BICOR system to the DIGITRON for direct data transfer and system steering.

Discussion

As can be seen from these examples, individually calculated triple orthogonal projections can be obtained with considerable improvement of the visualization of the stenotic segment.

The method is especially helpful in PTCA procedures for improved portraying of the stenosis to be dilated and for guiding of the intracoronary instrumentation. Other applications include coronary examinations where quantitative measurements are to be performed, especially densitometric measurements, where orthogonal projections are mandatory. Then — and only then — are such densitometric measurements reliable.

But even conventional diameter measurements can be improved using this approach: since the stenotic segment is located in the isocenter of the X-ray unit, the exact radiological magnification factor can be easily calculated and used for calibration purposes. By this approach there is no need for a scaling device such as the coronary catheter, which may be the source of considerable errors in quantitation.

Furthermore, this method allows for reproducible visualization in serial examinations, even if the anatomical orientation of the heart has changed, e.g. after bypass surgery or significant changes in body weight.

However, there are some limitations of this method induced by collision of the gantries with each other or with the cradle. This will happen, if the spatial orientation of the coronary segment is in the transverse plane. In case of such orientation, triple orthogonal projections cannot be performed due to system collision. However, in most of these cases, at least *double* orthogonal projections can be used, i.e. biplane projections orthogonal to the vessel segment, but not to each other.

In summary, using the geometric properties of biplane multidirectional X-ray equipment, the basic requirements for an optimal geometric visualization and for reliable quantitation of coronary lesions can be met by individually adjusted orthogonal projections.

References

1. Eldh P: Axial views. Cathet Cardiovasc Diagn 2: 315—317, 1976.

2. Taylor KW, McLoughlin MJ, Aldridge HE: Specification of angulated projections in coronary arteriography. Cathet Cardiovasc Diagn 3: 367—374, 1977.
3. Wollschläger H, Lee P, Zeiher A, Solzbach U, Bonzel T, Just H: Mathematical tools for spatial computations with biplane isocentric X-ray equipment. Biomed Tech 31: 101—106, 1986.
4. Wollschläger H, Lee P, Zeiher A, Solzbach U, Bonzel T, Just H: Derivation of spatial information from biplane multidirectional coronary angiograms. Med Prog Technol 11: 57—63, 1986.
5. Wollschläger H, Lee P, Bonzel T, Zeiher A, Just H: Biplane multidirectional angiocardiography: exact orthogonal positioning of the X-ray systems. (Laterally mounted C-Arm-L-Arm-Systems). Biomed Tech 29: 261—266, 1984.

3. Accurate densitometric quantification requires strict attention to the physical characteristics of X-ray imaging

J. MARTIN PFAFF, S. WHITING, N. E. EIGLER, and J. S. FORRESTER

SUMMARY. Densitometric evaluation of routine cardiac digital arteriographic images is influenced by sources of error which include image receptor response characteristics, X-ray scatter, image intensifier veiling glare, and beam hardening. In this study the magnitude of each of these errors was determined and correction techniques were developed for the most prevalent errors. The video camera/digital linearity was determined and a systematic approach developed for optimization. Phantom studies were used to resolve each component of densitometric error. Iodine and tissue beam hardening were evaluated under narrow beam geometry with 5—25 cm H_2O and 0—265 mg/cm^2 tin. The effect of beam energy was assessed for peak tube potentials of 60—90 kVp. Scatter and veiling glare were measured as a function of field size using small lead blocks to attenuate the primary beam. These studies demonstrated that errors in densitometric measurement of both absolute and relative iodine concentrations are substantial unless corrections are applied to the raw data. Practical densitometric corrections for scatter and veiling glare are presented and validated under simulated clinical conditions. These investigations suggest that strict attention to sources of nonlinearity combined with practical correction techniques allow accurate quantification of myocardial contrast parameters.

Introduction

Densitometric quantification of cardiac arteriograms for the extraction of physiologic parameters, such as coronary anatomy or regional myocardial perfusion, has received widespread research application, even though the errors inherent in the techniques used may be substantial [1—13]. It is well known, that the representation of tissue iodine concentrations as video-densities is subject to significant error introduced by the physical attributes of X-ray and light interaction with the detection system [14—21]. Specifically, nonlinear contributions from X-ray patient scatter, light scatter within the image intensifier phosphors (veiling glare) and camera lens, pincushion distortion, and beam hardening of the polychromatic X-ray flux due to iodine and tissue thickness complicate the simple exponential relationship between iodine concentration and image intensity [22—26]. System response characteristics such as video tube gamma and film characteristic curves

J. C. Reiber & P. W. Serruys (eds.), New Developments in Quantitative Coronary Arteriography,
22—33.

present additional potential nonlinearities between measured videodensities and their respective contrast concentrations [16, 17, 20]. The goal of this study, therefore, was to evaluate the prevalent components of densitometric error and to develop and validate correction algorithms to improve the accuracy for densitometric analysis of routine digital coronary arteriography.

Methods

Experimental setup

The X-ray system used for this study consisted of a Philips Maximus generator, Eimac 0.6 mm focal spot X-ray tube, Thompson-Houston tri-mode image intensifier, and a conventional 10 : 1 antiscatter grid.

The output from a pulsed progressive-readout video camera with a plumbicon (PbO) pickup tube was digitized into 512^2 matrices by an ADAC 4100C image processor. The 10 bit analog-to-digital (A/D) converter was adjusted to give a digitized value between 0 and 5 for the black level, and 1024 just below plumbicon saturation. A linear acquisition transformation map was applied to compress the 10 bit digitized range to the 8 bit (256 grey level) image intensities.

Since the atomic number of tin(50) is close to that of iodine(53), highly uniform tin foils with projected concentrations ranging from 8 to 265 mg/cm² were used in place of iodinated contrast material to avoid errors due to inadequate mixing of diluted iodine contrast agents.

Camera/digital response

The response of the TV-A/D converter subsystem was measured using a series of exposures at fixed kVp and mA with exposure times varying from 8 to 80 ms.

Narrow beam calibration

Projected 'tin concentrations from 8 to 265 mg/cm² were acquired under narrow beam geometry in which the X-ray beam was collimated to a 1 cm × 1 cm area by placing 2 mm thick lead sheets proximal to the tin and on the face of the image intensifier to minimize X-ray scatter. Aluminum filtration (3.8 cm) was added to simulate typical patient thickness. Individual effective attenuation coefficients (u_{eff}) for each tin concentration were then calculated by the following equation:

$$u_{eff} \, (cm^2/gm) = (Ln[I_0/I_1]/x) \times 1000 \, mg/gm$$

where I_1 and I_0 are the measured digital intensities with and without a projected tin concentration of x mg/cm^2. Since these values decrease slightly with increasing tin concentration due to beam hardening, an average attenuation was obtained by linear regression of multiple contrast thicknesses as a function of true projected tin concentration.

Beam hardening

Tin beam hardening was assessed by linear regression of u_{eff} as a function of tin concentration. Water (patient) beam hardening was evaluated in a similar manner by measuring changes in u_{eff} as a function of water thickness (5 to 25 cm in increments of 5 cm).

Beam energy

The effect of beam energy on tin attenuation was measured by varying the peak tube potential from 60 to 90 kVp. Aluminum filtration, 1.9 and 3.8 cm, was used to measure changes in energy sensitivity as a function of beam hardness.

Scatter and veiling glare

Broad beam geometry was used to assess the effects of scatter and veiling glare (SVG). A square lead attenuator ($4 \times 4 \times 2$ mm) was placed alongside the tin foils to attenuate 75 kVp X-rays by greater than 99% [27]. The measured intensity beneath the lead will serve as an estimate of the SVG contribution from adjacent regions.

Densitometric analysis of projected tin concentration consisted of calculating mean digital intensities within two 10×10 pixel regions of interest (ROI): one in the center of the tin 'shadow', and one beneath the lead attenuator positioned within 1 cm of the tin foil. Images were acquired and analyzed for each tin concentration to evaluate densitometric intensities with respect to known projected tin concentrations under clinically simulated situations.

Simulated clinical scatter

An anthropomorphic chest phantom was positioned in the 30 degree RAO projection with a 12.5 × 12.5 cm field size to simulate scatter and magnification conditions observed in routine clinical procedures. Iodine vials, containing concentrations from 0 to 100 mg/cm², in increments of 20 mg/cm², were then positioned individually in the center of the field just beneath the chest phantom for densitometric quantification.

Correction algorithms

Two correction techniques were investigated to compensate for densitometric error attributable to SVG. The first algorithm, the static correction, is independent of iodine contrast material and involves subtraction of the SVG intensity, measured with no iodine, from each of the measured iodine intensities prior to logarithmic transformation. The second algorithm, the dynamic correction, compensates for iodine dependent SVG variations by measuring and subtracting SVG estimates for each iodine containing image, followed by logarithmic transformation. The uncorrected data, compensated only for exponential attenuation, and the SVG corrected videodensities were then compared with the measured iodine attenuation obtained with narrow beam geometry.

Coronary quantification

The previous densitometric errors and correction techniques were evaluated with respect to quantitative coronary arteriography. Precision drilled lucite "vessels" filled with Renografin-76 (370 mg iodine/cm³), measuring 0.5 to 4 mm in diameter, were imaged under broad beam geometry traversing 15 cm of lucite with field sizes of 25 and 200 cm² to simulate patient beam hardening and scatter. Measurement of contrast cross-sectional area was achieved by integrating the videodensitometric intensities beneath a linearly interpolated background. The limits of integration were set 0.7 mm outside the true vessel edges to account for image unsharpness. The absolute area was then calculated by dividing the measured densitometric area by u_{eff} obtained under narrow beam geometry with 15 cm of lucite. Absolute areas, with and without SVG correction, were compared with known dimensions. Relative errors were assessed by fitting a 2nd-degree polynomial to the curves and calculating the maximum error incurred for stenoses between 0—100%.

Results

Camera response

Camera non-linearities, representing 20% variation in measured contrast, were present near the saturation point of the plumbicon video tube (0.8–1.2 mV). These errors were eliminated by increasing the tube gain resulting in stable contrast measurements and a linear tube gamma of 1.00, $r = 0.99$. The digitized black level was measured as an intensity of 4 and remained stable throughout the range of video intensities.

Narrow beam calibration

Figure 1 illustrates the logarithmic tin contrast ($Ln[I_0/I_1]$) as a function of true projected tin concentration. The linear regression of these data (dashed line) represents an average tin attenuation of 7.92 cm^2/gm. These data demonstrate a linear relationship between measured densitometric concentration and projected iodine concentration ($r > 0.992$) with no apparent decrease in u_{eff} over the 0–265 mg/cm^2 range.

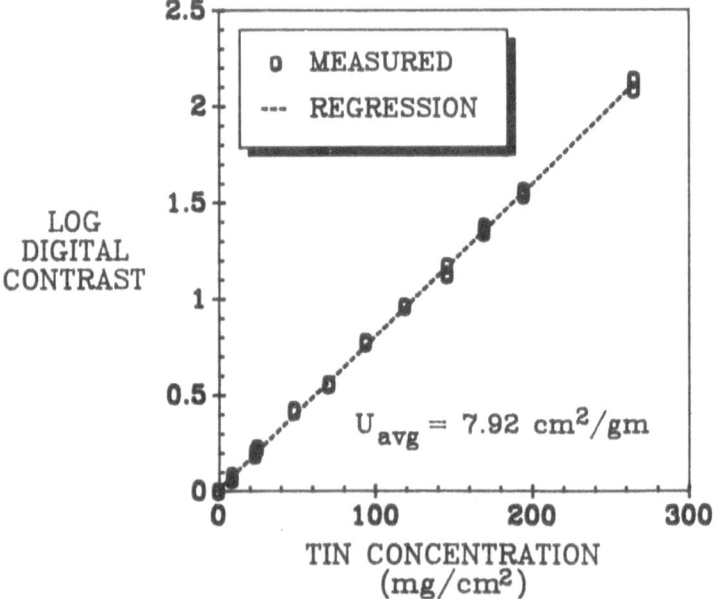

Figure 1. Narrow beam calibration: Measured tin contrast acquired with minimal scatter is plotted as a function of projected tin concentration. The dashed line represents the linear regression with an average attenuation (slope) of 7.92 cm^2/gm.

Beam hardening

The beam hardening component due to tin was statistically significant (slope $= -0.0035$ cm^2/gm per mg/cm^2 Sn, p(slope) < 0.02) suggesting that beam hardening errors due to variations in contrast material concentration are less than 4.5% in the 0–100 mg/cm^2 range.

The effect of water beam hardening on measurement of iodine or tin thickness is given in Table 1. Linear regression of these data demonstrate a decrease in u_{eff} with increasing water thickness (slope $= -0.077$ cm^2/gm per cm H$_2$O, y-intercept $= 10.9$ cm^2/gm, $r = -0.995$, p(slope) < 0.002). Thus, u_{eff} is reduced by about 4% with each 5 cm increase in patient thickness.

Table 1. Tin attenuation: effect of water beam hardening.

Water thickness (cm)	Tin effective attenuation coefficient (cm^2/gm)
5	10.5 ± 0.7
10	10.1 ± 0.5
15	9.6 ± 0.4
20	9.4 ± 0.3
25	9.0 ± 0.4

Beam energy

Figure 2 illustrates the decrease in the attenuation coefficient for tin with increasing peak tube potential (kVp). These data suggest a high dependence on effective beam energy which decreases with increasing energy. Increasing aluminum filtration from 1.9 to 3.8 cm does not significantly alter the variation in u_{eff} with respect to peak tube potential. For example, the decrease in tin attenuation coefficients due to an increase in energy from 70 to 80 kVp is 19% and 17% for aluminum filtration of 3.8 and 1.9 cm, respectively.

Scatter and veiling glare

Figure 3 shows the measured iodine contrast, under simulated scatter conditions, for the uncorrected, static and dynamic corrected data. The narrow beam calibration data, designated by the dashed line, represents an average iodine attenuation of 10.1 cm^2/gm. The uncorrected data demonstrate substantial error in measured iodine concentration. For example, the measured concentration for 80 mg/cm^2 was 35 mg/cm^2 representing a 56% error. The

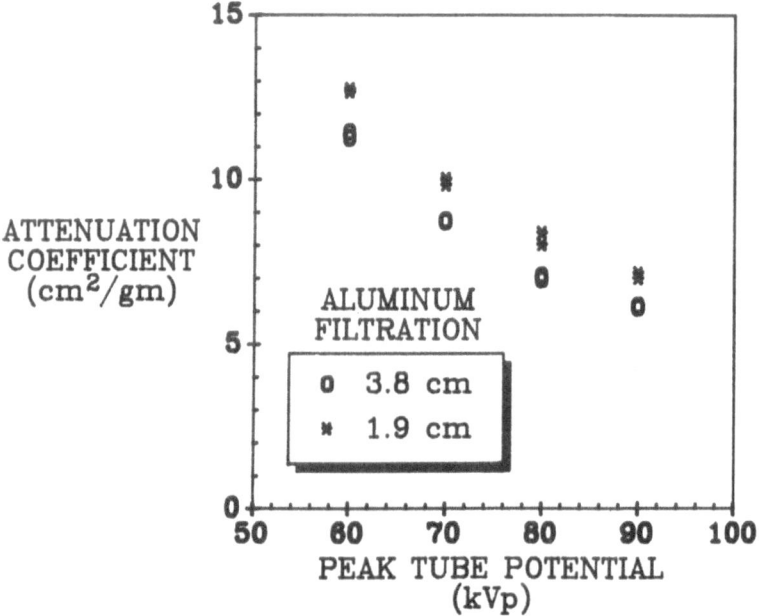

Figure 2. Beam energy: Measurements of tin attenuation are shown to decrease substantially with respect to increasing peak tube potential (kVp) for two aluminum filtrations.

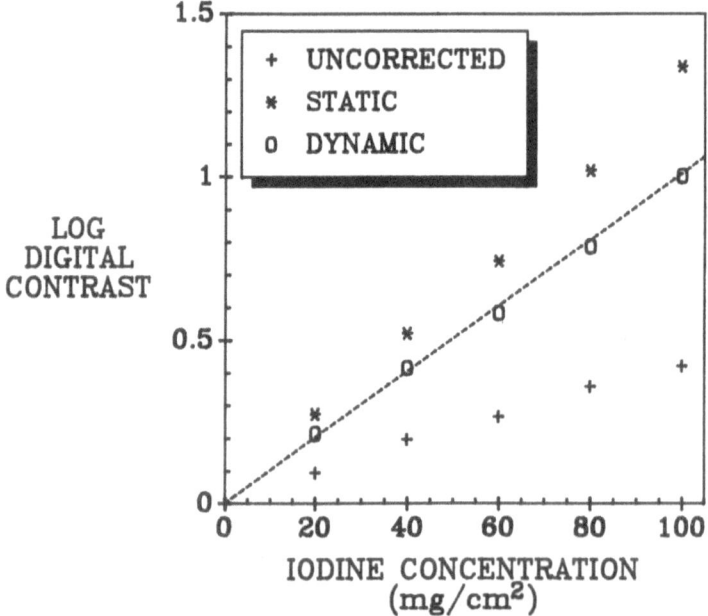

Figure 3. SVG Correction techniques: Uncorrected and corrected videodensitometric concentrations are shown as a function of true projected iodine concentration. Uncorrected iodine contrast demonstrates significant deviation from the narrow beam u_{avg} of 10.1 cm^2/gm designated by the dashed line. Both SVG corrections reduce the absolute error; however, the dynamic correction data correspond best with the narrow beam calibration.

static correction improves this error; however, the results now overestimate true projected iodine concentration by 29% at 80 mg/cm². Using the dynamic method, estimates of iodine concentration were corrected to within 4% over the entire range of iodine concentration.

Coronary quantification

The left-hand panel of Fig. 4 illustrates measured vessel cross-sectional area without SVG correction. These values show marked deviation from the line of identity which increases with field size. For example, a 3.25 mm (8.3 mm²) vessel will be underestimated by 46 and 16% for the 200 and 25 cm² field sizes, respectively. Relative errors for the calculation of percent stenosis were greatest between 40—60% narrowing and were 8.4 and 6.9% for the 200 and 25 cm² field sizes, respectively.

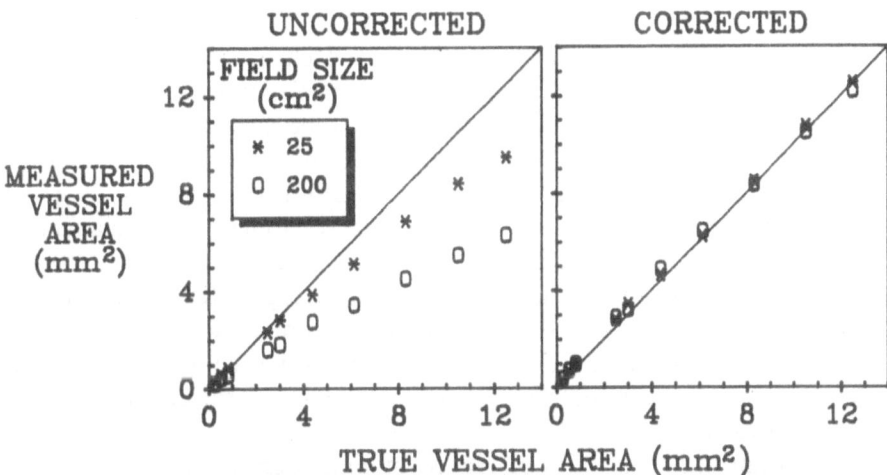

Figure 4. Coronary quantification: The left panel illustrates the measured cross-sectional area of cylindrical vessels without correction for SVG. The accuracy of absolute area calculations is shown to decrease with increasing field size. The right panel shows the same measurements corrected by the dynamic SVG correction technique.

The right hand panel of Fig. 4 demonstrates the previous vessel areas corrected for SVG by the dynamic method. Both field sizes agree well with known vessel dimensions (cumulative: slope = 0.99, y-intercept = 0.24 mm², SEE = 0.17 mm²). Relative errors are also reduced to 4.4 and 2.4% for the 200 and 25 cm² field sizes, respectively. These data suggest that iodine dependent SVG corrections allow accurate measurement of vessel cross-sectional area independent of field size.

Discussion

This study demonstrates that videodensitometric intensities are subject to substantial error due to digital system response characteristics, scatter, and veiling glare, which result in nonlinear underestimation of true projected iodine concentration. Nevertheless, our data also suggest that both absolute and relative densitometric accuracy may be dramatically improved by applying correction algorithms which compensate for these components of densitometric inaccuracy.

In contrast to previously published measurements of camera linearity [16, 28], our plumbicon video tube represented a significant source of error prior to gain correction. Not only did response linearity fail at medium to high intensities, we have observed this response to vary with temperature and length of operation. As much as 20% error may be incurred if these nonlinearities are ignored.

Variations in beam energy represent a significant source of error if studies are performed without constant X-ray techniques. Our data suggest that variations from 70 to 80 kVp will decrease iodine contrast by 18 percent. Stable X-ray energies are critical for studies which evaluate the temporal variations of contrast media such as myocardial perfusion or coronary blood flow. Pre-injection calibration techniques will also be incapable of predicting absolute iodine thickness if energy fluctuations persist throughout the exam.

Beam hardening due to contrast thickness (tin) was minimal, representing less than 5% error for a 3 mm coronary vessel which has a maximum projected iodine concentration of 111 mg/cm^2 (Renografin-76 = 370 mg iodine/cm^3). We also found that the use of an average attenuation calibration, obtained by linear regression of multiple contrast thicknesses resulted in only 2—5% error for quantification of vessel cross-sectional area. Larger errors will be present for ventriculography, since higher projected concentrations of contrast are present.

Water beam hardening also produced minimal densitometric error (4% error per 5 cm change in patient thickness). This component of densitometric error can be eliminated by obtaining a densitometric calibration near the region of analysis. Although regional densitometric error was not investigated in this study, it is well known that SVG, spatial linearity (pincushion distortion), and tissue thickness are spatially variant [22, 23, 25]. For example, if an iodine calibration is obtained over the lung field, and quantification of contrast thickness is performed over the mediasteinum or abdominal region, then considerable error may be accumulated. It is therefore recommended, that a calibration object and SVG estimate be obtained as close as reasonably possible to the region requiring quantification.

Narrow beam densitometric calibration of our system produced values of iodine and tin attenuation similar to those reported in the literature [14, 29].

From these values, we have shown that absolute vessel cross-sectional area may be obtained. Tables of u_{eff}, required for absolute measurements, could be obtained as a function of patient thicknesses, tube filtration, and beam energy; however, these would be impractical for clinical application since exact patient thickness along the path of the X-ray beam is not known. For routine application, iodine attenuation must be derived from a calibration object such as a cylindrical vessel with known dimensions and iodine concentration. Coronary arteries could provide internal calibration; however, three important criteria must be met: (1) the contrast filled lumen must be circular in cross-section; (2) precise measurements of diameter are necessary; and (3) the vessel may not be foreshortened with respect to the X-ray beam. The sources of error inherent in these requirements will be minimized by measuring a known calibration object positioned perpendicular to the X-ray flux, and therefore, a pre-injection calibration object containing several iodine concentrations is recommended.

Scatter and veiling glare were the predominant sources of densitometric error, comprising as much as 30 to 60% of the mean video intensity. The decreasing accuracy of measured vessel cross-sectional areas with increasing field size was a reflection of this SVG effect. For example, we observed a 16 and 46% underestimation of vessel area for the small and large field sizes, respectively. Relative measurements of myocardial washout parameters or percent stenoses will also be subject to error due to the non-linearity imposed by SVG contributions. Our data show 5—10% error in percent stenoses measurements which agree favorably with results predicted by Barrett and Boone [14].

The iodine independent SVG correction (static) reduced absolute densitometric error for all tin concentrations, although it did overestimate contrast thickness with respect to the narrow beam calibration. The dynamic correction technique, in contrast, resulted in absolute densitometric error of less than 4 percent. These results indicate that changes in the SVG component due to increased iodine concentration will affect densitometric accuracy corrected only by pre-contrast techniques. We conclude from these data, that correction techniques need to compensate for SVG variations due not only to imaging conditions (field size, air gap, patient thickness), but equally important, for variations due to iodine concentration.

Although data corrected by the dynamic method best represent those results obtained under well collimated conditions for a variety of field sizes, two limitations remain. The first is that lead disks may obstruct diagnostic information. This limitation is not critical in myocardial perfusion imaging, but some radiologic procedures may require the use of static SVG measurements acquired prior to the injection of contrast agent. The second limitation of our correction techniques is that they do not account for regional variations in SVG within a given image. Densitometric values obtained within the myocardial silhouette and corrected by a lead SVG estimate in the center of the region show approximately 5—10% variation; however, further investigation is necessary to determine the effects of collimation, projection, and dynamic range of the image. Several algorithms for correction of the regional components of SVG offer potential solution to this problem [22, 25].

We conclude from these investigations that videodensitometric iodine concentrations, both absolute and relative, contain substantial error which may be reduced by applying simple postprocessing scatter and veiling glare correction techniques. Although accurate densitometric analysis requires rigorous calibration and attention to densitometric details, the ability to detect absolute contrast concentrations in spite of the initial magnitude of densitometric error is encouraging. It is evident from these results, that quantification without regard for the previously defined densitometric errors will preclude accurate and reproducible measurement of physiologic parameters by videodensitometric techniques.

Acknowledgements

Supported in part by NIH SCOR grant # HL 27499.

References

1. Mancini GBJ, Simon SB, McGillem MJ, LeFree MT, Friedman HZ, Vogel RA: Automated quantitative coronary arteriography: morphologic and physiologic validation in vivo of a rapid digital angiographic method. Circulation 75: 452—460, 1987.
2. Simons MA, Kruger RA, Power RL: Cross-sectional area measurements by digital subtraction videodensitometry. Invest Radiol 21: 637—644, 1986.
3. Whiting JS, Drury JK, Pfaff JM, Chang BL, Eigler NL, Meerbaum S, Corday E, Nivatpumin T, Forrester JS, Swan HJC: Digital angiographic measurement of radiographic contrast material kinetics for estimation of myocardial perfusion. Circulation 73: 789—798, 1986.
4. Nichols AB, Brown C, Han J, Nickoloff EL, Esser PD: Effect of coronary stenotic lesions on regional myocardial blood flow at rest. Circulation 74: 746—757, 1986.
5. Reiber JHC, Kooijman CJ, Slager CJ, Gerbrands JJ, Schuurbiers JCH, Boer A den, Wijns W, Serruys PW, Hugenholtz PG: Coronary artery dimensions from cineangiograms-methodology and validation of a computer-assisted analysis procedure. IEEE Trans Med. Imaging MI-3(3): 131—141, 1984.
6. Barrett W, Seibert T, Hines H, Scheibe P: Automated detection of coronary arteries and quantitation of percent stenosis from DSA images: a comparison of geometric and videodensitometric techniques. Comput Cardiol: 123—126, 1984.
7. Serruys PW, Reiber JHC, Wijns W, Brand M vd, Kooijman CJ, Katen HJ ten, Hugenholtz PG: Assessment of percutaneous transluminal coronary angioplasty by quantitative coronary angiography: diameter versus densitometric area measurements. Am J Cardiol 54: 482—488, 1984.
8. Harrison DG, White CW, Hiratzka LF, Doty DB, Barnes DH, Eastham CL, Marcus ML: The value of lesion cross-sectional area determined by quantitative coronary angiography

in assessing the physiologic significance of proximal left anterior descending coronary arterial stenoses. Circulation 69: 1111—1119, 1984.

9. Bateman WA, Kruger RA: Blood flow measurement using digital angiography and parametric imaging. Med Phys 11(2): 153—157, 1984.

10. Spiller P, Schmiel FK, Pölitz B, Block M, Fermor U, Hackbarth W, Jehle J, Körfer R, Pannek H: Measurement of systolic and diastolic flow rates in the coronary artery system by X-ray densitometry. Circulation 68: 337—347, 1983.

11. Kruger RA: Estimation of the diameter of and Iodine concentration within blood vessels using digital radiography devices. Med Phys 8(5): 652—658, 1981.

12. Paulin Š, Sandor T: Densitometric assessment of stenoses in coronary arteries. SPIE 70: 337—340, 1975.

13. Rosen L, Silverman NR: Videodensitometric measurements of blood flow using cross-correlation techniques. Radiology 109: 305—310, 1973.

14. Barrett W, Boone J: The effect of beam hardening and scatter on videodensitometric determination of percent stenosis. Comput Cardiol: 15—20, 1985.

15. White KS, Baxter B, Nelson JA: Digital separation of primary and scatter components of chest radiographs. Invest Radiol 20: 854—859, 1985.

16. Nudelman S: Photoelectronic-digital radiology. Past, present, and future. In: Heintzen PH, Brennecke R (eds.): Digital imaging in cardiovascular radiology. Georg Thieme Verlag, Stuttgart 1983: pp 1—14.

17. Reiber JHC, Slager CJ, Schuurbiers JCH, Boer A den, Gerbrands JJ, Troost GJ, Scholts B, Kooijman CJ, Serruys PW: Transfer functions of the X-ray-cine-video chain applied to digital processing of coronary cineangiograms. In: Heintzen PH, Brennecke R (eds.): Digital imaging in cardiovascular radiology. Georg Thieme Verlag, Stuttgart 1983: pp 89—104.

18. Nalcioglu O, Roeck WW, Pearce JG, Gillan GD, Milne ENC: Quantitative fluoroscopy. IEEE Trans on Nucl Sci NS-28(1): 219—223, 1981.

19. Spears JR: Rotating step-wedge technique for extraction of luminal cross-sectional area information from single plane coronary cineangiograms. Acta Radiol Diagn 22: 217—225, 1981.

20. Baily NA: Video techniques for X-ray imaging and data extraction from roentgenographic and fluoroscopic presentations. Med Phys 7(5): 472—491, 1980.

21. Silverman N: Television fluorodensitometry: technical considerations and some clinical applications. Invest Radiol 5: 35—45, 1970.

22. Love LA, Kruger RA: Scatter estimation for a digital radiographic system using convolution filtering. Med Phys 14(2): 178—185, 1987.

23. Seibert JA, Nalcioglu O, Roeck WW: Characterization of the veiling glare PSF in X-ray image intensified fluoroscopy. Med Phys 11(2): 172—179, 1984.

24. Shaw C, Plewes DB: A real time scheme for correction of radiation scatter and veiling glare effects in quantitative DSA. Med Phys 11(3): 385, 1984.

25. Shaw C-G, Ergun DL, Myerowitz PD, Van Lysel MS, Mistretta CA, Zarnstorff WC, Crummy AB: A technique of scatter and glare correction for videodensitometric studies in digital subtraction videoangiography. Radiology 142: 209—213, 1982.

26. Burgess AE, Pate G: Voltage, energy and material dependence of secondary radiation. Med Phys 8(1): 33—38, 1981.

27. Radiological Health Handbook, U.S. Dept of Health, Education and Welfare: #017-011-00043-0, p 155, 1970.

28. Coulam, Erickson, Rollo, James: The physical basis of medical imaging. Appleton-Century-Crofts, New York, 1981, pp 84—86.

29. Shaw CG, Ergun DL, Van Lysel MS, Peppler WW, Dobbins JT, Zarnstorff WC, Myerowitz PD, Swanson DK, Lasser TA, Mistretta CA, Dhanani SP, Strother CM, Crummy AB: Quantitative techniques in digital subtraction videoangiography. SPIE Digital Radiography 314: 121—127, 1981.

4. Morphologic and densitometric quantitation of coronary stenoses; an overview of existing quantitation techniques

JOHAN H. C. REIBER

SUMMARY. Various groups are involved in the development and use of computer-based techniques for the assessment of quantitative measurements of coronary arterial dimensions. In this presentation an extensive overview of the different quantitative approaches will be given.

Key elements in these systems are the cine-digitizer for the 35 mm cinefilm approaches and the digital camera for the on-line approaches, the software for the semi- or fully-automated contour detection of a catheter segment (calibration) and of the coronary arterial segment (first-, second-derivative approaches or combination), and the software for the assessment of clinically relevant parameters. It is important to know whether the contour data are corrected for pincushion distortion, for the line-spread function of the X-ray system, and for the differential magnification between the catheter segment and the analyzed arterial segment. Furthermore, the question arises how the data from biplane analyses are being handled. Densitometric techniques have been developed for the assessment of absolute and relative cross-sectional area stenosis from a single angiographic view. In these cases data must be presented on calibration and correction procedures, since there are many nonlinear components in the densitometric image analysis chain.

A complete set of quantitative parameters should include obstruction and reference (how defined?) diameters and areas (circular, elliptical or densitometric approach), extent of obstruction, %-diameter and area stenosis, asymmetry of stenosis, area atherosclerotic plaque, the roughness of the arterial segment, and transstenotic pressure gradient at a given flow. Validation procedures must include data on the accuracy and precision of the edge detection technique based on (perspex) models with obstruction sizes ranging from 0.5 to 5 mm, as well as on *in-vivo* models. Furthermore, data on the results from repeated analyses of angiographic studies (reproducibility), and for the densitometric approach data on the variability from different views and under different X-ray system settings must be presented. It is proposed that the validation data are given in terms of the mean difference (accuracy) and standard deviation of the differences (precision) between corresponding measurements.

Introduction

At the present time there are about a dozen groups worldwide actively involved in the development of techniques for the objective and reproducible quantitative analysis of coronary angiograms. Such techniques

J. C. Reiber & P. W. Serruys (eds.), New Developments in Quantitative Coronary Arteriography,
34—88.

should provide, among others, absolute measurements on the minimal and reference diameters, extent and asymmetry of the obstructions, relative percent diameter and area stenosis, the area of the atherosclerotic plaque, the roughness of the coronary arterial segment, as well as data on the mean diameters of nonobstructed coronary segments, assessed from multiple projections. By combining all stenosis measurements, the functional pressure-flow effects of the stenosis, as well as coronary flow reserve can be assessed [1]. In those situations, where the obstructions are very asymmetric, such as post-PTCA where dissections frequently occur, and during and after thrombolytic therapy [2], the computation of relative and absolute cross-sectional narrowing by densitometry seems the ultimate goal to achieve.

The majority of the applications of quantitative coronary cineangiography require the comparison of the arterial dimensions either in a control group versus those in a treated group, or pre- versus post-intervention and possibly with the data from some later control-angiogram. The sample size of the number of patients that need to be investigated to demonstrate a certain effect is proportional to the variability of the measurement technique divided by the number of years between the angiograms squared [3]. From a viewpoint of the population size, duration and cost-effectiveness of a study, it is therefore of great importance to minimize the variability of the angiographic data acquisition and computer analysis procedures.

In general, the quantitative analysis of coronary obstructions is performed from 35 mm cinefilm. However, recent developments in digital cardiac imaging systems have been directed towards obtaining such measurements on-line during the catheterization procedure from video digitized images. With the present limitations in spatial resolution of these on-line digitized images, this approach is of particular interest as a tool for diagnostic and/or therapeutic decision making during the catheterization procedure. However, with the use of modern small field-of-view (FOV) image intensifiers (4" and 5" FOV) and the increase in data transfer rates such that 1024^2 images at 30 frames/s will become feasible, it may be possible in the near future to assess the effects of interventions on-line using the diameter and densitometric cross-sectional area measures mentioned above.

In this chapter an overview will be given of the different techniques that are now available for the quantitative morphologic and densitometric computer-aided analysis of the coronary obstructions [4, 5]. The majority of the techniques have been developed for cinefilm analysis; however, these are in the same or slightly modified format also applicable to the on-line digitally acquired data. All the data that is presented in this chapter have been obtained by sending a total of 12 widely known investigators a list with 25 questions on the different aspects of this topic. The summarized results presented in the tables of this chapter were sent to the individual investigators for approval.

Investigators

All twelve principal investigators returned the questionnaire; these are:

Brown — Univ. of Washington, Seattle, WA, USA
Collins — Univ. of Iowa, Iowa City, IA, USA
Doriot — Hôpital Cantonal Univ., Geneva, Switzerland
Kirkeeide — Univ. of Texas, Houston, TX, USA
Marchand — Thomson CGR, Buc, France
Nichols — Columbia Univ., New York, NY, USA
Parker — Univ. of Salt Lake City, Salt Lake City, UT, USA
Reiber — Erasmus Univ., Rotterdam, the Netherlands
Sanders — Stanford Univ., Palo Alto, CA, USA
Sandor — Harvard, Boston, MA, USA
Selzer — JPL, Los Angeles, CA, USA
Vogel — Univ. of Maryland, Baltimore, MD, USA

The following subjects will be discussed in more detail in the subsequent sections: image acquisition/ digitization of on-line digital cardiac systems; image acquisition and digitization of 35 mm cinefilm; contour detection approaches on the off-line and on-line systems; contour analysis approaches; validation procedures.

On-line digital cardiac systems (Table I)

The possibilities of presenting quantitative data about coronary morphology and functional significance immediately following an angiographic investigation is very attractive from the viewpoint of diagnosis and clinical decision making, particularly with the ever increasing application of recanalization techniques in the catheterization laboratory, such as PTCA [6—10], the use of thrombolytic agents [8, 11, 12], the introduction of the stent [13], and possibly in the near future laser [14, 15] and/or spark erosion techniques [16]. Therefore, we may expect in the coming years a dramatic increase in the development and use of on-line digital cardiac systems with more and more software packages of improved quality available for the quantitative analysis. The improvement in image quality of the on-line digital systems with pulsed fluoroscopy and real-time image enhancement techniques will also be very beneficial and necessary for the modern therapeutic procedures, such as the stent implementation and the subsequent follow-up angiographic studies [17].

A number of questions of the questionnaire were related to the description of the image acquisition and digitization part of the digital systems; the

Table I. Image acquisition/digitization on-line digital cardiac systems.

	Marchand	Doriot	Parker	Vogel
1. Name of Digital Cardiac System	CGR	Siemens Digitron II	Siemens Digitron II	ADAC
2. Limitations in matrix acquistion				
— Matrix size	512^2 1024^2	256^2 512^2	512^2	256^2 512^2 1024^2
— Max. frame rate in frames/s (f/s) (pulse duration)	512^2: 30 f/s 1024^2: 7.5 f/s	*Continuous X-ray* 256^2: 50 f/s (20 ms) 512^2: 25 f/s (40 ms) *Pulsed X-ray* 256^2: 25 f/s (<18 ms) 512^2: 12.5 f/s (<18 ms)	15 f/s at present; 30 f/s in near future	256^2: 60 f/s 512^2: 30 f/s 1024^2: 4 f/s
— Density resolution (bits)	10 bits	10 bits (both 256^2 and 512^2)	10 bits	8 bits
3. Type video camera	Primicon	Saticon	Saticon	Plumbicon
Size video tube	1″	1″	1″	1″
Interlaced or noninterlaced scanning mode	both interlaced and noninter- laced available	256^2: interlaced 512^2: noninterlaced	noninterlaced (both interlaced and noninter- laced available)	noninterlaced
4. 35 mm Cinefilm acquisition possible simultaneously with digital acquisition?	—	NOT YET, will be provided soon	YES	YES
If yes, what are the limitations?	—	—	X-ray dose is reduced with simultaneous cine and digital as compared to digital only	none

results are presented in Table I. The available software for quantitative analysis of the images will be discussed later.

At the present time there are only four groups (Doriot, Marchand, Parker, Vogel) actively involved in the development of state-of-the-art quantitative software packages for on-line coronary angiography. Doriot and Parker use the Siemens Digitron II system, Marchand the CGR system and Vogel the ADAC system (Table I, item 1); Vogel was the first one developing and using high quality software packages for the description of the morphologic and functional severity of coronary stenoses on an on-line digital system [18—20].

To quantitate the coronary morphology, the minimal requirement for image acquisition must be 512^2 matrices at a rate of 25 frames/s (Europe) or 30 frames/s (USA) with a density resolution of preferably 10 bits. In addition, pulsed X-ray radiation should be used to minimize motion blur in the images. From Table I, item 2, it appears that all three systems come close to meeting these specifications, although each of these fails at one or two minor points. Pulsed X-ray acquisition apparently is not available on the CGR and ADAC systems; in addition, ADAC uses only 8 bits of density resolution. Both CGR and ADAC allow acquisition at 1024^2 matrices, although at low frame rates of 7.5 f/s and 4 f/s, respectively. For the image acquisition all three systems use 1″ video cameras, with either a saticon, plumbicon, or primicon tube in the noninterlaced mode (Table I, item 3) [21].

At the present time there is still a lot of debate going on about the question whether the cinefilm-based systems can be replaced by the digital systems for the quantitative interpretation of intervention studies. A few centers have completely abolished cinefilm [22], but with the present resolution of the digital systems the cinefilm is still the preferred medium for the accurate assessment of changes in arterial dimensions in intervention studies [23]. Extensive studies need to be carried out to determine the advantages, disadvantages and the limitations of digital and cinefilm. Until those points have been resolved, one should be able to use 35 mm cinefilm simultaneous with the digital acquisition without any limitations (Table I, item 4).

Image acquisition and digitization of 35 mm cinefilm (Table II)

For the digitization of selected cineframes, two basic approaches have been adopted: (1) optical magnification by means of a cine-video projector with different lens systems and a video-camera; and (2) electronic magnification by means of a cine-digitizer with either a high resolution linear or area array CCD-camera (Table II, item 5). The video camera based systems vary from a customized system (Collins), a self-modified Tagarno-projector (Doriot), an Eyecom II from Spatial Data System (Kirkeeide), a video camera attachment to a standard Vanguard model XR-35 35mm projector (Nichols), a specially designed cine-to-video converter by Vanguard (Sanders [24], Vogel), to a GE CAP35 cineprojector modified by the addition of a 1000 line video camera (Selzer [25]), and finally to a second generation video based cine-digitizing system (CIVICO III), developed at the Erasmus University (Reiber [26]). In all but one of these systems standard 1″ video cameras have been used (Table II, item 6); in two systems plumbicon tubes were installed, in 5 systems a vidicon tube and in one system a pasecon tube. Selzer *et al.* have installed a 1000 line vidicon camera in their GE CAP35 projector.

Table II. Overview of items related to the image acquisition and digitization of 35 mm cinefilm. Items 9 concerns the hostcomputer as used both for the cinefilm systems and for the direct digital approach. NA = not applicable.

	Image acquisition/digitization (1a)					
	Brown	Collins	Doriot	Kirkeeide	Marchand	Nichols
35 mm cinefilm digitization						
5. Type cinefilm digitizing system	analog cinefilm projection system (Vanguard)	customized	Tagarno projector + self constructed imaging chain	Spatial Data Systems (Eyecom II)	NA	Vanguard XR-70 Coronary Analyzer
6. Type camera used	NA	Vidicon (1") Cohu model 8000	Plumbicon (1")	Vidicon	NA	Vidicon (Panasonic WV-1500)
7. Optical or electronic magnification factors available	analog magnification of 5.5×	optical, 4×	optical, 1—7×	optical, 1.8× (used in majority of cases) and 4×	NA	2×
8. For cine-digitizer with different optical lenses, is the lens selection manual or computer controlled?	NA	manual	single lens system, manual positioning of lens and video camera	manual	NA	manual
9. Host computer	– Vax-11/750	– MicroVax II	– Vax-11/750	– Vax-11/780	– 68010 Motorola	– 68008 Motorola
Image Processor	– NA	– DeAnza-Gould IP8500	– DeAnza-Gould IP6400	– none	– Vicom VDP	– only Graphics overlay
Operating System	– VMS	– VMS	– VMS	– VMS	– Versados	– Motorola VME/10 Development system
Computer Language	– Flex	– Fortran-77	– Fortran-77	– Fortran	– Pascal + Assembler	– C
10. Pixel size in digitized image at the usual magnification and referred to isocenter with the average focus/image intensifier (II) distances	NA, analog magnification 5.5× at 6" II	60 μm at 3.7× magnification and 7" II	25 μm at 3× magnification and 7" II	100 μm at 1.8× magnification and 7" II	–	140 μm at 2× magnification and 6" II

Table II (continued).

	Image acquisition/digitization (1b)					
	Parker	Reiber	Sanders	Sandor	Selzer	Vogel
35 mm cinefilm digitization						
5. Type cinefilm digitizing system	NA	two versions: a. CIVICO III (*Cine-Video-Converter*) b. Tagarno 35CX modified with high resolution optical chain	two versions: a. *at present*: Vanguard cine-to-video converter b. *converting to*: Siemens Cipro projector with CCD camera	video camera mounted in front of cinefilm projection system. Resulting optical magnification continuously adjustable.	GE CAP35 modified by addition of 1000 line video camera + digitizer	Vanguard/ADAC
6. Type camera used	NA	a. Pasecon (1″) b. CCD linear array	a. Vidicon (1″) (Sierra Scientific) b. Videk Megaplus CCD camera (1300 × 1000 pixels)	Vidicon (1″)	Vidicon (MegaVision, Inc.)	Plumbicon (1″)
7. Optical or electronic magnification factors available	NA	a. optical, 0.7, 1, 1.4, 2, 2.8, 4× b. 0.66, 1, 2×	optical 1, 3.7, 7×	0.7, 1, 1.4, 2, 2.8, 4× or more	optical: 1, 1.6, electronic: 2; both: 3.2	optical 1, 2, 4×
8. For cine-digitizer with different optical lenses, is the lens selection manual or computer controlled?	NA	both cine-digitizers are computer controlled	manual	manual	NA	manual

Table II (continued)

Image acquisition/digitization (2b)

	Parker	Reiber	Sanders	Sandor	Selzer	Vogel
9. Host computer	– 8086 (Siemens Digitron) – VAX-11/750 with Digitron I as display device	a. – PDP 11/44 – VTE – RSX-11M – Fortran-77 b. – LSI 11/73 – VIP 500 – RSX-11M+ – Fortran-77	*at present:* – HP 1000 – DeAnza-Gould – RTE – Fortran *converting to:* – HP Vectra – Data Translation – MS-DOS – C	– MicroVax II – ITI frame grabber + Warrior array processor – MVMS – Fortran	– MicroVax II – MegaVision 1024 XM – VMS – Fortran (JPL MiniVICAR Assembler used for I/O)	– PDP 11/73 – ADAC Array Processor – RT-11 – Fortran
Image Processor						
Operating System	– VMS					
Computer Language	– Fortran-77					
10. Pixel size in digitized image at the usual magnification and referred to isocenter with the average focus/image intensifier (II) distances	275 μm with 7″ II using on-line digital system; (magnification due to diverging X-ray beam ≈ 1.3X)	60 μm at 2.0X optical magnification and 5″ II (80 μm at 7″ II)	50 μm at 3.7X magnification and 6″ II	63–105 μm at 6″ II	80–100 μm at 1.6X magnification and 6″ II	65 μm at 4X magnification and 5″ II

Overall, the optical or electronic magnification factors that are available on these systems, range from 0.7 to 7× (Table II, item 7). However, in practice the 2× magnification factor is used most frequently. Selzer can use both optical (1, 1.6×) and electronic (2×) zooming, resulting in a maximal magnification of 3.2×. Brown *et al.* use a magnification factor of 5.5× with their analog projection system [27]. In all these cine-digitizers, except the ones developed at the Erasmus University in Rotterdam, the lens selection and camera positioning is done manually (Table II, item 8).

In the CIVICO III the cinefilm is mounted on a plateau with a film guiding system that can be moved under computer control left/right and upwards/downwards; the selected portion of the image is then projected onto a high resolution 1″ pasecon video camera (Fig. 1). The camera and the projection lens can be moved independently from each other under com-

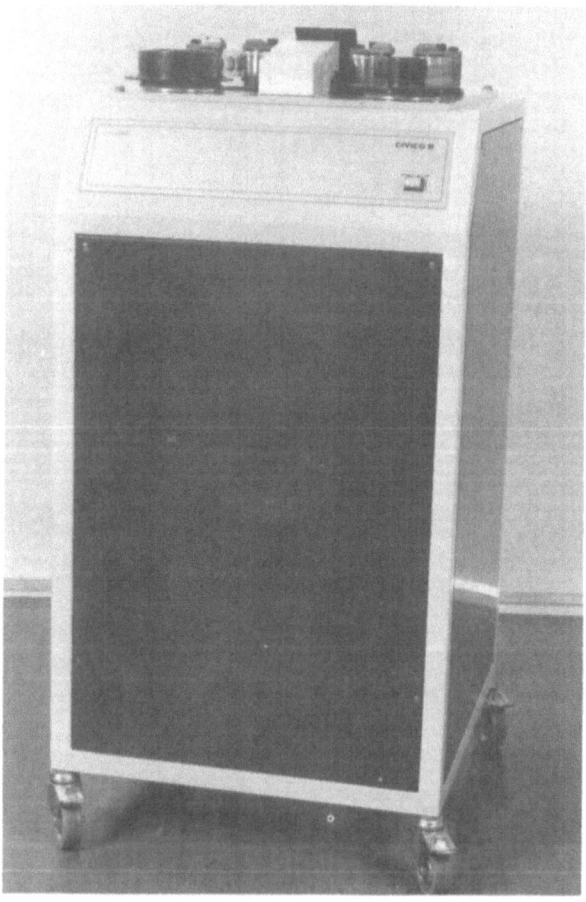

Figure 1. Photograph of 2nd generation video-based cine-digitizing system. (CIVICO III).

puter control, allowing the selection of the appropriate optical magnification (ranging from 0.7 to 4 in steps of $\sqrt{2}$). The light source consists of three light emitting diodes (LEDs) with a narrow light spectrum; the emitted amount of light can be linearly adjusted. A user-controlled, motor-driven diaphragm and automated light control system further provide for optimal image quality in the selected region of interest.

The CCD camera cinefilm digitizer developed by Reiber *et al.* is a standard cineprojector (Tagarno 35CX) with a field-installable modification package for high resolution digitization of a selected cineframe [5, 28]. This modification package consists of a film guiding system, a specially developed optical chain and a linear array (1728 elements) CCD camera; the array can be moved mechanically over a total of 2846 positions. The monochromatic light source consists of an array of four LEDs optimally suitable for densitometric analysis of the cinefilm with the present optical chain. Any area of 6.9 × 6.9 mm in a selected cineframe (size 18 × 24 mm) can be digitized by the CCD-camera with a resolution of 512 × 512 pixels with 8 bits of grey levels. Effectively, this means that the entire cineframe of size 18 × 24 mm can be digitized at a resolution of 1329 × 1772 pixels. A homogeneity in the brightness distribution over the entire digitized image of better than 5% has been achieved [29].

Sanders is building a new CCD-camera based cinefilm digitizer with a Siemens Cipro projector and a high resolution area type CCD-camera (Videk Megaplus, 1300 × 1000 pixels).

Computer hardware and software

A great variety of host computer systems has been used for the develop-ment of the quantitative software (Table II, item 9). These include VAX-11/780 (Kirkeeide), VAX-11/750 (Brown, Doriot), MicroVax II (Collins, Sandor, Selzer), PDP 11/44 (Reiber), PDP 11/73 (Reiber, Vogel), HP 1000 (Sanders), 8086 μP in Digitron II (Parker), HP Vectra personal com-puter (Sanders), and Motorola 68008 and 68010 microprocessors (Nichols, Marchand).

The video converted (cine)frames must be digitized and stored in an image processing system before any image processing functions can be applied. Here again the variety in complexity and thus cost is large: DeAnza Gould IP6400 (Doriot, Sanders) and IP8500 (Collins), Vicom VDP (Marchand), VTE DigitalVideo (Reiber), Pie Data VIP 500 (Reiber), Data Translation (Sanders), Imaging Technologies (Sandor), MegaVision-1024 XM (Selzer) and ADAC Array Processor (Vogel). In the system developed by Brown selected cineframes are projected with a standard cinefilm projector on a large writing tablet, allowing manual tracing of the boundaries of the arterial segment of interest; the coordinates of these boundary points are sent to the host computer for subsequent analysis. As a result, Brown does not need an image processor. Kirkeeide digitizes the selected frame and stores the data directly into the memory of the VAX-computer for subsequent analysis. Nichols only displays the analog video image and uses a graphics overlay for the display of alphanumeric characters, contours and lines on the screen. Parker uses a VAX-11/750 with the Digitron I as a display device.

With so many different host computer systems employed, the variety of Operating Systems is also large: VMS (7×), RSX-11M(+) (2×), RTE (1×), RT11 (1×), MS-DOS (1×), Versados (1×) and the Motorola VME/10 Development System (1×). Fortunately, there is much more consensus on the high level computer language in which the application software packages have been written. The great majority of the packages have been written in Fortran 77, while Marchand uses Pascal and assembly language, Brown uses Flex, and Nichols and Sanders use the modern language C.

The last item concerns the pixel size (μm) in the digitized image at the usual optical or electronic magnification and referred to the isocenter with the average focus-to-image intensifier distance (Table II, item 10). In other words, from this item the pixel density (number of pixels per mm) in the image can be calculated. The pixel density is linearly related to the selected magnification, and inversely linearly related to the image intensifier size. The data from Table II, item 10, are difficult to compare because of all the different magnifications and field-of-view sizes of the image intensifiers listed. If all the given pixel sizes are normalized to an image intensifier size of 6″ and a magnification of 2×, the following comparative data are obtained (Table III).

It is clear that the pixel size in the majority of the cinefilm based systems

Table III. Pixel size in digitized image (Table II, item 10) normalized to an image intensifier size of 6″ and an electronic or optical magnification of 2×.

Investigator	Pixel size (μm)
Collins	95
Doriot	32
Kirkeeide	77
Marchand	unknown
Nichols	140
Parker (Digital)	118
Reiber	72
Sanders	93
Sandor	magn. unknown
Selzer	64—80
Vogel (Digital)	156

is in the range of 64–95 μm or the pixel density ranges from 15.6–10.5 pixels/mm. Doriot uses an exceptionally small pixel size (32 μm) or high pixel density (31.3 pixels/mm), while Nichols' system and the two digital systems (Parker, Vogel) are characterized by large pixel sizes (118–156 μm) or low pixel density values (8.5–6.4 pixels/mm) as was to be expected. Marchand did not specify the pixel size for the CGR digital system.

It is of course true, that the higher the pixel density, the more pixels are available for contour detection; however, in general, one cannot state that a higher pixel density results in a more accurate edge detection performance. As the pixel density increases, the quantum mottle and film grain noise increase as well. As a result, an optimal value in pixel size must be found, which is in my opinion in the range of 64–80 μm/ pixel or pixel density of 15.6–12.5 pixels/mm.

Contour detection approaches (Table IV)

Items related to the contour detection approaches that have been developed for the various systems are presented in Table IV.

For the computer-assisted definition of the boundaries of a selected coronary segment, in general, the following steps can be distinguished:

(1) definition of coronary segment to be analyzed;
(2) edge definition;

The different implementations of these steps will be discussed in some more detail in the following paragraphs.

Definition of coronary segment to be analyzed (Table IV, item 11)

In general, the following four different approaches have been in use:

1. user indicates approximate borders of vessel (Sanders);
2. user-definition of windows over stenotic and normal segments (Doriot, Nichols);
3. user indicates number of center points in arterial segment to be analyzed (Collins, Marchand, Kirkeeide, Reiber, Sandor, Selzer);
4. automated centerline tracing (Parker, Vogel).

By the first approach, Sanders manually traces the approximate borders of the vessel and on the basis of these data the boundary positions are detected more accurately by means of edge detection techniques [30, 31].

Doriot and Nichols only place windows over the stenotic and normal

Table IV. Overview of specifications on the contour detection approaches of the various systems.

	Contour detection (1a)					
	Brown	Collins	Doriot	Kirkeeide	Marchand	Nichols
11. Definition of coronary segment to be analyzed	user manually traces boundaries of coronary segment on projected image	user indicates number of center points within coronary segment	user defines two rectangular windows, one on pre or post cross section and the other at the stenotic cross section	user indicates number of center points within coronary segment	user defines 2 points in the vessel	user positions cursor over stenotic and normal segments
12. Edge definition based on:	manual tracing	contour path determined in cost matrix based on weighted sum of 1st- and 2nd-derivative functions	max. value of 2nd-derivative function	max. value of 1st-derivative function along density profile with corrections based on phantom studies	1st semi-derivative function	full-width at half maximum (FWHM) of density profile
13. Edges corrected for line-spread function of X-ray system?	YES	NO	NO	YES	NO	NO
14. Edges corrected for pincushion distortion?	YES, radially symmetric parabolic correction function $\left(1 + \dfrac{R^2}{C}\right)$	NO	NO	YES, radially symmetric correction function	NO	NO

Table IV (continued)

	Contour detection (2b)					
	Parker	Reiber	Sanders	Sandor	Selzer	Vogel
					(approx. 10^2 squares over entire image); rubber sheet transform for entire image is optionally available (not used in current clinical trial)	
15. Method of calibration to convert pixel measurements to absolute sizes (mm)	analytically from geometric X-ray system settings in biplane images	manual or automated edge definition of catheter segment	Determine diameter of metallic marker on catheter	Automated edge definition of catheter segment	Automated edge definition of catheter segment	Automated edge definition of catheter segment
16. Correction procedure for differential magnification between catheter and arterial segment from biplane views available on your system?	NA	NO	YES, but not usually used	NO	NO	NO

Table IV (*continued*)

Contour detection (1b)

	Parker	Reiber	Sanders	Sandor	Selzer	Vogel
11. Definition of coronary segment to be analyzed	automated centerline tracking	user indicates number of center points within coronary segment	user indicates approximate borders of vessel	automated centerline tracking following manually definition of number of center points within coronary segment	user indicates number of center points within coronary segment	automated centerline tracking
12. Edge definition based on:	matched filter	contour path determined in cost matrix based on weighted sum of 1st- and 2nd-derivative functions; 2 iterations	max. 1st-derivative of density profiles perpendicular to initially manually defined borders	1st- and 2nd-derivative functions	max. of 1st-derivative function; 2 iterations	weighted sum of 1st- and 2nd-derivative functions
13. Edges corrected for line-spread function of X-ray system?	NO	NO	NO	NO	NO	NO
14. Edges corrected for pincushion distortion?	YES, quadratic approximation	YES, intersection points of cm-grid detected automatically; correction vector computed for each pixel using bilinear interpolation from 4 neighbors	YES, sometimes; assume radial symmetry of distortion	NO	YES, correction vectors autom. defined from cm-grid; edge coordinates corrected using bilinear interpolation over each grid square	YES, 'rubber sheet' vectorial pixel shift based on image of orthogonal array of bronze ball bearings

Table IV (continued)

Contour detection (2b)

	Parker	Reiber	Sanders	Sandor	Selzer	Vogel
					(approx. 10² squares over entire image); rubber sheet transform for entire image is optionally available (not used in current clinical trial)	
15. Method of calibration to convert pixel measurements to absolute sizes (mm)	analytically from geometric X-ray system settings in biplane images	manual or automated edge definition of catheter segment	Determine diameter of metallic marker on catheter	Automated edge definition of catheter segment	Automated edge definition of catheter segment	Automated edge definition of catheter segment
16. Correction procedure for differential magnification between catheter and arterial segment from biplane views available on your system?	NA	NO	YES, but not usually used	NO	NO	NO

segments and the widths of the arterial segment within these windows is computed with edge detection techniques [32—34].

If the edge positions of an entire coronary segment must be computed, the best approach is to detect these points along scanlines perpendicular to the local centerline direction of the segment. The third user-interactive approach requires that the operator defines a midline estimate for the arterial segment to be analyzed by indicating a few center points along the vessel by means of a sonic pen or writing tablet [5, 25, 35—37]. This centerline is then smoothed and defines the scanlines perpendicular to the local centerline directions for the computation of the edge positions. Reiber *et al.* and Selzer *et al.* have advocated updating this centerline by a new centerline computed from the contour positions once these have been detected and possibly corrected manually, and repeating the contour detection procedure [5, 25]. By means of this iterative approach the influence of the user definition of the center points on the detected contour positions can be minimized.

LeFree and Vogel *et al.* have developed an automated procedure for the definition of the centerline applied to digital cardiac images [18]. A polar coordinate search algorithm is used to identify the centerline of the artery, following operator assignment of the approximate center of the lesion and the diameter of a circle defining the region of interest within which the centerline is to be found.

Edge definition

To date there does not seem to be a generally accepted contour detection technique; each research group has developed and used its own algorithm. Basically, the following approaches can be distinguished:

1. Manual tracing (Brown).
2. 1st-derivative function (Kirkeeide, Sanders, Selzer).
3. 1st-semi-derivative function (Marchand).
4. 2nd-derivative function (Doriot).
5. 1st- and 2nd-derivative functions (Collins, Reiber, Sandor, Vogel).
6. Matched filter (Nichols, Parker).

The first approach based on manual tracing of the arterial boundaries is quite obvious and does not require computer-supported edge detection techniques [27].

In the approach described by Kirkeeide *et al.*, the 1st-derivative function along a scanline is computed according to a least squares convolution technique [37, 38]. Two parameters of the edge detection algorithm are important: the convolution kernel size and the edge threshold level in the first-derivative function. They have shown that the errors in the diameter detection are hyperbolically related to the kernel size, which can be corrected for by simple empirical formulas.

Sanders *et al.* determine the positions with maximal first-derivative response along lines perpendicular to manually traced margins to improve on these manually determined positions [30, 31].

Selzer *et al.* search for positions with maximal first-derivative response along scanlines perpendicular to the local direction of the earlier defined centerline [35, 36]. Marchand *et al.* use a 1st-semi-derivative function.

These positions defined by the maximal values of the first-derivative functions correspond with the inflection points of the brightness profiles along the scanlines. It has been our experience that such positions fit the arterial segments too tightly; if only the 1st-derivative response is used, certain correction factors should be employed such that the final contour positions are shifted towards the base of the brightness profiles.

Doriot uses the maximal values of the 2nd-derivative functions to determine the edge positions [32].

To simplify and speed up the edge enhancement and contour definition procedures Kooijman and Reiber *et al.* resample the digital data along the scanlines, resulting in a stretched version of the arterial segment [5, 39]. In this resampled matrix the centerline has become a straight vertical line, whereas the scanlines are oriented horizontally. Edge enhancement can now easily be achieved by applying simple one-dimensional gradient functions along the horizontal lines. Second-derivative values can be obtained by applying the gradient function to the first-derivative matrix. In Fig. 2a the resampled intensity matrix of a coronary arterial segment is shown; Fig. 2c is the cost matrix of this example, where the intensity value of a pixel is a measure for the inverse value of the weighted sum of the first- and second-derivative values for that pixel. The left and right contours are obtained by searching in a cost matrix from top to bottom for a minimal cost path (satisfying some connectivity constraints) to the left and right of the center column, respectively [39]. Figure 2d shows these minimal cost contours superimposed in the cost matrix, while these contours are shown superimposed in the stretched arterial matrix in Fig. 2b. The great advantage of this minimum cost contour detection algorithm is the fact that the edge positions are not determined per individual scanline, but that information gathered from all the other scanlines is also taken into account. As a result, this approach is less sensitive to intervening structures such as branches and overlying structures, than the local approach. The contour detection procedure is performed iteratively; following the first iteration of the contour detection and possibly the manual correction of erroneous contour points, a new centerline is computed as the midline of the detected points and the contour detection procedure is repeated, resulting in the final arterial contours.

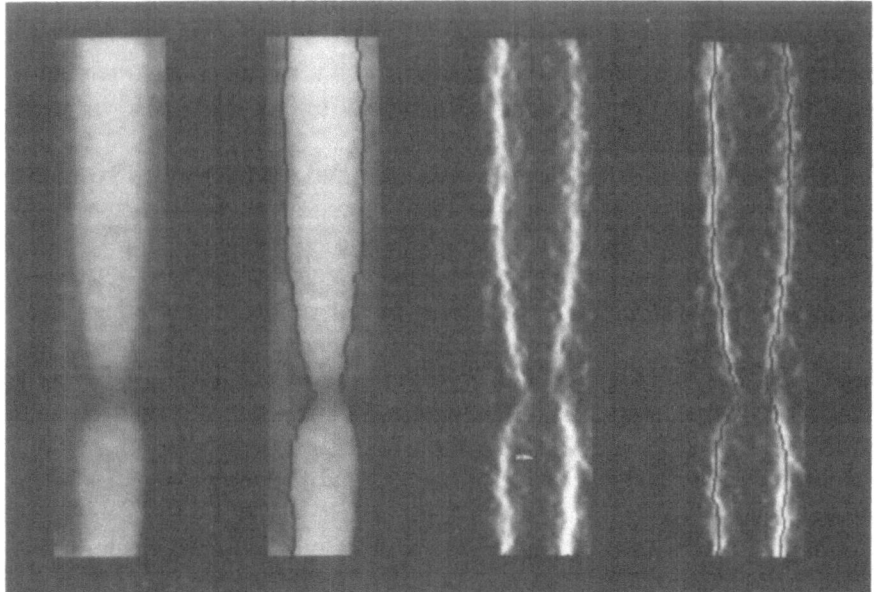

Figure 2. Minimal cost contour detection procedure ((a)—(d) from left to right). (a) Transformed intensity matrix; (b) Transformed intensity matrix with contours superimposed; (c) Cost matrix; (d) Cost matrix with contours superimposed.

Collins *et al.* also search for minimum cost paths in resampled matrices, initially applying a Sobel operator over the entire image in 2 passes (horizontal and vertical) to determine the edge strength of individual pixels [40], but later they have changed to a weighted sum of 1st- and 2nd-derivative functions.

In the technique described by LeFree and Vogel *et al.* automatic edge detection is accomplished in two passes over the scanlines [18]. During the first pass the edge points are chosen between the locations defined by the extrema of the first (inflection point) and second (base point) derivatives of the arterial profile, such that the brightness level of the edge points equals 75% of the brightness difference at the inflection and base points, above the brightness level at the base point. Those initial edge points with a distance from neighboring edge points greater than an empirically determined distance are marked as not falling on the true arterial edge contour. During the second pass the threshold values for the profiles corresponding to these spurious edge points are discarded and replaced by linear interpolation from the intensities at neighboring valid edge points. The final edge points thus use local gradient and intensity information.

Nichols *et al.* define the width of the arterial segment by the full-width-at-half-maximum (FWHM) of the video-densitometric profile measured along a scanline [34].

Parker *et al.* apply a matched filter kernel to the density profiles defined perpendicular to the automatically detected centerline of the vessel to obtain a likelihood matrix [41, 42]. Dynamic programming techniques are then applied to the likelihood matrix to find the optimal paths and thus the optimal boundaries of the vessel.

Only Brown and Kirkeeide correct the arterial boundary positions for the line-spread function (Table IV, item 13) of the X-ray system [27, 43].

Pincushion distortion and correction (Table IV, item 14)

It is well known that particularly the older types of image intensifiers introduce a geometric distortion, the so-called pincushion distortion. This results in selective magnification of an object near the edges of the image as compared to its size in the center of the field. These differences need to be corrected for, if absolute diameter measurements are to be derived from coronary angiograms. The standard procedure to assess the degree of distortion present is to film a centimeter grid which is positioned against the input screen of the image intensifier. This needs to be done only once for a given image intensifier tube at each of the available magnification modes.

A number of approaches to correct for pincushion distortion have been implemented. Theoretically, pincushion distortion is radially symmetric about the central X-ray beam, because of the rotational symmetry of the curved image intensifiers input screen and its internal fields [44]. The first approach makes the assumption that the distortion is indeed radially symmetric about the center of the image intensifier and that relative magnification can be determined from the distance of the pixel under consideration from the center of the image intensifier. An empirically determined analytical function of the radius is then used to correct for the distortion. This approach has been implemented by Brown [27] and Kirkeeide [38].

The second method is also based on radial symmetry, but relative magnification factors for a single radial line are stored in the memory of the computer system. The relative magnification for each distance was obtained by averaging the four values measured in the four quadrants of the centimeter-grid image. Hence, no analytical function is employed; this approach has been taken by Sanders *et al.* [30, 31].

The third method, which is in use in our center as well as by Selzer, makes no assumption about the geometrical distribution of the distortion, but stores the relative magnifications of all the intersection points of the centimeter grid [5, 35, 36, 39]. We have developed a procedure that allows the fully automated detection of the wires and intersection points in the 1 : 1

projected cineframe. For a given point in the image which does not coincide with one of the displayed intersection positions, the correction vector is determined by means of bilinear interpolation between the correction vectors of the four neighboring intersection points; Selzer also uses bilinear interpolation.

In their digital cardiac system, LeFree and Vogel *et al.* have implemented a somewhat similar approach, except for the fact that they correct the entire image by piecewise linear warping and not only the contour positions of the catheter and arterial segment ('rubber sheet' transform) [18]. For these purposes a 1 cm spaced orthogonal array of bronze ball bearings is imaged at the image intensifier input screen. The 'rubber sheet' transform is also optionally available from Selzer.

In five institutes (Collins, Doriot, Marchand, Nichols and Sandor) the detected contour positions are not corrected for the pincushion distortion.

Calibration (Table IV, item 15)

To compute absolute sizes of the arterial segment analyzed, a calibration factor needs to be determined. Basically, two different approaches have been in use for the coronary arteries: (1) analytically from geometric X-ray system parameters; (2) on the basis of the known diameter of the contrast catheter or of the known size or distance of markers on the catheter. Following the first approach, the size of an object in the plane through the center of rotation of the X-ray system (isocenter) and parallel to the image intensifier input screen can be determined from simple geometric principles from the height levels of X-ray tube and image intensifier. However, for objects above or below the center of rotation a slightly more complicated analysis must be carried out, requiring a second, preferably orthogonal view of the object. Wollschläger *et al.* have developed a method to calculate the exact radiological magnification factors for each point in the fields of view of biplane multidirectional isocentric X-ray equipment [45, 46]. By this approach they avoid two error sources: contour detection of the catheter segment, and the differential magnification of the scaling device and the arterial segment. Parker also determines the calibration factors from the geometric X-ray system settings in biplane images; one of the options of Kirkeeide's method is also based on this approach.

If the catheter is used as a scaling device, the contours of a short segment of the tip or shaft may either be manually defined with a writing tablet, or contour detection techniques similar to those used for the coronary segments may be applied. The manual approach in biplane images is used by Brown [27]; Collins and Reiber allow both for manual and automated definition of a catheter segment. Most authors apply the same kind of automated edge detection technique to the catheter as used for the coronary segment (Collins, Doriot, Kirkeeide, Nichols, Reiber, Sandor, Selzer, Vogel). In our routine practice, the catheter is magnified optically or electronically with a factor of $2\sqrt{2} : 1$ or $2 : 1$, respectively and *a priori* information is included in the iterative edge detection procedure, based on the fact that the selected part of the catheter is the projection of a cylindrical structure. It should be realized that the size of the catheter as given by the manufacturer, in general, will deviate from its true size, especially for disposable catheters. Therefore, for intervention studies it may be advisable to measure the size of the catheter following the catheterization procedure with a micrometer [47, 48].

Some time ago, several new types of catheters with cardiomarker rings have been designed on the request of a number of investigators. Kirkeeide determines the distance between the cardiomarker rings (1 cm spacing) in biplane angiograms, while Sanders measures the diameter of a metallic marker on the catheter. Because of the high contrast of the marker in the X-ray images, the edges can be defined relatively reliably.

If the known size of the catheter in a single angiographic view is used for calibration purposes, the computed calibration factor is only applicable to objects in the plane of the catheter parallel to the image intensifier input screen. The change in magnification for two objects located at different points along the X-ray beam axis is about 1.5% for each centimeter that separates the objects axially with the commonly used focus-image intensifier distances. For coronary segments lying in other planes corrections to the calibration factor can be assessed from other views. Brown, Kirkeeide, Sanders and Wollschläger provide the means on their systems to correct for the differential magnification from biplane angiograms.

From the above, it is clear that for the measurement of truly absolute sizes of coronary segments, two views, preferably but not necessarily orthogonal to each other, are required. However, if one is only interested in the changes in sizes of coronary segments as a result of short- or long-term interventions, excellent results can be achieved from single-plane views. For these situations one must make sure that for the repeat angiogram the X-ray system is positioned in exactly the same geometry as during the first angiogram. This requires registration of the angles and height levels of the X-ray system, preferably on line with a microprocessor-based geometry read-out system [47]. Although the calibration factor used for a particular coronary arterial segment is then only an approximation of the true calibration factor, the same systematic error will be present for the first and repeat angiograms.

Contour analysis approaches (Table V)

From the contours of the analyzed arterial segment, following smoothing,

Table V. Overview of specifications on the contour analysis approaches of the various systems.

	Contour analysis (1a)					
	Brown	Collins	Doriot	Kirkeeide	Marchand	Nichols
17. Reference for %-D stenosis measurement	user-defined	user-defined	user-defined	both user-defined and computer estimations of pre-disease dimensions at obstruction are available; computer estimate is first displayed; user can subsequently manually correct or define other reference sections	—	user-defined
18. Do you calculate roughness measure of arterial segment as an indication for diffuse atherosclerosis?	NO	NO	NO	NO	NO	NO
19. Do you perform densitometric analysis of cross-sectional data from one angiographic view? Your technique is based on the following transfer functions:	NO	YES,	YES, intensity profiles of the 2 cross sections corrected for beam hardening	NO, use density information only when orthogonal biplane views are available	YES,	YES
– X-ray absorption from X-ray source to image intensifier (II)	—	– Lambert-Beer Law	– assessed by their own second order polynomial model (kV, conc. dependent)	– Lambert-Beer Law	– Lambert-Beer Law	– Lamber-Beer Law

Table V (continued)

	Contour analysis (2a)					
	Brown	Collins	Doriot	Kirkeeide	Marchand	Nichols
– from output II to brightness level in digitized image	—	– assessed from digitized sensitometric strip	– this transfer function has proven to be sufficiently linear	– uses linear portion of D vs log E-curve, regularly checked with digitized sensitometric strip	– linear transfer function	– logarithmic transformation and use of characteristic curve of cinefilm
20. Derived parameters coronary arterial segment	– obstruction diam. – obstruction area (elliptical cross sections) – reference diam. – %-D stenosis – %-Area stenosis (elliptical cross sections) – length of obstruction – area atherosclerotic plaque – transstenotic pressure gradient (mmHg) at given flow	– obstruction diam. – obstruction area (densitometric) – reference diam. – %-D stenosis – %-Area stenosis (densitometric)	– obstruction area (densitometric) – reference diam. – %-D stenosis – %-Area stenosis (densitometric)	– obstruction diam. – obstruction area (elliptical cross sections) – reference diam. – %-D stenosis – %-Area stenosis (elliptical cross sections) – length of obstruction – transstenotic pressure gradient (mmHg) at given flow	– %-Area stenosis (densitometric)	– obstruction diam. – obstruction area (densitometric) – reference diam. – %-D stenosis – %-Area stenosis (densitometric)
21. What do you do with the results from biplane analyses?	combine the results in a 3D-presentation using elliptical cross sections	use as separate items	until to date uses only single plane images (however with densitometric analysis)	combine the results in a 3D-presentation using elliptical cross sections	—	only use single plane analyses with densitometry

Table V (continued)

Contour analysis (1b)

	Parker	Reiber	Sanders	Sandor	Selzer	Vogel
17. Reference for %-D stenosis measurement	—	— user-defined — interpolated technique for estimation 'normal' vessel dimensions (tapering vessel allowed)	user-defined	user-defined	computer estimation defined by 90 percentile of diam. profile (no tapering); protocol requires that tracking does not proceed past a branch	user-defined
18. Do you calculate roughness measure of arterial segment as an indication for diffuse atherosclerosis?	NO	YES, each coronary segment is sub-divided into subsegments of ≈ 5 mm length. Per subsegment, ratio of standard deviation of diam.-values and (max-min) value determines degree of roughness	YES, measure variation σ of vessel diameters, although not usually used	NO	YES, fit least squares straight line to vessel width profile and use residual variance as roughness measure	NO
19. Do you perform densitometric analysis of cross-sectional data from one angiographic view? Your technique is based on the following transfer functions:	YES,	YES,	NO	NO	YES	YES, optionally available; not used in current clinical trial
— X-ray absorption from X-ray source to image intensifier (II)	— Lambert-Beer Law	— Lambert-Beer Law	— NA	— NA	— Lambert-Beer Law	— Lambert-Beer Law

Table V (continued)

Contour analysis (2b)

	Parker	Reiber	Sanders	Sandor	Selzer	Vogel
– from output II to brightness level in digitized image	– linear transfer function	a. transfer function determined from 21 homogeneously exposed density frames generated on each patient film b. linear transfer function	– NA	– NA	– linear, validity checked with digitized sensitometric strip	– linear transfer function
20. Derived parameters	– obstruction area (densitometric) – other parameters under development	– obstruction diam. – obstruction area (densitometric) – reference diam. – %-D stenosis – %-Area stenosis (densitometric) – length of obstruction – symmetry of stenosis – area atherosclerotic plaque – transstenotic pressure gradient (mmHg) at given flow	– obstruction diam. – reference diam. – %-D stenosis – area atherosclerotic plaque	– obstruction diam. – reference diam. – %-D stenosis – length of obstruction	– obstruction diam. – reference diam. – %-D stenosis – %-Area stenosis (circular) – area atherosclerotic plaque	– obstruction diam. – obstruction area (densitometric) – reference diam. – %-D stenosis – %-Area stenosis (densitometric) – length of obstruction – symmetry of stenosis – area atherosclerotic plaque

Table V (continued)

Contour analysis (3b)

	Parker	Reiber	Sanders	Sandor	Selzer	Vogel
21. What do you do with the results from biplane analyses?	average the results from the two views	— use as separate items — average the results from the two views	— use as separate items — combine the results in a 3D-presentation using elliptical cross sections	combine the results in a 3D-presentation using elliptical cross sections	average the results from the 2 views; option: reconstruct 3D image, assuming elliptical cross sections and calculate cross-sectional areas, %-A stenosis and hemodynamic data	combine results in a 3D-presentation using elliptical cross sections

pincushion correction and calibration, a diameter function can be determined by computing the distances between the left and right edges. From these data a number of parameters may be calculated such as: minimal obstruction diameter; obstruction area; extent of the obstruction; percentage diameter stenosis; percentage area stenosis; symmetry of the stenosis; area of the atherosclerotic plaque; hemodynamic parameters of the obstruction; and mean diameter of a nonobstructive coronary segment. Particularly the minimal obstruction diameter is of great importance as it is present to the inverse fourth power in the formulas describing the pressure loss over a coronary obstruction. Moreover, to determine the effect of interventions on the severity of coronary obstructions, one should compute the changes in minimal obstruction diameter and not those in percentage diameter narrowing, as the reference position in general will also be affected by the intervention [9]. The different approaches to measuring these and other parameters will be described in the following paragraphs.

Reference for %-D stenosis measurement (Table V, item 17)

Although the absolute minimal obstruction diameter is one of the parameters of choice to describe the changes in the severity of an obstruction as a result of an intervention, percentage diameter narrowing in an individual case is intuitively a very pleasant parameter to work with.

The usual way to determine percentage diameter stenosis of a coronary obstruction, requires the user to indicate a reference position. A reference diameter is then usually computed as the average value of a number of diameter values in a symmetric region with center at the user-defined reference position. This or a similar approach which is denoted the user-defined reference technique has been taken by Brown, Collins, Doriot, Kirkeeide, Nichols, Reiber, Sanders, Sandor and Vogel.

However, it is clear that this computed %-D narrowing of an obstruction depends heavily on the selected reference position. In arteries with a focal obstructive lesion and a clearly normal proximal arterial segment, the choice of the reference region is straightforward and simple. However, in cases where the proximal part of the arterial segment shows combinations of stenotic and ectatic areas, the choice may be very difficult. To minimize these variations, alternative methods have been developed which are not dependent on a user-defined reference region [5, 35, 36, 39]. By these methods an estimate of the normal or pre-disease arterial size and luminal wall location is obtained on the basis of the computed centerline and the 90th percentile of the diameter values [Selzer, 25, 35, 36], or on the basis of a first-degree polynomial computed through the diameter values of the proximal and distal portions of the arterial segment followed by a translation to the 80th percentile level (reference diameter function) [Reiber, 5, 39]; tapering of the vessel to account for a decrease in arterial caliber associated with branches is taken care of in this last approach. In this last case, the proximal and distal boundaries of the obstruction are determined from the diameter function on the basis of significant maxima in curvature using variable degrees of smoothing. If the user does not agree with either one or both of the proximal and distal obstruction boundaries, these can be corrected manually. The reference diameter is now taken as the value of the reference diameter function at the location of the minimal obstruction diameter. This approach is denoted the interpolated or computer-defined reference technique. Kirkeeide *et al.* also estimate the pre-disease dimensions at the obstruction [1].

The interpolated or computer-defined percentage diameter stenosis is computed by comparing the minimal diameter value at the obstruction with the corresponding value of the reference diameter. An example of our technique is shown in Figure 3 for an obstruction in the mid-portion of the LAD in the RAO-projection. The actual contours as well as the estimated pre-disease reference contours of the arterial segment are superimposed in the image. The difference in area between the reference and the detected

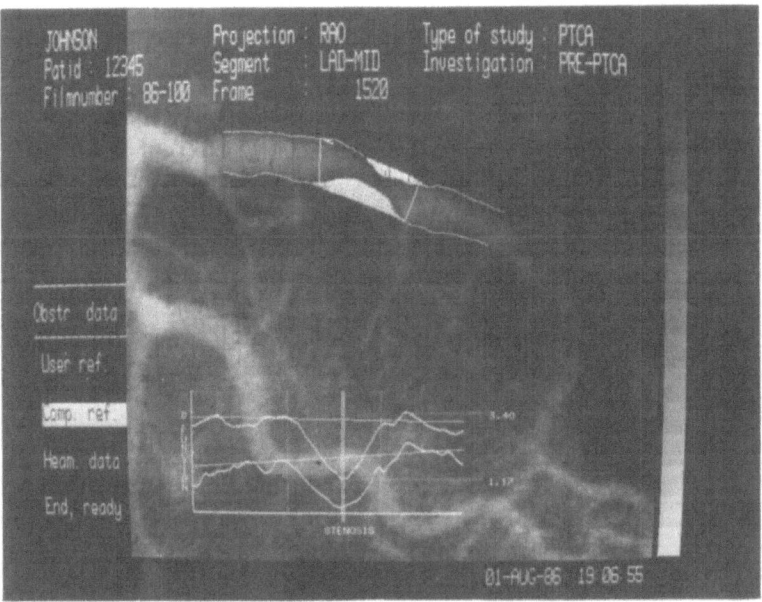

Figure 3. Example of the automatically detected luminal boundaries of the mid LAD-segment and the estimated pre-disease dimensions of the vessel at the site of the obstruction (reference edges). The upper function is the diameter function with the straight line through it being the reference diameter function; the lower function is the densitometric area function with the estimated reference area function (straight line).

luminal contours is marked over the obstructive lesion; this area is a measure for the atherosclerotic plaque in this particular angiographic view. The upper function is the diameter function with the straight line being the reference diameter function; the lower function is the densitometric area function (see section on Densitometry).

In addition, this interpolated or computer-defined reference diameter technique allows the assessment of the symmetry or asymmetry of the lesion in a given view with respect to a reconstructed centerline. Vessel midpoints for the proximal and distal "normal" portions are found by averaging the coordinates of the left and right contour points. For the obstructive region the vessel midpoints are obtained by interpolation between the proximal and distal vessel midpoints with a second-degree polynomial. The symmetry measure is given as a value between 0 and 1, with 1 representing a concentric lesion and 0 the most severe case of asymmetry or eccentricity. In addition to the fact that the interpolated technique provides data about the area of the atherosclerotic plaque and the lesion's symmetry in a given view, there is another very practical advantage. By this technique, knowledge about the exact location of a reference, either proximal or distal to the stenosis, is not required for the analysis of repeated angiograms.

From the available morphological data of the obstruction, the Poisseuille and turbulent resistances at different flows and thus the resulting transstenotic pressure gradients can be computed on the basis of the well-known fluid-dynamic equations [1, 5, 49].

For the example of Figure 3, the following quantitative measurements were obtained:

extent obstruction	:	7.51 mm
reference diameter	:	3.16 mm
obstruction diameter	:	1.17 mm
reference area (assuming circular cross sections)	:	7.86 mm^2
obstruction area (densitometric)	:	0.84 mm^2
area atherosclerotic plaque	:	9.90 mm^2
symmetry measure	:	0.53
diameter stenosis	:	63.1 %
area stenosis (densitometric)	:	89.4 %
transstenotic pressure gradient at mean flow of 1 ml/s	:	3.04 mmHg

The mean diameter of a nonobstructive coronary segment can easily be determined from the diameter data by requesting the user to indicate with the writing tablet, lightpen or similar device the proximal and distal boundaries of the desired segment; the length of the segment in mm is usually also provided. For intervention studies coronary branch points may be used to define the boundaries of the segment, as these can be determined fairly reproducibly.

64

Roughness measure of arterial segment (Table V, item 18)

Information about the 'roughness' of the arterial segment and thus about diffuse coronary artery disease may be obtained by subdividing the coronary segment into an integer number of subsegments with a length of about 5 mm and calculating for each subsegment the minimal, maximal, mean diameter and the standard deviation of the diameter value [5]. On the basis of the quotient of the standard deviation value and the difference between minimal and maximal diameter, it can be determined whether a subsegment is focally or diffusely diseased, or normal. However, clinical validation procedures need to be carried out to determine the true value of this parameter Fig. 4 shows the four subsegments for the example of Fig. 3; the derived sub-segmental data are given in Table VI.

Sanders uses the variation of the vessel diameters as a measure for diffuse atherosclerosis, while Selzer *et al.* fit a least squares straight line through the vessel width profile and use the residual variance as a roughness measure. Crawford *et al.* have developed various edge roughness measures for femoral arteries [50]; two edge roughness measures were defined by the root-mean-square differences between two sets of edge coordinates obtained by the use

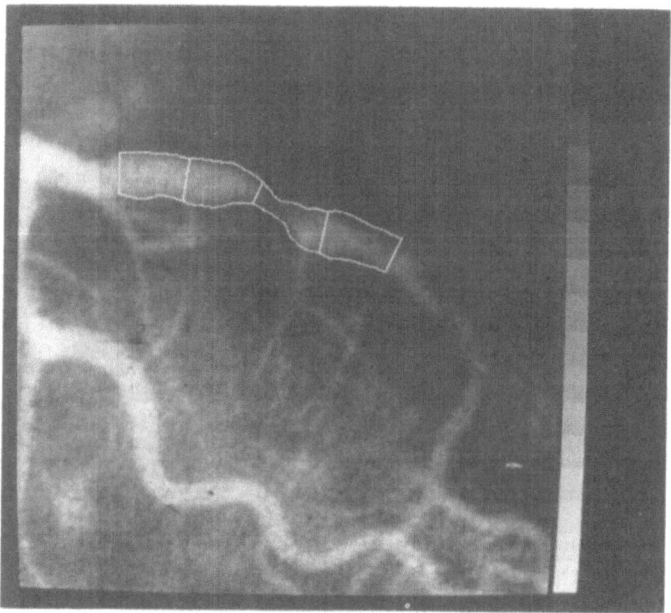

Figure 4. To obtain information about the 'roughness' (irregularities) of the arterial segment, the segment is subdivided into an integer number of subsegments with lengths of approximately 5 mm and for each subsegment the standard deviation with respect to the mean value is computed. The subsegmental data for this example is presented in Table VI.

Table VI. Subsegmental data for the example of Fig. 4. Segment no. 1 is the most proximal segment.

Segment	1	2	3	4
Length (mm)	5.51	5.51	5.51	5.51
Minimal diam. (mm)	2.92	1.74	1.17	2.68
Maximal diam. (mm)	3.29	3.27	3.03	3.40
Mean diam. (mm)	3.04	2.85	2.02	2.99
Standard dev. (mm)	0.12	0.48	0.69	0.24
Focal or Diffuse Disease	NO	YES	YES	NO

of filters of different lengths. The other investigators do not calculate a roughness measure as an indication for diffuse atherosclerosis.

Densitometry (Table V, item 19)

Since the luminal cross section at a coronary obstruction is frequently irregular in shape, percentage diameter reduction measured in a single angiographic view is of limited diagnostic value [2]. The hemodynamic resistance of an obstruction is determined to a great extent by the minimal cross-sectional area. Computation of this cross-sectional area reduction from the percentage diameter reduction measured in a single view requires the assumption of, e.g., circular cross sections, an assumption which hardly ever holds. This is particularly true post-PTCA, where dissections may occur [6, 51]. The resulting error may be reduced by incorporating two orthogonal projections and computing elliptical cross sections. However, with the often occurring eccentric lesions even this last approach may yield inaccurate results.

The edge detection techniques described above, in general are based on the measurement of changes in the brightness profiles along scanlines perpendicular to local centerline segments. Therefore, if one could constitute the relationship between the path lengths of the X-rays through the artery and the absolute brightness values in the digitized image, one would obtain the information required to compute the cross-sectional areas from a single view (Fig. 5). It is clear that a homogeneous mixing of the contrast agent with the blood must be assumed for the measurement to have any meaning. This approach is called the densitometric measurement technique. An additional advantage of the densitometric technique is that the stringent requirements on the accuracy of the edge detection can be diminished. If the detected boundaries are outside of the true edges and if the background correction procedure (see later) works well, then the true cross-sectional area can still

66

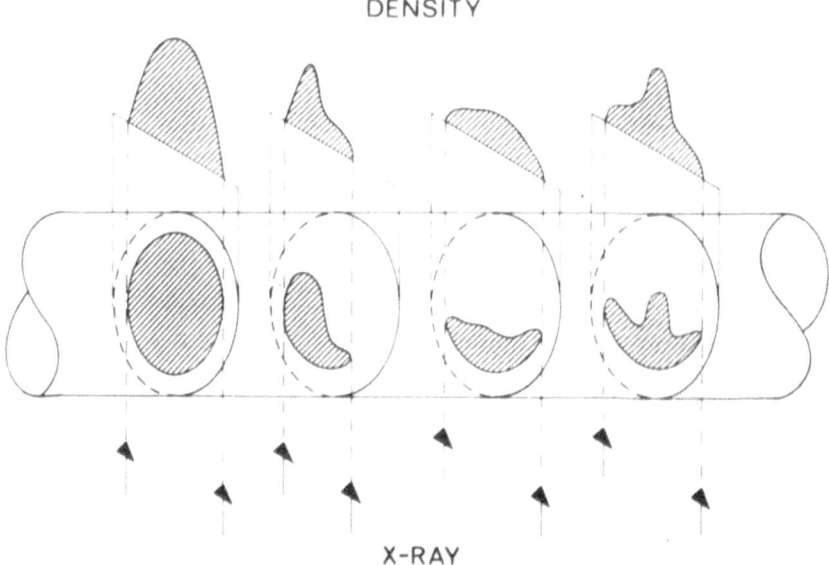

DENSITY

X-RAY

Figure 5. Schematic illustration of the relationship between the irradiated object thickness and the brightness level in the digitized angiographic image.

be computed with the necessary accuracy. Table V shows that nine investigators (Collins, Doriot, Marchand, Nichols, Parker, Reiber, Selzer, Vogel) perform densitometric analysis of cross-sectional data from one angiographic view; Kirkeeide uses the density information only when orthogonal biplane views are available. The common approaches and the differences between the various techniques will be discussed briefly in the following paragraphs.

A simplified block diagram of a complete X-ray/cine acquisition and analysis system is shown in Figure 6A. In a digital cardiac system the video camera at the output screen of the image intensifier (Fig. 6B) is connected directly to the Image Processor via the analog-to-digital (A/D) converter. The image data are stored on a digital disk for later retrieval and analysis.

Constitution of the relationship between path length and brightness values requires detailed analysis of the complete imaging system. In a simplified approach, we are only interested in the static properties of the system. Analysis of the static transfer function of each link in the chain reveals that computation of the complete transfer function is very difficult. There is a large number of parameters involved, many of which are spatially variant [5, 52]. In practice, a number of simplifications are introduced to arrive at usable techniques.

Eight of the nine investigators assume that the X-ray absorption process, comprising the first part of the imaging chain from X-ray source to the image intensifier input screen, can be described by the Lambert-Beer law. Despite

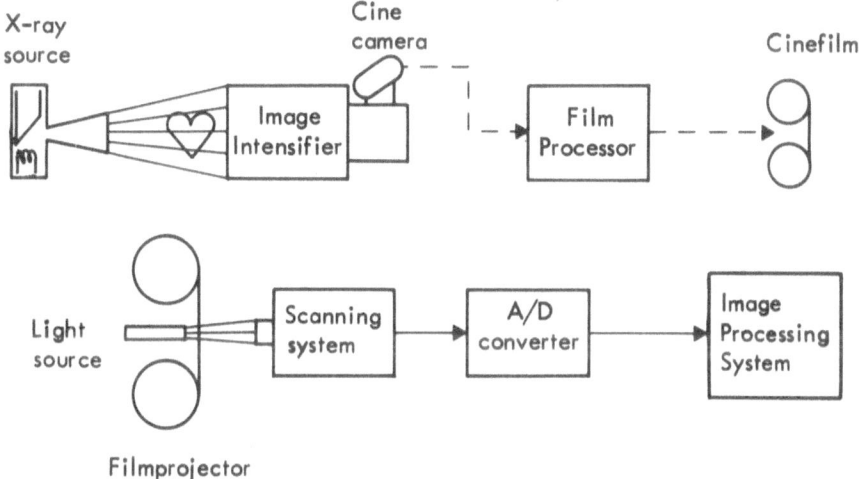

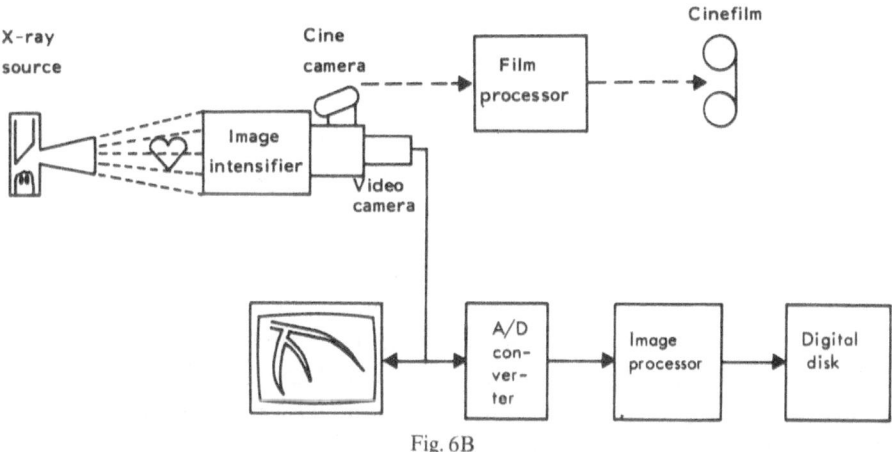

Figure 6. Block diagrams of an off-line X-ray/cine acquisition and analysis system (Fig. 6A) and of an on-line digital cardiac system (Fig. 6B).

many potential sources of error in the absorption process (nonmonochromatic X-ray spectrum, beam hardening, scattering, etc.) it has indeed been demonstrated by Bürsch and Heintzen that by the use of appropriate filters and scatter grids the Lambert-Beer law is applicable for densitometric measurements in clinical studies to a sufficient degree of accuracy [53, 54].

On the other hand, Doriot *et al.* have indicated that the Lambert-Beer absorption law cannot account for the nonlinear relationship between the densitometric signal and logarithmic X-ray transmission through the lumen of an opacified coronary artery [32, 55]. Therefore, they have developed a physical model which takes the polychromasy and scattered radiation into account and have shown that this relation can be approximated by a 2nd-order polynomial. The coefficients of this polynomial depend primarily on the voltage applied to the X-ray tube and on the iodine concentration of the injected contrast medium. For a particular X-ray system the coefficients of the polynomial can simply be obtained once by means of a linear wedge filled with contrast material. They have shown that the errors in the assessment of the densitometric percent area stenosis and obstruction area by the conventional densitometric technique (using the Lambert-Beer Law and possibly compensating for the nonlinearity introduced by the cinefilm) depend on the actual size and shape of the intact and stenotic lumens, on their rotational orientation with respect to the incident X-rays, on the kV-level of the X-ray tube and on the iodine concentration of the injected contrast medium [55].

However, in general, for the remaining subsystems of the cinefilm imaging chain comprising the image intensifier, the cinefilm exposure and development process, and the film sampling process which may be achieved via video and A/D conversion, with a CCD camera or other device, simplified formulas relating measured brightness levels with the irradiated object thicknesses are used neglecting the influence of spatially nonhomogeneous responses. By this approach the response of film exposure, the density D versus log(exposure) curve, is being linearized (linear transfer function). Kirkeeide, Reiber and Selzer have implemented this approach [1, 38, 56]. Nichols *et al.* assume a logarithmic transformation based on the photo-electric measurement technique of the light from the projector; they also make use of the characteristic curve of the cinefilm. Collins *et al.* determine the transfer function on the basis of a sensitometric strip [57].

We have also implemented a more complicated approach in an attempt to correct for the nonlinearities in the D versus $\log(E)$ plot and for the daily variations in the cinefilm processing [5, 52]. For this purpose, a special sensitometer has been developed which allows 21 full cineframes covering the entire densitometric range of the film to be exposed on each film cassette before it is mounted on the image intensifier of the X-ray system (Fig. 7). The color temperature of the light source is the same as the one from the output screen of the image intensifier. The analysis procedure of a coronary cineangiogram therefore starts with the digitization of these 21 sensitometric frames, allowing the assessment of a nonlinear transfer function.

By means of this calibration procedure many nonlinear, both temporally and spatially variant effects in the film-processing and the film-video or film-CCD camera system are taken into account. It has indeed been shown that this sensitometric approach improves the accuracy of the cross-sectional area measurements as compared to the linear approach [29, 56].

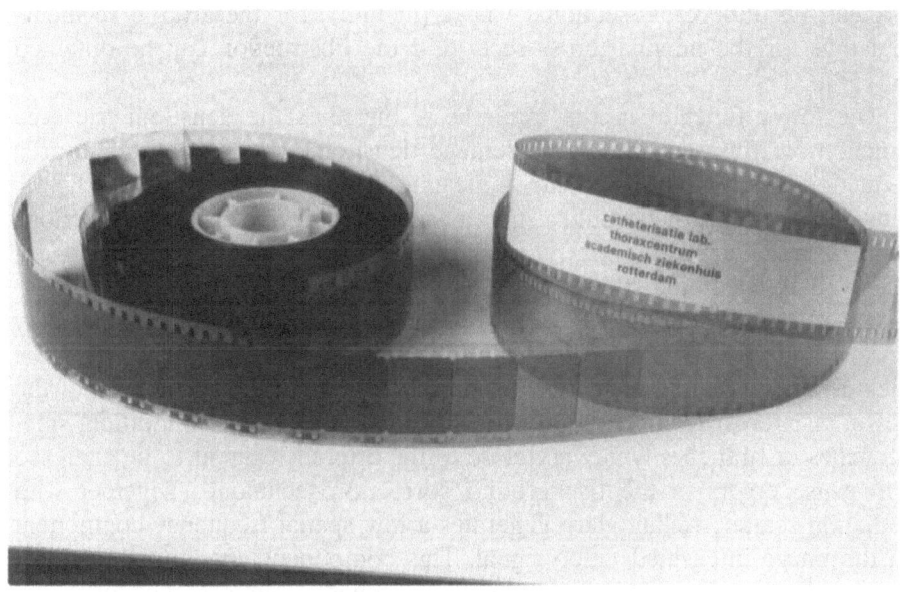

Figure 7. Example of cinefilm with sensitometric strip of 21 homogeneously exposed cine-frames.

In a digital cardiac system, the transfer function from the output of the image intensifier up to the digitized image can be approximated accurately by a linear function (Doriot, Marchand, Parker, Vogel).

The basic steps in the densitometric procedure to compute percentage cross-sectional area reduction of a selected lesion can be summarized as follows. The contours of a selected arterial segment are detected as described before. On each scanline perpendicular to the centerline, a profile of brightness values is measured. This profile is transformed into an absorption profile by means of the computed transfer functions (linear or nonlinear depending on the technique used). The background contribution is estimated by computing the linear regression line through the background points directly left and right of the detected contours. Subtraction of this background portion from the absorption profile within the arterial contours yields the net cross-sectional absorption profile. Integration of this function results in a measure for the cross-sectional area at the particular scanline. By repeating this procedure for all the scanlines, the cross-sectional area function $A(i)$ is obtained. Percentage area reduction of an obstruction is determined by comparing the minimal area value at the obstruction with the mean value at a selected reference position. The earlier mentioned interpolated approach can also be applied for the estimation of the pre-disease area values. If we assume that the cross section at the reference position is circular, absolute cross-sectional values (in mm^2) for the arterial segments and thus for the minimal cross section at the obstruction can be obtained [51, 58].

The lower function in the example of Fig. 3 is the densitometric area function for this segment. A percentage densitometric cross-sectional area reduction of 89.4% was found, indicating that the obstruction is slightly more severe than one would estimate by assuming circular cross sections (86% area reduction).

It will be clear that the densitometric analysis of coronary arterial segments is a difficult problem because of all the potential problems that may arise. In addition to all the possible error sources mentioned above, these include veiling glare and scatter, beam hardening and the orientation of the vessel of interest with respect to the X-ray beam [41, 59]. In addition, side-branches or branches lying very close to the arterial segment to be analyzed will cause errors in the background correction technique. Together with radiation scatter, veiling glare generates a low spatial frequency component in the image intensified video signal. This component nonuniformly biases the black level in video angiography. In general, the presence of X-ray scatter and glare causes a suppression of contrast in the intensified image. A technique using a digital convolution algorithm has been proposed by Shaw *et al.* to approximate and correct for the scatter and glare [60].

Pfaff *et al.* have corrected for scatter and veiling glare by measuring the intensity beneath a 4 mm lead disk and subtracting it from each of the pixel intensities prior to logarithmic transformation [61]. They concluded that errors in densitometric measurement of both absolute and relative iodine concentrations are substantial unless corrections are applied to the raw data.

Although various phantom studies have been published on densitometric analysis of obstructions, until to date to my knowledge only two *in-vivo* validation studies have been published. Wiesel *et al.* described a study with closed-chest dogs in which 10 plastic cylinders with precisely machined circular and irregular lumina were inserted into the coronary arteries. Minimal cross-sectional area of the stenosis was determined by the edge-detection technique from two orthogonal views (ellipse method) and by densitometry from one view. They concluded that the ellipse method is more accurate for circular stenoses, while the irregular stenoses were better quantitated by the video density method with an average absolute difference of 0.50 mm^2 and an SEE = 0.47 [58]. Collins *et al.* have performed the *in-vivo* validation study by comparing the densitometric data with the results from intra-operative high frequency epicardial echocardiography [57].

A further demonstration of all the possible problems with densitometry can be given by the fact, that only few investigators have been able to demonstrate so far, that the densitometric results from different views of the same vessel agree very closely, which must be a requirement if densitometry really works as well as we would hope [62].

Derived parameters coronary arterial segment (Table V, item 20)

The investigators were requested to list all the parameters that they compute and use to describe a coronary obstruction. For Table V, item 20, the following list with the frequency of use indicated can be derived:

Derived parameters coronary arterial segment	*frequency*
— Obstruction diameter (mm)	(9×)
— Obstruction area (mm²)	
* circular	
* elliptical	(2×)
* densitometric	(6×)
— Reference diameter (mm)	(10×)
— %-D stenosis (%)	(10×)
— %-A stenosis (%)	
* circular	(1×)
* elliptical	(2×)
* densitometric	(6×)
— length of obstruction (mm)	(5×)
— symmetry of stenosis	(2×)
— area atherosclerotic plaque (mm²)	(5×)
— transstenotic pressure gradient (mmHg) at given flow	(3×)

Thus, almost all investigators use the 'simple' parameters obstruction diameter, reference diameter, %-D stenosis, obstruction area and %-A stenosis assessed by different techniques. Less frequently used are the length of the obstruction, the area of the atherosclerotic plaque, the symmetry of the stenosis and finally the transstenotic pressure gradient at a given flow.

What do you do with the results from biplane analyses? (Table V, item 21)

In general, coronary obstructions are analyzed from at least two, preferably orthogonal, angiographic views, because of the eccentricity of lesions and because of the fact that the obstruction may be much better visible in one view than in another due to foreshortening or overlap with other vessels or branches. According to the responses, six of the investigators (Brown, Kirkeeide, Sanders, Sandor, Selzer (optionally), Vogel) compute elliptical cross sections from the biplane data, requiring that the two views be matched such that the images of the stenosis in both views coincide [27]. It is generally assumed, that the points of minimum diameter in both views correspond to the same site in the artery. However, such an assumption can be a potential source of error. Collins, Reiber and Sanders also use the data as separate items. On the other hand, Parker, Reiber and Selzer, average the results from the two views. Finally, Doriot and Nichols only perform single-plane analyses with densitometry.

Measurement variabilities and validation procedures

Although different approaches on the morphologic and densitometric analysis of coronary obstructions have been published in the literature as described above, it is very difficult if not impossible at this point in time to compare these systems quantitatively, i.e. the question how well all these systems work with routinely obtained coronary angiograms cannot be answered. Data about the accuracy and precision of the edge detection and analysis procedures, the success scores under different image qualities, computation time, etc. are usually not provided in the publications; if they are provided, different parameters to describe the validation results have been used making comparisons very difficult [63]. Recently, discussions among several groups active in this field have taken place in an attempt to define commonly accepted validation procedures for the quantitative coronary angiography analysis systems. In my opinion the following validation procedures should be carried out:

1. *Assessment of accuracy edge detection and densitometric techniques*

— Phantom studies of coronary obstructions with dimensions from 0.5 to 5.0 mm under different imaging conditions (various concentrations of the contrast agent, different kV-levels covering the routinely used range) and under static and dynamic flow conditions [64].
— In vivo animal studies with hollow plastic cylinders of various luminal shapes and sizes inserted in the coronary arteries [65—67].
— For densitometric studies the hypothesis that the results are independent of the angiographic views in which these studies were acquired, must be tested.

2. *Reproducibility*

— Repeated analysis of a set of clinical coronary angiograms obtained under various imaging conditions to assess inter- and intra-observer variabilities.

Parameters describing the validation results

It is suggested to describe the results from the validation studies in terms of the mean differences and the standard deviations of the signed differences (measurement 1 — measurement 2; not absolute differences) between the true and measured values or between the values from repeated measurements.

Approaches towards standardization in angiographic data acquisition and analysis

It has been shown that the variabilities in the arterial measurements can be decreased by standardizing on the angiographic data acquisition and analysis procedures [47, 68]. In summary, the following measures have been proposed:

— Precise registration of the angulations of the X-ray system for the different angiographic views, so that the repeat angiographies can be performed in the same views.
— Administration of vasodilative drug immediately prior to angiographic investigations.
— Use of modern isoviscous and iso-osmolar contrast agents.
— Administration of contrast medium preferably by ECG-triggered injector.
— Selection of contrast catheter constructed of such material that high quality image results (high angiographic image contrast and edge gradient) [48].
— Measurement of actual size catheter with micrometer following catheterization procedure.

The results from the questionnaires regarding the validation procedures performed are described in detail in Table VI. The different items will be discussed in more detail in the following paragraphs.

Accuracy diameter measurements based on edge detection technique (Table VI, item 22)

As described in the previous section on measurement variabilities, the first validation study to test a particular design and implementation of a quantitative coronary angiographic system should be concerned with the accuracy of the actual edge detection technique based on phantom studies of coronary obstructions. Brass model or models made of any other material with a very high X-ray absorption coefficient should not be used, since these do not mimick the clinical situation. Only six investigators have presented results on the accuracy and precision of these techniques. The models used have indeed been perspex models of various sizes (range 0.3—5 mm) (Collins, Kirkeeide, Nichols, Reiber, Vogel) and brass arteries (Brown). The results

Table VI. Overview of the results from all the validation procedures performed by the different investigators.

	Validation procedures (1a)					
	Brown	Collins	Doriot	Kirkeeide	Marchand	Nichols
22. Accuracy diameter measurements based on edge detection technique						
Model used for assessment accuracy edge detection technique.	brass artery of known diameter	perspex model with obstruction diameters ranging from 0.47 to 4.1 mm	—	perspex model with obstruction diameters ranging from 0.5 to 5.0 mm	perspex model with obstruction diameters ranging from 1 to 16 mm	perspex model with obstruction diameters ranging from 0.30 to 2.51 mm
Accuracy diameter measurement (mean difference between true and measured values).	0.030 mm	0.017 mm	—	0.01 mm	—	—
Precision diameter measurement (standard deviation of the differences).	0.080 mm	0.043 mm	—	0.08 mm; numbers represent absolute differences from regression analysis	—	0.12 mm (SEE); $r = 0.99$
These values were assessed at the following kV-levels:	—	66 kV	—	70, 90 kV	50—90 kV	—
and concentrations of the contrast agent:	100%	100%	—	75, 100%	5—320 mg/ml	75%
23. In vivo validations Have you done any in vivo validations?	YES, postmortem arteries pressure injected with barium gelatin. Histologic planimetry of lesion at site of cine-analysis	YES, comparison of lesion cross-sectional area data by densitometry and by high-frequency epicardial echo measurements	—	YES, comparison of measured in-vivo pressure drop and CFR in dogs to predicted values	NO	YES, comparison of densitometrically determined severity of stenosis from coronary cine-angiogram with areas of acrylic resin casts.

Table VI (continued)

	Brown	Collins	Doriot	Kirkeeide	Marchand	Nichols
Validation procedures (2a)						
Mean differences	—	—	—	—	—	—
s.d. of differences	$r = 0.94$	$r = 0.86$	—	—	—	Area stenosis 0.71 mm^2 (SEE); $r = 0.99$
24. Variability repeated analyses (not densitometric)						
Variability in repeated analysis of the same angiographic studies.						
Mean differences:						
Obstruction diam. (mm)	0.10	—	—	0.08	—	—
%-D stenosis	3.0	—	—	−1.6 (single plane)	—	—
%-A stenosis	4.0	—	—	−0.2 (biplane)	—	—
S.d. of differences:						
Obstruction diam. (mm)	0.10	0.32 (SEE); $r = 0.88$ vs. Brown/Dodge	—	0.18	—	—
%-D stenosis	2.5	—	—	6.2 (single plane)	—	—
%-A stenosis	5.5	—	—	4.1 (biplane)	—	5.34% (SEE); $r = 0.96$
25. Validation DENSITOMETRIC technique						
Model used:	NA	Comparison with high-frequency epicardial echo measurements of lesion cross-sectional area	—	Plexiglass models (0.5–5.0 mm in diameter) with circular and crescent cross sections	Perspex model (see [22])	Perspex model (see [22])

Table VI (continued)

	Brown	Collins	Doriot	Kirkeeide	Marchand	Nichols
Validation procedures (3a)						
Accuracy and precision densitometric technique:						
Mean differences:						
Diameter (mm):	—	—	—	—	—	—
%-A stenosis:	—	—	—	0.3	7%	—
Area-stenosis (mm²):	—	—	—	−0.01	—	—
S.d. of differences:						
Diameter (mm):	—	—	—	—	—	—
%-A stenosis:	—	$r = 0.86$ (area measures proportional to absolute area)	—	1.8	5%	4.1% (SEE); r = 0.98
Area stenosis (mm²):	—		—	0.24	—	0.32 mm² (SEE); r = 0.99
Repeated analysis:						
Mean differences:						
%-A stenosis:	—	—	—	—	—	—
Area-stenosis (mm²):	—	—	—	—	—	—
S.d. of differences:						
%-A stenosis:	—	Results on area-stenosis (proportional to absol. area): *Interobserver var., same frame* $r = 0.88$; *Intraobserver var., 2 consecutive frames* $r = 0.98$	—	—	—	*Interobserver var.* 5.3% (SEE); r = 0.96
Area stenosis (mm²):	—		—	—	—	*Interobserver var.* 2.6% (SEE); r = 0.99 0.26 mm² (SEE); r = 0.99

Table VI (continued)

	Validation procedures (4a)					
	Brown	Collins	Doriot	Kirkeeide	Marchand	Nichols
Variability densitometric analysis of obstructions assessed from different angiographic views:				Have found that results are highly variable depending on whether or not other vessels become super-imposed on vessel of interest image. View selection is critical!		
Mean differences:						
%-A stenosis:	—	—	—		2%	—
Area stenosis (mm²):	—	—	—		—	—
S.d. of differences:						
%-A stenosis:	—	—	—		1%	—
Area stenosis (mm²):	—	$y = 1.04x + 0.002$; $r = 0.94$; for LAO vs. RAO analyses	—		—	0.11 mm² (SEE); $r = 0.98$

Table VI (continued.)

Validation procedures (1b)

	Parker	Reiber	Sanders	Sandor	Selzer	Vogel
22. Accuracy diameter measurements based on edge detection technique						
Model used for assessment accuracy edge detection technique.	polyethylene tubing and teflon rods	perspex model with obstruction diameters ranging from 1.5 to 5.0 mm	polyethylene tubing of varying diameters	vessel phantom of size 0.8—6 mm filled with various concentrations of Renografin 76	plexiglass block with 14 drilled holes (0.3 mm—5.0 mm), filled with different conc. of contrast	perspex model with obstruction diameters ranging from 0.5 to 5.0 mm
Accuracy diameter measurement (mean difference between true and measured values).	—	− 0.03 mm	—	—	in the phase of redoing extensive validation studies with their new equipment. Particularly interested in frame-to-frame variability.	—
Precision diameter measurement (standard deviation of the differences).	—	0.09 mm	—	—	—	0.135 mm (s.d. of absolute differences)
These values were assessed at the following kV-levels:	70—90 kV	60—110 kV	—	70—100 kV	—	70 kV
and concentrations of the contrast agent:	50%	50, 100%	—	25—100%	—	100%

Table VI (continued)

	Validation procedures (3b)					
	Parker	Reiber	Sanders	Sandor	Selzer	Vogel
23. In vivo validations						
Have you done any *in vivo* validations?	NOT YET	NO	NO	NO	NO	YES, *in vivo* canine model stenoses 0.84—1.83 mm in size
Mean differences	—	—	—	—	—	—
S.d. of differences	—	—	—	—	—	obstr. diam. 0.09 mm (SEE); *r* = 0.98
24. Variability repeated analyses (not densitometric) Variability in repeated analysis of the same angiographic studies.						
Mean differences:						
Obstruction diam. (mm)	—	0.00	0.02	—	—	—
%-D stenosis	—	−2.08% (interpol.)	0.1%	—	—	—
%-A stenosis	—	—	—	—	—	—
S.d. of differences:						
Obstruction diam. (mm)	—	0.10	0.06	0.5% for 6.26 mm vessel; 7.3% at 0.88 mm	—	*r* = 0.999
%-D stenosis	—	3.94% (interpol.)	3.4%	—	—	—
%-A stenosis	—	—	—	—	—	—

Table VI (continued)

| | Validation procedures (4b) | | | | | |
	Parker	Reiber	Sanders	Sandor	Selzer	Vogel
25. Validation DENSITOMETRIC technique						
Model used:	polyethylene tubing and Teflon rods	perspex models with obstruction diameters from 0.3 to 6.0 mm filled with 50% and 100% contrast and filmed at 4 kV-levels	—	—	Concentric (10 holes) and eccentric asymmetric holes phantom inside and outside enbalmed chest; validation study currently in progress.	—
Accuracy and precision densitometric technique:						
Mean differences:						
Diameter (mm):	0.3 mm	*Sensitometric*: —	—	—	—	—
%-A stenosis:	—	2.79% (absolute error) —	—	—	—	—
Area-stenosis (mm²):	—	*Logarithmic*: — 5.64% (absolute error) —	—	—	—	—

Table VI (continued)

Validation procedures (5b)

	Parker	Reiber	Sanders	Sandor	Selzer	Vogel
S.d. of differences:		*Sensitometric:*				
Diameter (mm):	0.3 mm	—	—	—	—	—
%-A stenosis:	—	1.76%	—	—	—	2.16%
Area stenosis (mm²):	—	—	—	—	—	—
		Logarithmic:				
		—				
		3.05%				
		—				
Repeated analyses:						
Mean differences:						
%-A stenosis:	—	—	—	—	—	
Area-stenosis (mm²):	—	—	—	—	—	
S.d. of differences:						
%-A stenosis:	—	—	—	—	—	$r = 0.999$
Area stenosis (mm²):	—	—	—	—	—	—
Variability densitometric analysis of obstructions assessed from different angiographic views:						
Mean differences:						
%-A stenosis:	—	—	—	—	—	—
Area stenosis (mm²):	—	—	—	—	—	—
S.d. of differences:						
%-A stenosis:	—	—	—	—	—	13.3%
Area stenosis (mm²):	—	—	—	—	—	—

on the accuracy of the different techniques are all very good, ranging from 0.01 mm to 0.03 mm. However, due to the fact that different definitions have been used to describe the precision (absolute differences, true differences, standard error of the estimate), the numbers given cannot be compared easily. These problems have also been discussed by D. Herrington in his chapter in this book [63]. In general, the studies mentioned above were performed at different kV-levels ranging from 50—110 kV, and at different concentrations varying from 50% to 100%. Apparently, nobody has performed a dynamic phantom study with contrast agent pumped through the model with a roller pump. It will be of tremendous interest to see the results under those dynamic conditions.

In vivo validations (Table VI, item 23)

The next question was concerned with *in vivo* validations of the technique. Four investigators (Brown, Collins, Nichols and Vogel) responded with YES to this question. Brown and Nichols used postmortem material and found correlation coefficients of 0.94 and 0.99, respectively; in Nichols' study the SEE (area stenosis) was 0.71 mm². Collins *et al.* compared the lesion cross-sectional area data by densitometry (which is in their case proportional to the absolute area; not calibrated in mm²) with the data by high-frequency epicardial echo measurements, and found a correlation coefficient of $r = 0.86$ [57]. Vogel and Mancini performed a truly *in-vivo* study with dogs instrumented with precision-drilled, plastic cylinders to create intraluminal stenoses; the stenosis diameters ranged from 0.83 to 1.83 mm [66, 67]. With their on-line digital system, they found an SEE $= 0.09$ mm ($r = 0.98$) for the obstruction diameter.

Finally, Kirkeeide *et al.* have compared *in-vivo* pressure drop and coronary flow reserve measurements with predicted values; unfortunately, no results were presented.

Variability repeated analyses (nondensitometric data) (Table VI, item 24)

This question was concerned with the variability in repeated analysis of the same angiographic study. Limited data is only available from seven investigators (Brown, Collins, Kirkeeide, Nichols, Reiber, Sanders and Sandor). The mean differences (accuracy) in the obstruction diameter ranged from 0.00 to .0.10 mm, in the %-D stenosis from 0.1% to 3%, and in the %-A stenosis from −0.2 to 4%. The values for the standard deviation of the differences (precision) in the obstruction diameters ranged from 0.06 mm to 0.18 mm, in the %-D stenosis from 2.5% to 6.2%, and in the %-A stenosis from 4.1 to 5.5%. Again we must be very careful in comparing these numbers, since different definitions may have been used. Collins *et al.* compared their minimal lumen diameters by automated edge detection techniques with those obtained by the Brown/Dodge method (manual tracing on optically magnified images) and found $r = 0.88$ and SEE = 0.32 mm.

Validation densitometric technique (Table VI, item 25)

Question 25 was concerned with the validation of the densitometric technique. The first portion of this question was related to the accuracy and precision of the technique, i.e. how large are the differences with truly known values. Only Collins, Kirkeeide, Marchand, Parker and Reiber responded with some limited data. The validation data from Collins have been described already under the In-vivo Validation-section (Table VI, item 23). Parker used polyethylene tubing and Teflon rods for his experiments, the others used perspex models. The one parameter that three out of five investigators measured was the accuracy of %-A stenosis, which ranged from 0.3% to 7%. The precision in %-A stenosis ranged from 1.76% to 5%, which is a very acceptable result. Kirkeeide and Nichols also determined the precision in the absolute area stenosis measurement by densitometry and found values of 0.24 and 0.32 (SEE) mm^2, respectively. Selzer *et al.* use a model with concentric (10 holes) and eccentric asymmetric holes placed inside and outside of an embalmed chest; this validation study is currently in progress.

Only Collins, Nichols and Vogel have studied the variability in repeated analyses of densitometric studies. Collins found correlation coefficients in the cross-sectional area measurements for interobserver variations on the same frames of $r = 0.88$, and for intraobserver variations on 2 consecutive frames of $r = 0.98$. Nichols found inter- and intra-observer variabilities in %-A stenosis of 5.3% (SEE) and 2.6% (SEE) with correlation coefficients of 0.96 and 0.99, respectively. The intra-observer variability in absolute area stenosis was found to be 0.26 mm^2 (SEE) with $r = 0.99$. Vogel found a correlation coefficient of $r = 0.999$ in the repeated analysis of %-A stenosis.

Finally, we have looked at the variability of densitometric measurements of the same obstructions, but assessed from different angiographic views. It was discussed earlier that the results should be independent of the angiographic view if the technique works well. Five investigators, Collins, Kirkeeide, Marchand, Nichols and Vogel responded. Collins found a correlation coefficient of 0.94 between the cross-sectional area data from RAO and LAO views; the relation between the data could be described by $y =$

$1.04x + 0.002$. Kirkeeide responded that the view selection is critical; in his experiences the results are highly variable depending on whether or not other vessels become superimposed on the vessel of interest; this has been confirmed by other investigators. Marchand found an extremely good accuracy and precision in %-A stenosis of 2% and 1%, respectively. Nichols found a precision of 0.11 mm² (SEE) with $r = 0.98$ in the absolute area measure, while Vogel found a precision in %-A stenosis of 13.3%.

Concluding remarks

In this chapter an extensive overview of the major developments in off- and on-line quantitative coronary arteriography have been presented. It is clear from the text and from the details listed in the Tables, that the developments are rather heterogeneous. However, this should not only be seen as a negative point. As long as optimal results have not been achieved in certain areas, there is a need for competition and new ideas to come up with the best approaches. However, there is one area of great concern and that is the validation of the techniques. The data in this chapter clearly demonstrate that the validation data of most systems is still very incomplete and that the individual results are described in different terms, such that intercomparison of the data is very difficult if not impossible. There must be a consensus on which validation studies to perform and particularly which parameters to use for the description of the results. Best would be if certain phantoms and sets of films and digital data would be distributed to the investigators so that all validation studies can be performed on the same image data.

Acknowledgements

The author wishes to thank Mrs. E. F. van den Ende and Mrs M. J. Kanters-Stam for their secretarial assistance in the preparation of this manuscript. In addition, he wishes to acknowledge the cooperation of all eleven investigators in the field of quantitative coronary arteriography who have responded to his questionnaire and provided all the details of the individual approaches.

References

1. Gould KL, Kirkeeide RL: Assessment of stenosis severity. In: Reiber JHC, Serruys PW (eds): State of the art in quantitative coronary arteriography. Martinus Nijhoff Publishers, Dordrecht/Boston/Lancaster, 1986, pp 209–228.
2. Brown BG, Gallery CA, Badger RS, Kennedy JW, Mathey D, Bolson EL, Dodge HT: Incomplete lysis of thrombus in the moderate underlying atherosclerotic lesion during

intracoronary infusion of streptokinase for acute myocardial infarction: quantitative angiographic observations. Circulation 73: 653—661, 1986.

3. Blankenhorn DH, Brooks SH: Angiographic trials of lipid-lowering therapy. Arteriosclerosis 1, 242—249, 1981.

4. Reiber JHC, Kooijman CJ, Slager CJ, Gerbrands JJ, Schuurbiers JCH, Boer A den, Wijns W, Serruys PW: Computer assisted analysis of the severity of obstructions from coronary cineangiograms: a methodological review. Automedica 5: 219—238, 1984.

5. Reiber JHC, Serruys PW, Slager CJ: Quantitative coronary and left ventricular cineangiography; methodology and clinical applications. Martinus Nijhoff Publishers, Boston/Dordrecht/Lancaster, 1986.

6. Serruys PW, Reiber JHC, Wijns W, Brand M van den, Kooijman CJ, Katen HJ ten, Hugenholtz PG: Assessment of percutaneous transluminal coronary angioplasty by quantitative coronary angiography: diameter versus densitometric area measurements. Am J Cardiol 54: 482—488, 1984.

7. Serruys PW, Geuskens R, Feyter P de, Brand M vd, Deckers J, Katen H ten, Reiber H: Incidence of restenosis 30 and 60 days after successful PTCA: A quantitative coronary angiographic study in 200 consecutive patients (Abstract). Circulation 72 (Supp. III): III—140, 1985.

8. Serruys PW, Wijns W, Brand M van den, Ribeiro V, Fioretti P, Simoons ML, Kooijman CJ, Reiber JHC, Hugenholtz PG. Is transluminal coronary angioplasty mandatory after successful thrombolysis? A quantitative coronary angiographic study. Br Heart J 50: 257—265, 1983.

9. Beatt KJ, Luijten HE, Reiber JHC, Serruys PW: Early regression and late progression in coronary artery lesions in the first 3 months following coronary angioplasty. (Chapter 11 in this volume).

10. Luyten HE, Beatt KJ, Feyter PJ de, Brand M vd, Reiber JHC, Serruys PW: Angioplasty for stable versus unstable angina pectoris: are unstable patients more likely to get restenosis? A quantitative angiographic study in 339 consecutive patients. Int J Cardiac Imaging (in press).

11. Serruys PW, Arnold AER, Brower RW, Bono DP de, Rutsch W, Uebis R, Vahanian A: Quantitative assessment of the effect of continued rt-PA infusion on the residual stenosis after initial recanalisation in acute myocardial infarction (Abstract). Circulation 74: II—368, 1986.

12. Serruys PW, Arnold AER, Brower RW, Bono DP de, Bokslag M, Lubsen J, Reiber JHC, Rutsch W, Uebis R, Vahanian A, Verstraete M: Effect of continued rt-PA administration on the residual stenosis after initially successful recanalization in acute myocardial infarction — a quantitative coronary angiography study of a randomized trial. Eur Heart J 8: 1172—1181, 1987.

13. Sigwart U, Puel J, Mirkovitch V, Joffre F, Kappenberger L: Intravascular stents to prevent occlusion and restenosis after transluminal angioplasty. N Engl J Med 316: 701—706, 1987.

14. Isner JM, Clarke RH: Laser angioplasty: unraveling the Gordian Knot. J Am Coll Cardiol 7: 705—708, 1986.

15. Lee G, Garcia JM, Chan MC, Corso PJ, Bacos J, Lee MH, Pichard A, Reis RL, Mason DT: Clinically successful long-term laser coronary recanalization. Am Heart J 112: 1323—1325, 1986.

16. Slager CJ, Essed CA, Schuurbiers JCH, Bom N, Serruys PW, Meester GT: Vaporization of atherosclerotic plaques by spark erosion. J Am Coll Cardiol 5: 1382—1386, 1985.

17. Bakker J: Digital imaging in cardiovascular applications. Int J Cardiac Imaging (submitted).

18. LeFree M, Simon SB, Lewis RJ, Bates ER, Vogel RA: Digital radiographic coronary artery quantification. Comput Cardiol: 99—102, 1985.

19. Hodgson JMcB, LeGrand V, Bates ER, Mancini GBJ, Aueron FM, O'Neill WW, Simon SB, Beauman GJ, LeFree MT, Vogel RA: Validation in dogs of a rapid digital angio-

graphic technique to measure relative coronary blood flow during routine cardiac catheterization. Am J Cardiol 55: 188—193, 1985.

20. Mancini GBJ, Simon SB, McGillem MJ, LeFree MT, Friedman HZ, Vogel RA: Automated quantitative coronary arteriography: morphologic and physiologic validation in vivo of a rapid digital angiographic method. Circulation 75: 452—460, 1987.

21. Kruger RA, Riederer SJ: Basic concepts of digital subtraction angiography. GK Hall, Medical Publishers, Boston, 1984.

22. Tobis J, Nalcioglu O, Iseri L, Johnston WD, Roeck W, Castleman E, Bauer B, Montelli S, Henry WL: Detection and quantitation of coronary artery stenoses from digital subtraction angiograms compared with 35-millimeter film cineangiograms. Am J Cardiol 54: 489—496, 1984.

23. Arntzenius AC, Kromhout D, Barth JD, Reiber JHC, Bruschke AVG, Buis B, Gent CM van, Kempen-Voogd N, Strikwerda S, Velde EA van der: Diet, lipoproteins, and the progression of coronary atherosclerosis. The Leiden Intervention Trial. N Engl J Med 312: 805—811, 1985.

24. Sanders WJ, Alderman EL, Harrison DC: Coronary artery quantitation using digital image processing. Comput Cardiol: 15—20, 1979.

25. Selzer RH, Shircore A, Lee PL, Hemphill L, Blankenhorn DH: A second look at quantitative coronary angiography: some unexpected problems. In: Reiber JHC, Serruys PW (eds): State of the art in quantitative coronary arteriography. Martinus Nijhoff Publishers, Dordrecht/Boston/ Lancaster, 1986, pp 125—143.

26. Reiber JHC: Morphologic and densitometric analysis of coronary arteries. In: Heintzen P (ed): Progress in Cardiovascular Angiography. Martinus Nijhoff Publishers, Dordrecht, 1987 (in press).

27. Brown BG, Bolson E, Frimer M, Dodge HT: Quantitative coronary arteriography. Estimation of dimensions, hemodynamic resistance, and atheroma mass of coronary artery lesions using the arteriograms and digital computation. Circulation 55: 329—337, 1977.

28. Reiber JHC, Kooijman CJ, Slager CJ, Ree EJB van, Kalberg RJN, Tijdens FO, Plas J van der, Frankenhuyzen J van, Claessen WCH: Taking a quantitative approach to cineangiogram analysis. Diagn Imag 7: 87—89, 1985.

29. Kooijman CJ, Kalberg R, Slager CJ, Tijdens FO, Plas J van der, Reiber JHC: Densitometric analysis of coronary arteries. In: Young IT, Biemond J, Duin RPW, Gerbrands JJ (eds): Signal Processing III: Theories and Applications. North-Holland, Amsterdam/New York/Oxford/ Tokyo, 1986, pp 1405—1408.

30. Alderman EL, Berte LE, Harrison DC, Sanders W: Quantitation of coronary artery dimensions using digital imaging processing. In: Brody WR (ed): Digital Radiography. SPIE 314, 1982, pp 273—278.

31. Ellis S, Sanders W, Goulet C, Miller R, Cain KV, Lespérance J, Bourassa MG, Alderman EL: Optimal detection of the progression of coronary artery disease: comparison of methods suitable for risk factor intervention trials. Circulation 74: 1235—1242, 1986.

32. Doriot P-A, Pochon Y, Rasoamanambelo L, Chatelain P, Welz R, Rutishauser W: Densitometry of coronary arteries — an improved physical model. Comput Cardiol: 91—94, 1985.

33. Nichols AB, Gabrieli CFO, Fenoglio Jr JJ, Esser PD: Quantification of relative coronary arterial stenosis by cinevideodensitometric analysis of coronary arteriograms. Circulation 69: 512—522, 1984.

34. Nichols AB, Brown C, Han J, Nickoloff EL, Esser PD: Effect of coronary stenotic lesions on regional myocardial blood flow at rest. Circulation 74: 746—757, 1986.

35. Selzer.RH, Blankenhorn DH, Crawford DW, Brooks SH, Barndt R: Computer analysis of cardiovascular imagery. Proc Caltech/JPL Conf on Image Processing Techn, Data Sources and Software for Comm and Scient Appl, Pasadena, 1976, pp 1—20.

36. Ledbetter DC, Selzer RH, Gordon RM, Blankenhorn DH, Sanmarco ME: Computer

quantitation of coronary angiograms. In: Miller HA, Schmidt EV, Harrison DC (eds): Noninvasive Cardiovascular Measurements, SPIE 167, 1978, pp 17—20.

37. Kirkeeide RL, Fung P, Smalling RW, Gould KL: Automated evaluation of vessel diameter from arteriograms. Comput Cardiol: 215—218, 1982.

38. Wong W-H, Kirkeeide RL, Gould KL: Computer applications in angiography. In: Collins SM, Skorton DJ (eds): Cardiac Imaging and Image Processing. McGraw-Hill Book Company, New York, 1986, pp 206—238.

39. Kooijman CJ, Reiber JHC, Gerbrands JJ, Schuurbiers JCH, Slager CJ, Boer A den, Serruys PW: Computer-aided quantitation of the severity of coronary obstructions from single view cineangiograms. First IEEE Comp Soc Int Symp on Medical Imaging and Image Interpretation, IEEE Cat No 82 CH1804-4, 1982, pp 59—64.

40. Fleagle SR, Johnson MR, Skorton DJ, Marcus ML, Collins SM: Geometric validation of a robust method of automated edge detection in clinical coronary arteriography. Comp Cardiol: 197—200, 1987.

41. Parker DL, Pope DL, Petersen JC, Clayton PD, Gustafson DE: Quantitation in cardiac video-densitometry. Comput Cardiol: 119—122, 1984.

42. Pope DL, Parker DL, Clayton PD, Gustafson DE: Left ventricular border recognition using a dynamic search algorithm. Radiology 155: 513—518, 1985.

43. Kirkeeide RL, Gould KL, Parsel L: Assessment of coronary stenoses by myocardial perfusion imaging during pharmacologic coronary vasodilation. VII. Validation of coronary flow reserve as a single integrated functional measure of stenosis severity reflecting all its geometric dimensions. J Am Coll Cardiol 7: 103—113, 1986.

44. Lavayssière B, Liénard J, Marchand JL: RII geometrical distortion modelling and calibration. In: Lemke HU, Rhodes ML, Jaffee CC, Felix R (eds). Computer Assisted Radiology. Springer-Verlag, Berlin, 1987, pp 225—229.

45. Wollschläger H, Lee P, Zeiher A, Solzbach U, Bonzel T, Just H: Improvement of quantitative angiography by exact calculation of radiological magnification factors. Comput Cardiol 1985: 483—486.

46. Wollschläger H, Zeiher AM, Lee P, Solzbach U, Bonzel T, Just H: Optimal biplane imaging of coronary segments with computed exact triple orthogonal projections (Chapter 2 in this volume).

47. Reiber JHC, Serruys PW, Kooijman CJ, Slager CJ, Schuurbiers JCH, Boer A den: Approaches towards standardization in acquisition and quantitation of arterial dimensions from cineangiograms. In: Reiber JHC, Serruys PW (eds): State of the Art in Quantitative Coronary Arteriography. Martinus Nijhoff Publishers, Dordrecht/Boston/Lancaster, 1986, pp 145—172.

48. Reiber JHC, Kooijman CJ, Boer A den, Serruys PW: Assessment of dimensions and image quality of coronary contrast catheters from cineangiograms. Cathet Cardiovasc Diagn 11: 521—531, 1985.

49. Siebes M, D'Argenio DZ, Selzer RH: Computer assessment of hemodynamic severity of coronary artery stenosis from angiograms. Comput Methods and Programs in Biomedicine 21: 143—152, 1985.

50. Crawford DW, Brooks SH, Selzer RH, Barndt Jr. R, Beckenbach ES, Blankenhorn DH: Computer densitometry for angiographic assessment of arterial cholesterol content and gross pathology in human atherosclerosis. J Lab Clin Med 89: 378—392, 1977.

51. Tobis J, Nalcioglu O, Johnston WD, Qu L, Reese T, Sato D, Roeck W, Montelli S, Henry WL: Videodensitometric determination of minimum coronary artery luminal diameter before and after angioplasty. Am J Cardiol 59: 38—44, 1987.

52. Reiber JHC, Slager CJ, Schuurbiers JCH, Boer A den, Gerbrands JJ, Troost GJ, Scholts B, Kooijman CJ, Serruys PW: Transfer functions of the X-ray-cine-video chain applied to digital processing of coronary cineangiograms. In: Heintzen PH, Brennecke R (eds): Digital Imaging in Cardiovascular Radiology. Georg Thieme Verlag, Stuttgart, 1983, pp 89—104.

88

53. Bürsch J, Jo̱ R, Heintzen P: Validity of Lambert-Beer's law in roentgendensitometry of contrast material (Urografin) using continuous radiation. In: Heintzen PH (ed): Roentgen-, Cine and Videodensitometry: Fundamentals and Applications for Blood Flow and Heart Volume Determinations. Georg Thieme Verlag, Stuttgart, 1971, pp 81–84.

54. Heintzen P, Moldenhauer M: X-ray absorption by contrast material using pulsed radiation. In: Heintzen PH (ed): Rcentgen, Cine- and Videodensitometry: Fundamentals and Applications for Blood Flow and Heart Volume Determinations. Georg Thieme Verlag, Stuttgart, 1971, pp 73–81.

55 Doriot PA, Rutishauser W: On the accuracy of densitometric measurements of coronary artery stenosis based on Lambert-Beer's absorption law. (Chapter 7 in this volume).

56. Reiber JHC, Kooijman CJ, Slager CJ, Boer A den, Serruys PW: Improved densitometric assessment % area-stenosis from coronary cineangiograms (abstract). X World Congress of Cardiology, Washington, 1986, pp 39.

57. Johnson MR, McPherson DD, Fleagle SR, Hunt M, Hiratzka L, Kerber RE, Marcus ML, Collins SM, Skorton DJ. Videodensitometric analysis of human coronary stenosis: in vivo validation using intra-operative high frequency epicardial echocardiography. Circulation 77: 328–336, 1988.

58. Wiesel J, Grunwald AM, Tobiasz C, Robin B, Bodenheimer MM: Quantitation of absolute area of a coronary arterial stenosis: experimental validation with a preparation in vivo. Circulation 74: 1099–1106, 1986.

59. Seibert JA, Nalcioglu O, Roeck WW: Characterization of the veiling glare PSF in X-ray image intensified fluoroscopy. Med Phys 11: 172–179, 1984.

60. Shaw CG, Ergun DI, Van Lysel MS, Peppler WW, Dobbins JT, Zarnstorff WC, Myerowitz PD, Swanson DK, Lasser TA, Mistretta CA, Dhanani SP, Strother CM, Crummy AB: Quantitation techniques in digital subtraction videoangiography. In: Brody WR (ed): Digital Radiography. SPIE 314: 121–129, 1982.

61. Pfaff JM, Whiting JS, Eigler NE, Forrester JS: Accurate densitometric quantification requires strict attention to the physical characteristics of X-ray imaging. (Chapter 3 in this volume)

62. Johnson MR, McPherson DD, Hunt MM, Hiratzka LF, Marcus ML, Kerber RE, Collins SM, Skorton DJ: Videodensitometry is independent of angiographic projection and lumen shape. J Am Coll Cardiol 9: 183A, 1987 (Abstract).

63. Herrington DM, Walford GA, Pearson TA: Issues of validation in quantitative coronary angiography. (Chapter 10 in this volume).

64. Simons MA, Kruger RA, Power RLB: Cross-sectional area measurements by digital subtraction videodensitometry. Invest Radiol 21: 637–644, 1986.

65. Block M, Bove AA, Ritman EL: Coronary angiographic examination with the dynamic spatial reconstructor. Circulation 70: 209–216, 1984.

66. Mancini GBJ, Simon SB, McGillem MJ, LeFree MT, Friedman HZ, Vogel RA: Automated quantitative coronary arteriography: morphologic and physiologic validation in vivo of a rapid digital angiographic method. Circulation 75: 452–460, 1987.

67. Mancini GBJ: Morphologic and physiologic validation of quantitative coronary arteriography utilizing digital methods. (Chapter 8 in this volume)

68. Reiber JHC, Serruys PW, Kooijman CJ, Wijns W, Slager CJ, Gerbrands JJ, Schuurbiers JCH, Boer A den, Hugenholtz PG: Assessment of short-, medium- and long-term variations in arterial dimensions from computer-assisted quantitation of coronary cineangiograms. Circulation 71: 280–288, 1985.

5. Intravenous digital coronary angiography — a review of technical considerations and recent results

EDWARD J. TOGGART, W. PEPPLER, N. HANGIANDREOU, and
C. MISTRETTA

SUMMARY. Although intravenous (IV) digital subtraction angiography (DSA) techniques are successfully used for the diagnosis of peripheral, carotid, and aortic vascular disease, satisfactory images of the coronary arteries are much more difficult to obtain because of unique imaging problems. These include vessel and soft tissue motion, large scene dynamic range, and overlap of simultaneously opacified cardiac and noncardiac structures. Because early DSA systems were not well suited for addressing these problems, it was soon concluded that the coronary arteries could not be adequately imaged by intravenous techniques. Although it remains a difficult problem, we have recently readdressed IV DSA coronary angiography, using a system which includes several improvements relative to the early DSA systems. This chapter describes the major imaging problems associated with IV coronary DSA and presents our current approach and most recent attempts to image the coronary arteries by intravenous techniques.

Introduction

Because of the many imaging problems posed by the coronary arteries it is unlikely that the intravenous technique will replace selective coronary angiography as a means of detailed anatomic evaluation of the coronary arteries. However, if adequate images could be obtained reliably, the intravenous approach might play a role as a screening test for coronary artery disease or in the follow-up of post-surgical or post-angioplasty patients. This chapter reports our recent progress in the investigation of these possibilities. After reviewing the special problems associated with IV coronary artery imaging, we will summarize the improvements in apparatus and processing techniques which have led to our most recent results.

Imaging problems

Present IV DSA techniques have been developed that are capable of producing noncardiac vascular images of diagnostic quality. Examples of vessels

J. C. Reiber & P. W. Serruys (eds.), New Developments in Quantitative Coronary Arteriography,
89–99.

that can be satisfactorily imaged after IV injection include the carotid arteries, aortic arch, abdominal aorta, iliac and femoral arteries. These vessels have certain characteristics in common which make them suitable for present IV DSA techniques. These include: (1) relatively little intrinsic soft tissue or vessel motion, (2) relative anatomic isolation, and (3) relatively homogeneous surrounding soft tissues. In the case of intravenous coronary angiography, none of these conditions are present, resulting in the problems discussed below.

Soft tissue and vessel motion

In static imaging situations, temporal subtraction provides excellent cancellation of confusing background structures and allows for optimal simultaneous display of all portions of the image. Even outside the heart, however, motion of bone or soft tissue structures can lead to disturbing artifacts. Examples of this are swallowing artifacts frequently encountered in carotid artery imaging and bowel artifacts experienced in abdominal imaging. These can generally be dealt with using remasking or pixel shifting techniques. Dual energy techniques can also be used which permit formation of tissue cancelled or bone cancelled images [1].

In the heart, motion caused by cardiac contraction can lead to significant tissue misregistration signals. Some of the first DSA algorithms employed blurred mask subtraction in which the preinjection mask image was averaged over an entire cardiac cycle. Although this was sufficient to permit enhancement of iodine by a factor of 8 in the subtracted iodine display, further improvement can be achieved using phase matched subtraction, in which a separate mask is recorded and used for each phase of the cardiac cycle. The success of this procedure depends on the absence of other significant *non-cardiac* motion, for example, respiratory motion.

The motion of the coronary vessels poses a serious limitation on the maximal signal-to-noise ratio which can be achieved in IV coronary angiography. It is well known that cineradiographic exposures on the order of 5 ms or less are preferred in order to prevent vessel blurring. This is particularly true in the systolic portions of the cardiac cycle. Because the concentration of iodine delivered using intravenous injection is probably 10 to 20 times lower than in conventional intra-arterial angiography, signal-to-noise ratio is a serious limitation. Image noise would be reduced by delivering a large X-ray exposure. However, even with the present state of the art X-ray equipment, operated at maximal current, it is difficult to deliver adequate X-ray exposures in 5 ms. Although increased exposure is available at elevated tube voltages, this is accompanied by an undesirable decrease in iodine contrast and overall signal-to-noise ratio.

Because of these problems unique to IV coronary DSA, exposure sequences and processing modes must be designed to optimize integration of all available quantum statistical information and to display it in a format that optimizes vessel perception.

Overlap of iodinated structures

Within the image plane, depending on the projection, the coronary arteries overlap the left and right ventricles, both atria and the pulmonary vasculature. Although the temporal characteristics of the contrast pass curve for each of these structures is not identical to the coronaries, considerable overlap exists. This results in the presence of iodinated *noncoronary* structures in the image which spatially overlap with and impair visual interpretation of the coronary signal. The problems produced by large structures such as the left ventricle and aorta, may be overcome to some extent through the use of high-pass spatial filtration. However, decreased transmission through these structures and elevated scatter fractions in these regions further reduce the already marginal signal-to-noise ratio.

Standard first-order remasking techniques do not provide good separation of coronary and pulmonary veins because of the temporal near coincidence of peak contrast in these structures. Lee has reported an adaptive temporal filtration technique in which a correlation image was formed using the aorta as a reference region [2]. Pixels which temporally correlated poorly with the aortic signal were suppressed. This technique served to completely suppress pulmonary structures resulting in a less complex image, but generated artifacts in regions where pulmonary and coronary vessels overlapped. Recently we have had promising results with a second-order subtraction technique which is described later in this chapter.

Excessive scene dynamic range

In general, failure to provide adequate equalization filters to create a more uniform scene transmission is one of the leading causes of poor image quality in intravenous angiography. In the case of cardiac imaging, the use of some form of X-ray beam equalization is even more critical. The heart and associated structures are surrounded in the chest cavity by the pulmonary parenchyma which is highly aerated. Pulmonary tissue is much more transmissive than the fluid filled heart and circulatory structures. In the presence of such large variations in transmission, camera noise reduces the effective utilization of X-ray information in the poorly penetrated regions of the image field. For example, assuming a maximal detected exposure of 1 mR and a dynamic range of 10, detective quantum efficiency (DQE) is reduced by a factor of three behind the opacified left ventricle. Iodine contrast is also reduced in low transmission areas due to cross scatter and glare from more transmissive regions.

We are presently developing a means for computer controlled printing of a patient specific filter for beam compensation [3]. This method is not yet available. Presently, we attempt to simulate its benefit as much as possible using shaped aluminum filters.

Recent developments

Since our earliest attempt at IV DSA coronary angiography in late 1980, several potential improvements have been investigated in the area of image acquisition and processing. These include:

(1) Progressive video scanning,
(2) Real time digital data storage,
(3) Real time convolution filters,
(4) Integrated phase matched subtraction,
(5) Dual energy subtraction,
(6) Adaptive temporal filtration,
(7) ECG-gated diastolic data acquisition,
(8) Second-order subtraction of pulmonary vasculature,
(9) Single cycle blurred mask subtraction.

We will briefly comment on each of these including those which have not been found to be beneficial.

1. Progressive video scanning involves the readout of the television camera from top to bottom in one continuous scan, as opposed to conventional interlaced scanning in which two fields, one of odd and one of even lines, are used to form the image. In coronary artery imaging, the time interval between the odd and even fields, leads to a double artery image seen as a sawtooth contour of the vessel edge. This happens because detectable vessel motion occurs during the time interval between scanning of adjacent lines. With progressive scanning, all nearby portions of the artery are imaged at approximately the same time, leading to a more exact representation in the image. Relating the improved temporal characteristics of progressive scanning to the dose/exposure time problem of coronary imaging, we conducted a subjective study of three dynamic imaging modes all acquired at 30 frames/second using identical fluoroscopic exposure levels. The first mode used a 1 ms X-ray exposure followed by progressive camera scanning. The second mode used continuous (33 ms) exposure with a progressive readout. The third mode used continuous exposure (33 ms/frame) with interlaced

readout. The three modes were compared with respect to subjective image quality of selective intra-arterial coronary angiograms from a canine preparation. Three experienced angiographers judged the interlaced mode to be inferior to either of the two progressive scan modes. When static images were viewed, the continuous exposure progressive scan images were considerably less sharp than the 1 ms exposure images. This was especially true for systolic frames. However, when viewed in a dynamic display, perceived vessel sharpness for the continuous exposure mode was considered comparable to the pulsed exposure mode. We concluded, that the progressive scan mode increases the upper limit of exposure time for coronary angiography particularly if images are viewed in a dynamic display. We presume that the eye-brain system uses the dynamic display to form a reprocessed image sequence in which some compensation for motion blurring is performed.

Based on these results we decided to apply the continuous exposure progressive scan mode to intravenous coronary angiography using a series of several contiguous 33 ms exposure frames acquired in diastole which, after processing, could be dynamically displayed. This mode permits a substantial increase in the detected X-ray exposure per image resulting in an improved signal-to-noise ratio. This has been used in four of our most recent human subjects.

2. Early DSA systems used analog storage on video disc or videotape to achieve 30 frames/s imaging rates. When an optimized imaging algorithm was present on the real-time video processor, an adequate amount of signal amplification could be used prior to recording such that recording noise was not noticeable. This was an inflexible system characterized by a limited ability to reprocess the image sequence. Data recorded and stored in a digital form, however, provides a far more flexible means of optimizing processing to fully exploit acquired data. This recording method also facilitates the dynamic display mode described elsewhere in this chapter.

3. Reduction of the dynamic range of the displayed *iodine* signal is necessary for optimal display of vessels crossing the opacified aorta or ventricle. For this purpose a real-time high-pass filter circuit has been constructed [4] and used in conjunction with the dynamic display.

4. In order to remove misregistration artifacts due to cardiac motion, phased matched image pairs are used. Either preinjection or postopacification frames are used for forming the subtraction mask. Typically, because of the patient motion associated with injection of contrast, late masks are more suitable. When several cycles are available in which coronary opacification is small, the subtraction mask is formed as a sum of all available late masks. This improves signal-to-noise ratio by approximately 1.4. Frames containing opacified coronary vessels cannot be summed because of minor cycle-to-cycle variations in the spatial location of the coronary arteries. This is

probably more noticeable with coronary arteries because of their relatively small diameter, making even small degrees of misregistration significant.

5. We recently reported a mode providing 15 dual energy images per second which we plan to use in a study of exercise ventriculography [5, 6]. In this mode, 10 ms X-ray exposures at 60 and 120 kVp are separated by 33 ms. Sequential high and low energy frames are then combined to form images in which soft tissue structures are cancelled. This mode was tested in a canine model as a potential means of motion immune intravenous coronary angiography [5]. A maximum 10 ms exposure is required to maintain no more than a 33 ms separation between high and low energy images. This exposure time per image is 1/3 that available in the 33 ms (continuous exposure) mode mentioned above. Additionally, tube current is limited to approximately 1/2 that available for temporal subtraction. Together this reduces the available X-ray exposure to approximately 1/6 that available with the temporal subtraction mode. Signal-to-noise ratio is marginal even in the most optimal temporal subtraction images. Further reductions produced by the dual energy mode suggest, that it is not an appropriate technique for intravenous coronary artery imaging.

6. Two forms of adaptive temporal filtration have been used. That based on the temporal phase correlation with the aorta has already been described. A second mode uses a selective recursive filter. Information is integrated continuously in static pixels, defined as those pixels which do not exceed a threshold change in gray scale from one frame to the next. Dynamic pixels, in which gray scale changes occur above the predetermined threshold, are merely updated with the current pixel value. With the next frame, a new integration cycle is initiated. This mode produces significant reductions in noise at the expense of reducing vessel sharpness. By varying the decision threshold used to detect motion, minor improvements may be achieved. However, noise fluctuations and motion are difficult to distinguish.

7. Due to the desire to: (a) concentrate patient exposure into the portion of the cardiac cycle when vessel motion is minimal; (b) acquire frames from several cardiac cycles; and (c) limit patient X-ray dose, ECG-gating is used to initiate a series of 6 or 7 contiguous 33 ms diastolic exposures for 6 to 7 cardiac cycles at or about the time of peak left ventricular opacification (Fig. 1).

8. Recently we have had success in suppressing pulmonary vessels using a second-order subtraction technique. This mode uses images from a series of previously phase-matched subtraction images. In this procedure, which is illustrated in Fig. 1, early images containing pulmonary vein opacification but little coronary opacification are weighted by a factor (W) typically between 0.2 and 0.5 and subtracted from frames with optimal coronary opacification. Because unopacified background anatomy has previously been subtracted in the phase-matched sequence, the unbalanced subtraction of

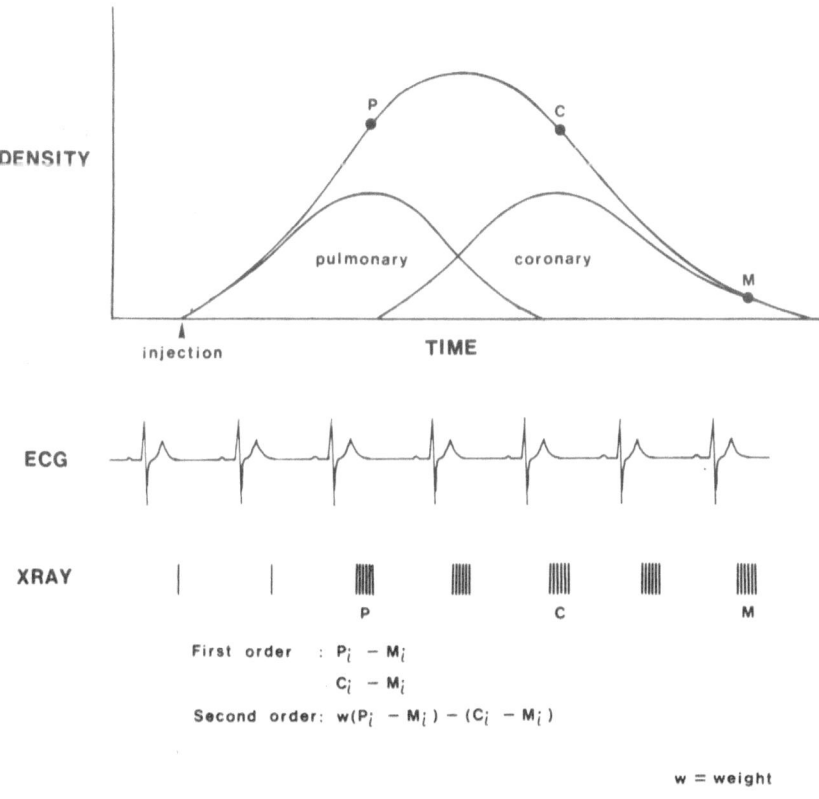

SECOND ORDER SUBTRACTION

First order : $P_i - M_i$
$C_i - M_i$
Second order: $w(P_i - M_i) - (C_i - M_i)$

w = weight
i = phase

Figure 1. Schematic representation of the image acquisition sequence. The single X-ray pulse/beat phase is used to follow the iodine bolus through the right heart and lungs. The six exposures/beat phase begins at about the LV contrast maximum. Equations are shown for the first- and second-order subtraction modes.

pulmonary and coronary images does not reintroduce unopacified background structures.

9. In a recent patient study, the image acquisition sequence (which is manually initiated while viewing a 1 frame/cycle subtraction display) was begun too early and all five cardiac cycles were obtained near peak coronary opacification. Because suitable early or late masks were not available, data from the most opacified cycle was processed using a mode in which each frame was subtracted from a mask consisting of the sum of all other frames of the same cardiac cycle (Fig. 2). Segments of vessels which moved appreciably in the imaging plane (projection angle = 15° RAO) were well visualized, including a small right ventricular branch of the right coronary artery which,

96

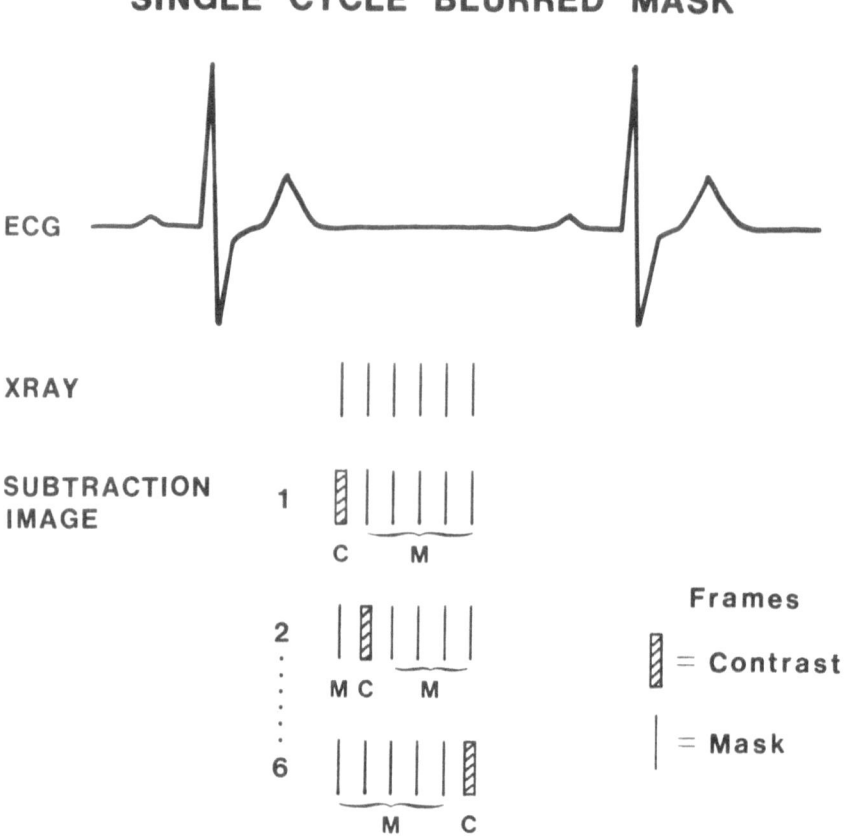

SINGLE CYCLE BLURRED MASK

Figure 2. Single cycle blurred mask mode. The data is acquired similarly to that shown in Figure 1. The contrast image is repetitively stepped back and forth through the images from one beat while the mask is composed of all the remaining images.

in the dynamic display, could be seen coursing to the cardiac apex. Although the image quality in this mode is inferior to second- order subtraction as described above, it could be a useful mode for examinations in which the timing of data acquisition is suboptimal.

Imaging procedures and results

Optimal projections for visualizing all the major epicardial branches of coronary arteries have not been determined. A specific projection can be tailored to optimally visualize a desired branch, the selection of which might be based on complementary clinical data such as the results of exercise tolerance tests, thallium scintigraphy, prior coronary angiography or prior angioplasty (see below). Currently, for pilot studies, we are using a shallow right anterior oblique projection (10—20° to the right of perpendicular on the anterior chest wall) with cranial or caudal angulation. This allows for examination of the mid and distal left anterior descending, circumflex, mid and distal right coronary artery. This type of projection also minimizes the patient thickness along the X-ray beam path. Transmission throughout the X-ray field is equalized with bolus material to improve DQE. This is crucial, particularly since long segments of the coronary arteries overlie the ventricles, which contain significant iodine signal during coronary image acquisition. Forty to fifty ml of standard ionic contrast material (370 mg of iodine/ml) at 20 ml/s is injected into the right atrium. The transit of contrast material is followed through the right heart, pulmonary circulation and left heart chambers using a single exposure per cardiac cycle after right atrial injection. This is done triggering the X-ray exposure from the electrocardiogram. As the aortic contrast density increases and LV density peaks, the imaging mode is entered. Six to seven consecutive 33 ms frames are obtained during diastole for each of 5 to 7 cardiac cycles. Frames are digitally stored on the video rate digital disk for processing.

We have used several approaches to processing raw image data including various forms of mask mode subtraction (discussed previously), recursive and high-pass spatial filtration combined with a repetitive dynamic display.

Generally, we have found it necessary to perform phase matched subtraction of noniodinated masks from iodinated frames as a starting point in the post-acquisition processing. Masks are either single frame or integrated phase matched frames. We have found that mask frames obtained early after iodine injection or after peak coronary contrast can produce subtraction images in which the coronary arteries are most pronounced. As mentioned earlier, because of minor patient motion associated with breath holding and the subjective sensation of dye injection, late masks generally produce superior subtraction. Most recently, we have employed the second-order subtraction technique described earlier in this chapter which significantly reduces overlying pulmonary signals. Figure 3 contains a phase matched subtraction frame and a second-order subtraction image from a human volunteer. Note the suppression of the pulmonary artery overlying the proximal circumflex after second-order subtraction.

As also can be seen from the still frames in Fig. 3, signal-to-noise is still low and a significant iodine signal in noncoronary structures is present. Because the present acquisition mode obtains 6—7 consecutive frames in diastole, these frames can be displayed as a consecutive series of frames in a repetitive fashion. Because there is a minor degree of coronary motion during diastole particularly in relation to pulmonary structures, when the images are viewed repetitively in sequence, the coronary arteries are much more easily identifiable. During the dynamic display real-time convolution

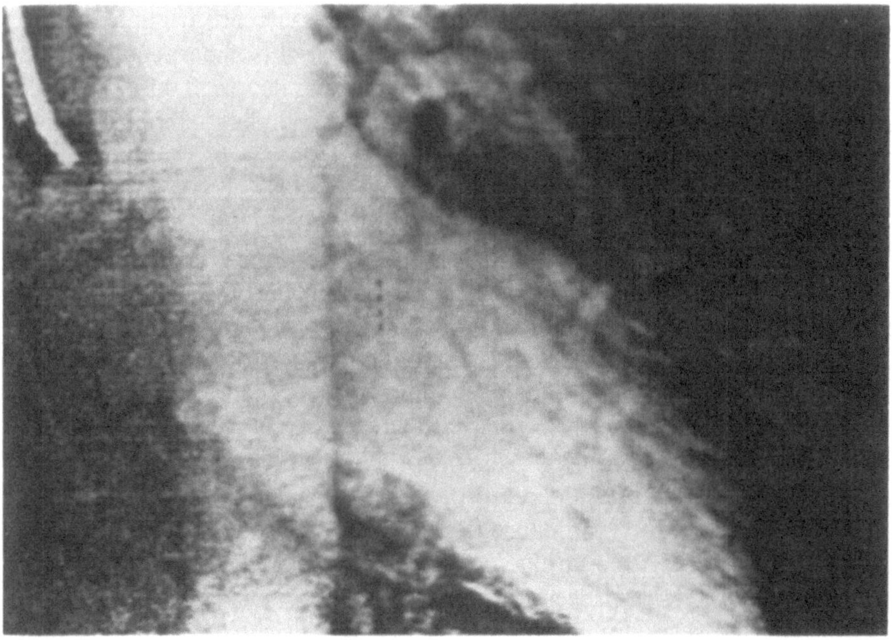

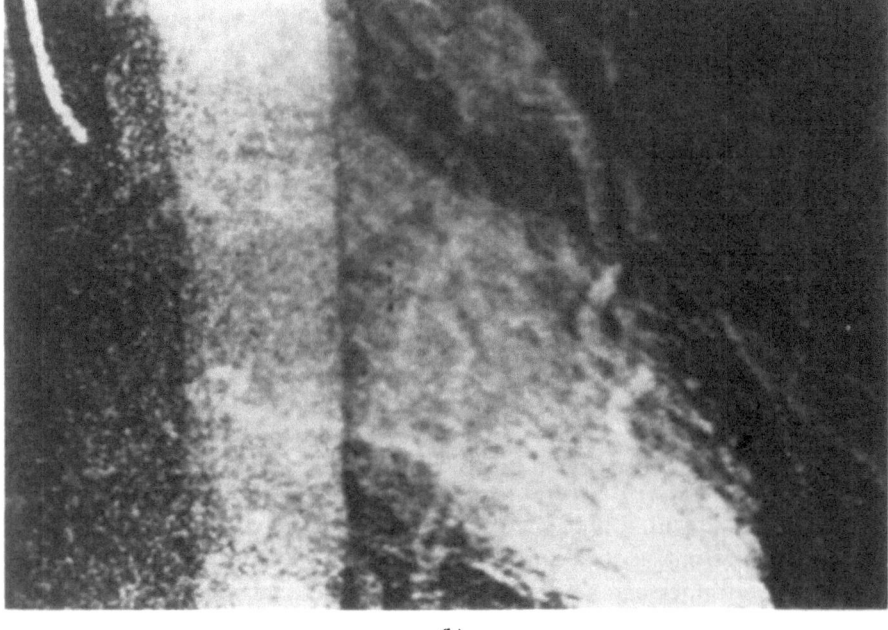

(a)

(b)

Figure 3. Comparison of first-order (a) subtraction and second-order (b) subtraction images from a human volunteer. 50 ml of standard contrast medium (370 mg/ml) were injected into the right atrium at 20 ml/s. Notice the suppression of the pulmonary artery overlying the proximal circumflex after second-order subtraction (b).

filters can be employed to optimize display of vessels overlying the opacified left ventricle.

Presently, the quality of intravenous DSA coronary angiography does not compare to that obtainable by direct intra-arterial injections. We are optimistic, however, that these techniques may be useful as a screening test with visual interpretation directed by the results of other cardiac studies, such as exercise tolerance test, thallium scintigraphy, radionuclide angiography, or previous angiography. We are currently initiating a prospective study to determine the efficacy of the current IV imaging mode in identifying recurrent stenosis after coronary angioplasty.

In summary, intravenous coronary DSA utilizing present technology may have the capacity to function as a screening test for diagnosis and follow up of coronary artery disease.

References

1. Van Lysel MS, Dobbins III JT, Peppler WW, Hasegawa BH, Lee CS, Mistretta CA, Zarnstorff WC, Crummy AB, Kubal W, Bergsjordet B, Strother CM, Sackett JF: Work in progress: hybrid temporal-energy subtraction in digital fluoroscopy. Radiology 147: 869—874, 1983.
2. Lee C-SR, Peppler WW, Van Lysel MS, Cusma JT, Folts JD, Zarnstorff WC, Mistretta CA, Dobbins III JT, Hasegawa BH, Naimuddin S, Molloi S, Hangiandreou N, Lancaster JC: Adaptive processing algorithms for intravenous digital subtraction coronary angiocardiography. In: Application of Optical Instrumentation in Medicine XIII. SPIE 535: 369—377, 1985.
3. Hasegawa BH, Naimuddin S, Dobbins JT, Mistretta CA, Peppler WW, Hangiandreou NJ, Cusma JT, McDermott JC, Kudva BV, Melbye KM: Digital beam attenuator technique for compensated chest radiography. Radiology 159: 537—543, 1986.
4. Dobbins III JT, Van Lysel MS, Hasegawa BH, Pepper WW, Mistretta CA: Spatial frequency filtering in digital subtraction angiography (DSA) by real-time digital video convolution. In: Applications of Optical Instrumentation in Medicine XI. SPIE 419: 111—121, 1983.
5. Molloi S, Peppler WW, Folts JD, Toggart EJ, Miller WP, Van Lysel MS, Mistretta CA: High-pass filtered dual-energy coronary angiography. Circulation 74: II-484, 1986.

6. Assessment of the anatomic and functional severity of coronary arterial stenosis: new measuring techniques using high-frequency epicardial echocardiography and Doppler ultrasound

RICHARD E. KERBER, D. D. McPHERSON, S. J. SIRNA,
M. L. MARCUS, L. F. HIRATZKA, and R. A. KIESO

SUMMARY. Presently available methods for the study of the coronary circulation have relied primarily on silhouette techniques (angiography). Such techniques are unable to visualize the coronary arterial wall and therefore cannot define the extent of disease in the wall. Although lumen diameters can be delineated, true lumen area measurements can only be obtained from angiograms by using specialized reconstruction techniques.

High-frequency epicardial echocardiography overcomes these disadvantages. We use a high-frequency ultrasonic transducer (12 MHz, Surgiscan, Biosound, Inc) with a nominal resolution of 0.1—0.2 mm to image the coronary arteries in short- and long-axis cross-sectional planes. Images are obtained by placing the hand-held gas-sterilized probe directly on the exposed epicardial coronary arteries in open-chest animals or patients undergoing cardiac surgery. Filling the pericardial cradle with saline provides the necessary coupling material. Ultrasonic images can then be analyzed for lumen area and arterial wall thickness measurements; atherosclerotic plaques are easily visualized.

We initially validated lumen area and wall thickness measurements from frozen frame images of animal coronary arteries with data obtained from dynamic techniques (sonomicrometers) and from static images (histologic sections of pressure-fixed coronary arteries). The high-frequency epicardial echocardiographic technique was then taken to the operating room, where we are presently collecting data on patients undergoing cardiac surgery. Initial clinical experience has demonstrated that coronary atherosclerosis is a diffuse process which tends to be underestimated by angiographic analysis. Coronary arteries even with only a single severe stenosis tend to be diffusely diseased, a process often not adequately visualized angiographically.

The high-frequency epicardial echocardiographic technique has also been of use in delineating anastomosis between grafts and native vessels; technical errors in graft insertion can be demonstrated and the adequacy of the anastomotic opening evaluated.

We have also performed comparisons of high-frequency echo-delineated coronary stenosis and measurements of coronary flow reserve using suction Doppler probes fixed to the coronary arteries. Coronary reserve is estimated by the assessment of the reactive hyperemic response following a brief (20 second) coronary occlusion. Blunting of the expected hyperemia confirms functional significance of an anatomic lesion. Lesions which appeared anatomically severe (small lumen, very thick arterial wall) by the high-frequency echo technique were associated with impaired Doppler-demonstrated flow reserve, thus demonstrating a good correlation between anatomic assessment and functional significance.

High-frequency epicardial echocardiography is a valuable tool in assessing the extent, severity and functional significance of coronary artery disease.

J. C. Reiber & P. W. Serruys (eds.), New Developments in Quantitative Coronary Arteriography,
100—114.

Introduction

At present the study of the coronary circulation relies heavily on angiography. This is a silhouette technique which is unable to visualize the coronary arterial wall directly. In addition, it estimates the extent of narrowing of the coronary lumen by comparison to putatively normal adjacent areas which pathologic studies suggest are actually not normal. True lumen area measurements can only be obtained from coronary angiograms using specialized reconstruction techniques.

In order to overcome these limitations, we have explored the use of high-frequency (12 MHz) epicardial echocardiography techniques for the direct visualization of coronary arterial lumen and wall. Such techniques were stimulated by initial studies by Rogers *et al.*, who used standard two-dimensional echo systems with signal processing to demonstrate coronary arterial calcifications in proximal vessels [1]. Unfortunately, standard echocardiography uses frequencies in the 2.25 to 5 MHz range. Two-point structural resolutions in using such instrumentation is inadequate to visualize the fine detail of the coronary arterial wall, which is frequently not more than 0.2 mm in diameter.

High-frequency (12 MHz) ultrasonic images were initially used by vascular surgeons performing peripheral vascular surgery (i.e., endarterectomy). Such high-frequency ultrasound transducers have nominal two-point structural resolution of 0.1—0.2 mm. Unfortunately, the loss in penetration demanded by using high-frequency transducers results in imaging field depths of only 1 or 2 cm. However, this limitation is less important if the transducer is used intraoperatively. Sahn *et al.* [2] introduced the concept of coronary arterial imaging using such high-frequency ultrasonic transducers. They demonstrated that arteries could be visualized and that atherosclerosis and atherosclerotic shadowing of distal structures due to calcification could be demonstrated [3].

Validation of echocardiographic measurements

Our initial studies using high-frequency epicardial echocardiography concentrated on validating measurements of coronary arterial lumen and wall made from echocardiographic images [4]. We used a 12 MHz transducer made commercially by Biosound Corp., Indianapolis, Indiana (Fig. 1). Initially, we studied animals (calves, sheep, dogs) with coronary arteries of varying sizes. The hand-held probe was placed directly on the exposed epicardial coronary artery and images were acquired. Figure 2 shows a typical coronary artery in cross-section along with an accompanying coronary vein which outlines the arterial wall. The wall and lumen are well seen. We made measurements of

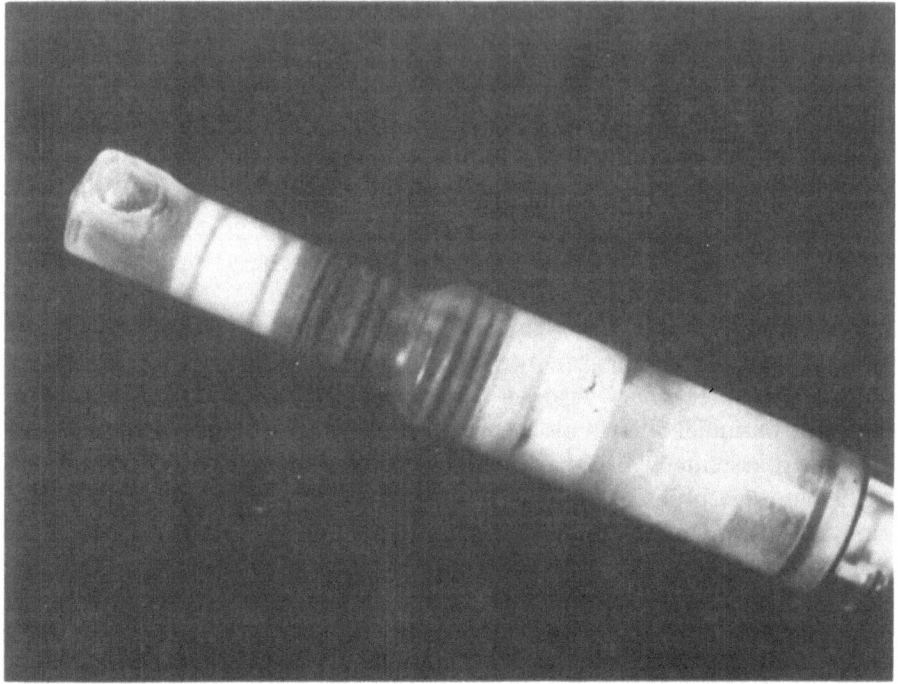

Figure 1. High-frequency echocardiographic probe (12 MHz) manufactured by Biosound Corp. The probe is 20 cm in length. The hand-held probe is placed on the exposed coronary artery by the surgeon. A fan of ultrasound emerges perpendicular to the lens cap at the distal end of the probe which is placed directly over the coronary artery. Reproduced from McPherson and Kerber, Echocardiography 3: 371—381, 1986, by permission.

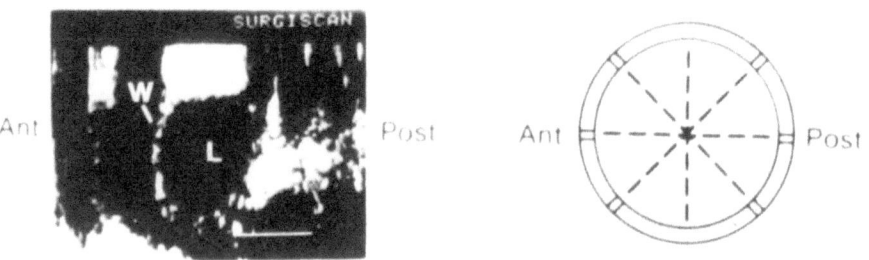

Figure 2. High-frequency epicardial echocardiographic recording of a calf circumflex coronary artery (left). The calibration bar indicates 3 mm. W = wall. L = arterial lumen. A coronary vein is adjacent to the artery on the left and outlines the wall. To the right is the convention used 'for echocardiographic and histologic comparisons. Reproduced from McPherson *et al.*, JACC 8: 600—606, 1986, by permission.

arterial wall and lumen according to a fixed convention. Subsequently, we compared these measurements to histologic diameter measurements made from the same arterial segments that had been imaged. For this purpose, it is crucial to pressure-distend and fix the arteries to the same pressure as was recorded during life in order to obtain physiologically accurate comparisons. Figure 3 shows an excellent correlation of histologic lumen diameter and echo lumen diameter in 68 coronary arteries from various animals.

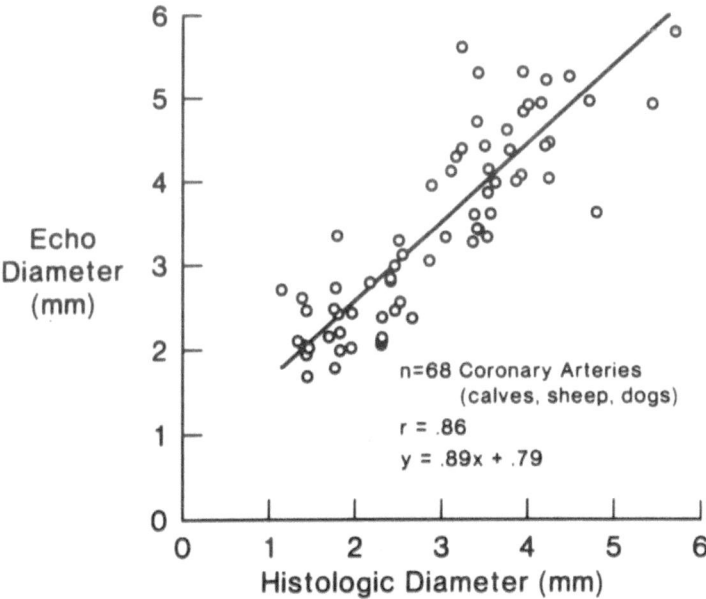

Figure 3. Comparisons of arterial diameters by high-frequency echocardiography and histology. Reproduced form McPherson *et al.*, JACC 8: 600–606, 1986, by permission.

We also used a dynamic technique — sonomicrometry — to further validate the echo diameter measurements [4]. In this technique, 2 piezo-electric crystals are sewn on either side of the coronary artery. When excited by an electrical pulse one transducer emits a burst of ultrasound which is received by the opposite transducer. This instantaneous time dimension gauge allows dynamic comparisons of arterial diameter measurements from echo vs. sonomicrometers, as can be seen in Fig. 4; an excellent correlation ($r = 0.94$) was obtained.

Further, we examined human coronary arterial segments obtained fresh from the morgue in patients who had recently died of various causes [4]. The arterial segments were distended, imaged by high-frequency echo in a water bath and subsequently, again, pressure fixed, and histologic comparisons were made. Figure 5 demonstrates the lumen diameter wall thickness measurements by high-frequency echocardiography and by histology in 13 such coronary segments; once again, an excellent correlation was obtained.

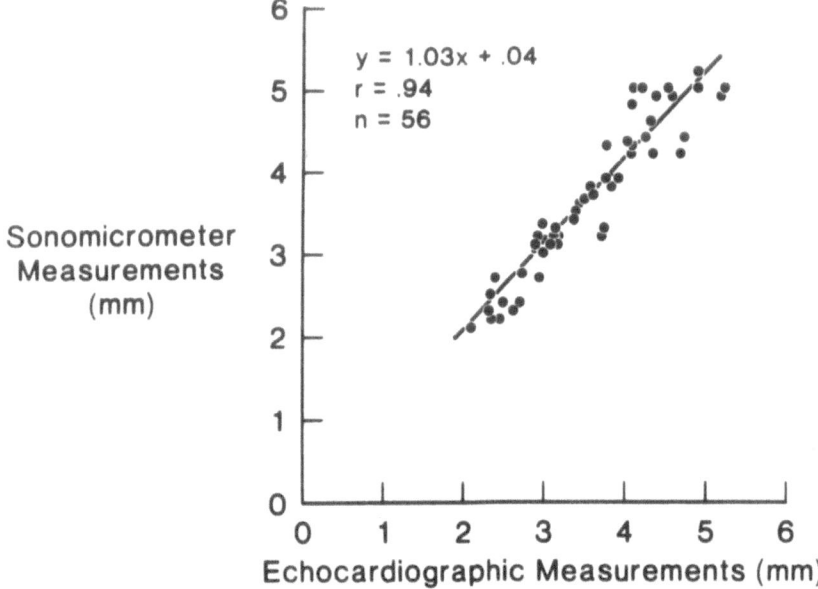

Figure 4. Comparisons of arterial diameters by high-frequency echocardiography and sono-micrometry. Reproduced from McPherson *et al.,* JACC 8: 600–606, 1986, by permission.

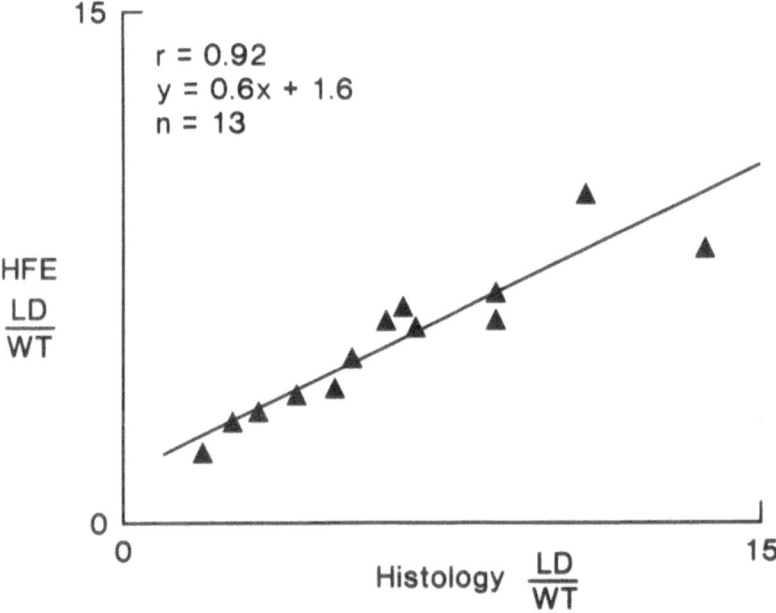

Figure 5. Comparisons of lumen diameter to wall thickness ratios by high-frequency echo-cardiography and histology in 13 fresh coronary arterial segments obtained from the autopsy room. Reproduced from McPherson *et al.,* JACC 8: 600–606, 1986, by permission.

Intraoperative applications of high-frequency epicardial echocardiography

A. Imaging of coronary arteries

Having successfully completed our validation studies we took the technique to the operating room. The gas-sterilized probe was held by the surgeon and scanned along the exposed artery; the pericardial well was filled with saline for coupling. Figure 6 demonstrates typical images obtained from three different types of coronary arteries. Normal coronary arteries show a thin wall, large lumen and no atherosclerosis. Typically, when the echo probe is placed by the surgeon over a stenosis, which has been demonstrated angiographically, marked initial atherosclerotic thickening is shown with severe reduction in the residual lumen [5]. Most interestingly, even when coronary angiography suggests there is no coronary disease in a specific area of a vessel, if there is disease elsewhere in the vessel then usually the whole artery shows some disease. This is seen in Fig. 6 (Group 3), where an artery which had an angiographic stenosis remote from the echo region but which appeared angiographically normal in the region imaged, actually had a markedly but symmetrically thickened intima and reduced lumen. In a large group of patients we examined lumen diameter to wall thickness ratios for arterial segments. We showed that these ratios were high, as expected, for patients with no angiographic evidence of coronary disease anywhere in the coronary circulation, and low for patients where there was significant angiographically demonstrated stenosis in the region echoed (the lumen diameters were reduced and the walls were thick, leading to a low ratio). Of particular interest, however, was the demonstration that in a group with angiographic stenosis remote from the echo region, the lumen diameter to wall thickness ratio was usually low, again indicating the presence of diffuse disease in vessels having angiographic evidence of stenosis anywhere within that vessel, and again pointing out the tendency of angiography to underestimate disease in many areas of coronary circulation [5]. This is demonstrated in Fig. 7. Figure 8 demonstrates an example of a coronary angiogram which appears to show only minimal irregularity of the right coronary artery (arrow), whereas the high-frequency echocardiographic image obtained from the same location shows diffuse thickening of the arterial wall.

B. Imaging of anastomosis of coronary artery bypass grafts and native vessels

An important application of the high-frequency epicardial echocardiographic technique is to assist in coronary artery surgery — specifically, anastomosis between vein grafts or internal mammary arteries and native vessels. The technique can be used to scan the artery and locate a site most free of

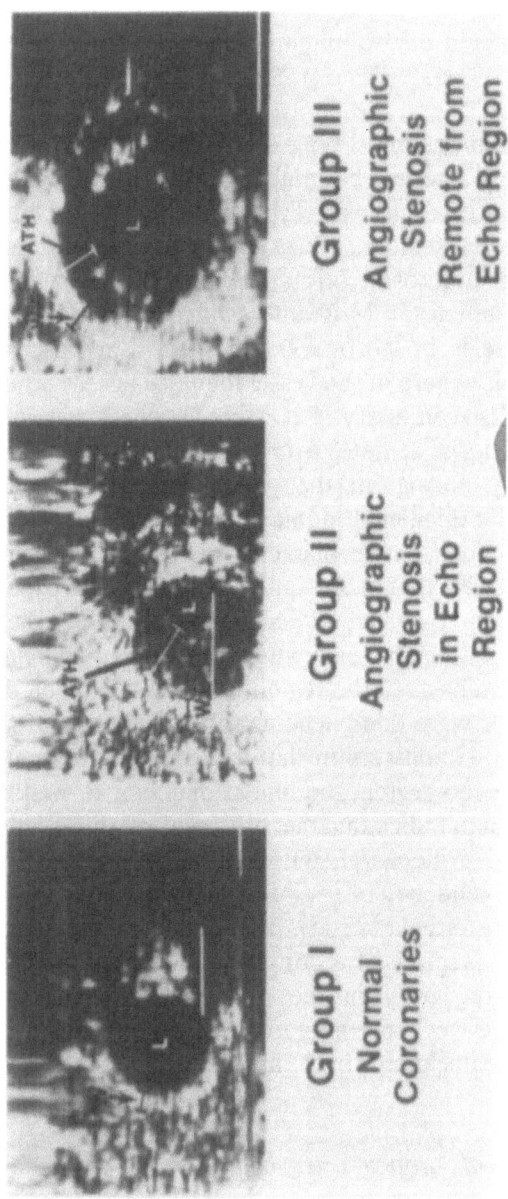

Figure 6. Typical coronary images (stop-frame videotape) from coronary arteries having varying degrees of atherosclerosis. L = lumen. W = wall. ATH = atherosclerotic intimal plaque. Notice that in the Group 3 illustration (angiographic stenosis remote from the echo region), there is severe atherosclerotic thickening which could not be appreciated angiographically. Calibration bars = 3 mm. Reproduced from McPherson *et al.*, N Engl J Med 316: 304—309, 1987, by permission.

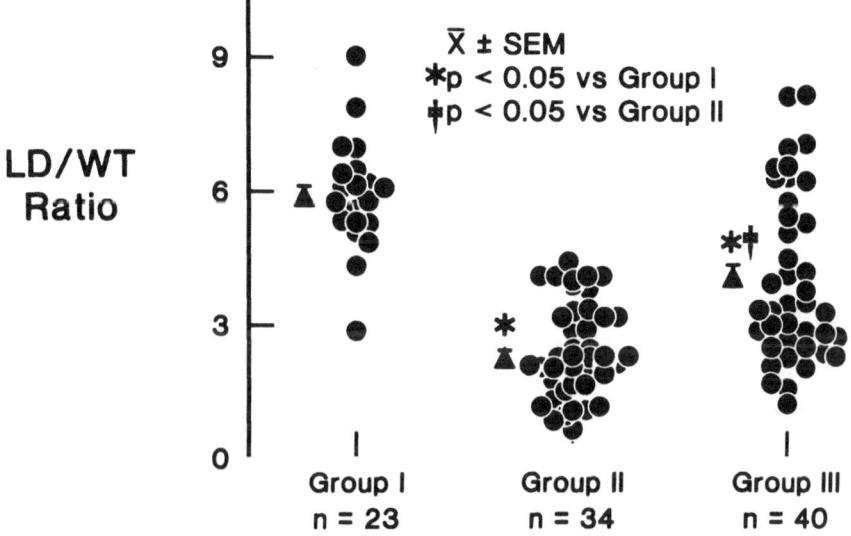

Figure 7. Lumen diameter-wall thickness ratios in three groups of patients (Group 1 = normals, Group 2 = angiographic stenosis in the echo region, Group 3 = angiographic stenosis remote from the echo region). The lumen diameter-wall thickness ratio is significantly lower in Group 2 and Group 3. Thus, diffuse atherosclerotic thickening is demonstrated by high-frequency echocardiagraphy (HFE) in segments of vessels that appear angiographically normal. Reproduced from McPherson *et al.*, N Engl J Med 316: 304—309, 1987, by permission.

atherosclerotic disease and therefore most suitable for graft implantation. Following the cessation of the suturing and termination of cardiopulmonary bypass, the quality of the graft-native vessel anastomosis can be inspected. We initially performed experimental studies where vein grafts were implanted into coronary arteries of dogs. Deliberately technical errors were created, so we could determine the appearance of such deliberate errors using high-frequency epicardial echocardiography [6]. Figure 9 shows an example of such an error; a venous flap was deliberately incorporated into the anastomosis and was easily visualized by the echocardiographic technique. We also compared measurements of the anastomotic size by high-frequency echo (HFE) and correlated them with histologic measurements, again using pressure-fixed distended specimens; an excellent correlation was found ($r = 0.92$, HFE = 0.8 histological size +0.3, $n = 12$).

Having learned the appearance of technical errors and also validated these measurements of anastomosis size, we have subsequently used the technique for the intraoperative evaluation of vein graft anastomosis [6]. The hand-held probe is placed with the contact area adjacent to the anastomosis to record both longitudinal and short-axis images. Figure 10 shows an

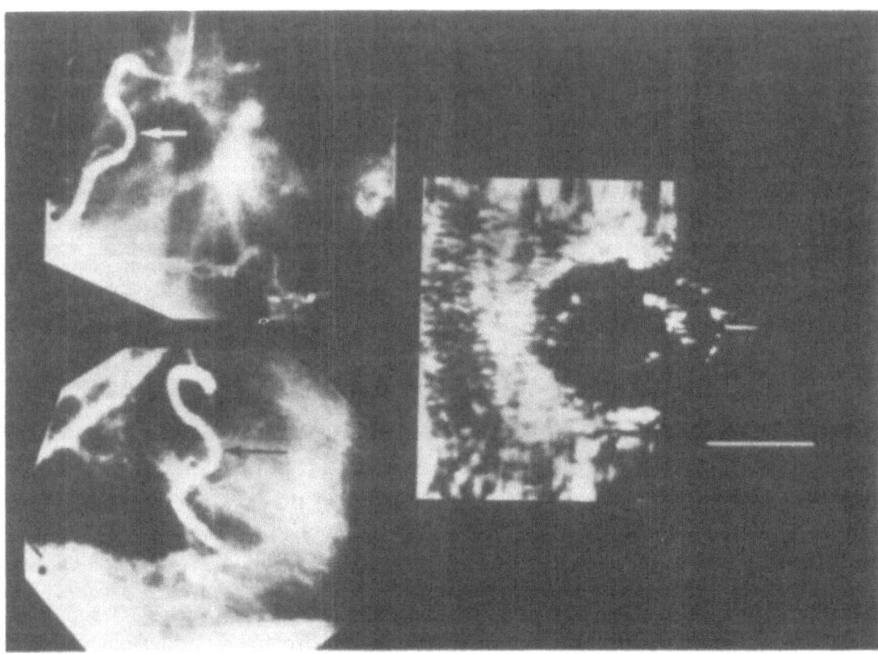

Figure 8. Echocardiographic image (same as Group 3 in Figure 6) of a right coronary artery with only minimal angiographic irregularities (arrows) and high-frequency epicardial echocardiographic image of the same location. Echocardiography reveals diffuse arterial wall thickening which was underestimated angiographically. Reproduced from McPherson *et al.*, N Engl J Med 316: 304—309, 1987, by permission.

example of a satisfactory anastomosis: the anastomotic opening is wide and the left anterior descending coronary artery, to which the anastomosis is made, is free of disease. A septal perforator is also visualized. Figure 11 shows an example of a less satisfactory side-to-side anastomosis. The anastomotic opening is smaller than the native vessel and atherosclerotic plaque is visible right at the site of the anastomosis. In some cases demonstration of such an unsatisfactory result has prompted our surgeons to reinstitute cardiopulmonary bypass and revise the anastomosis until the appearance is more satisfactory. We have also learned that side-to-side anastomoses, of the type demonstrated in Fig. 11, tend to result in less wide anastomotic openings then end-to-side anastomosis [6].

Evaluation of the functional significance of coronary stenosis by high-frequency echo and Doppler techniques

This paper has, so far, concentrated on anatomical images and correlations

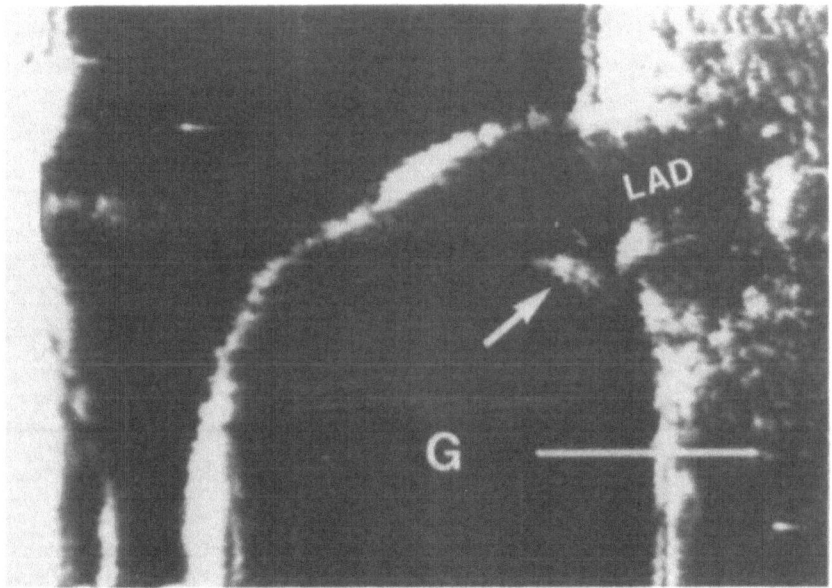

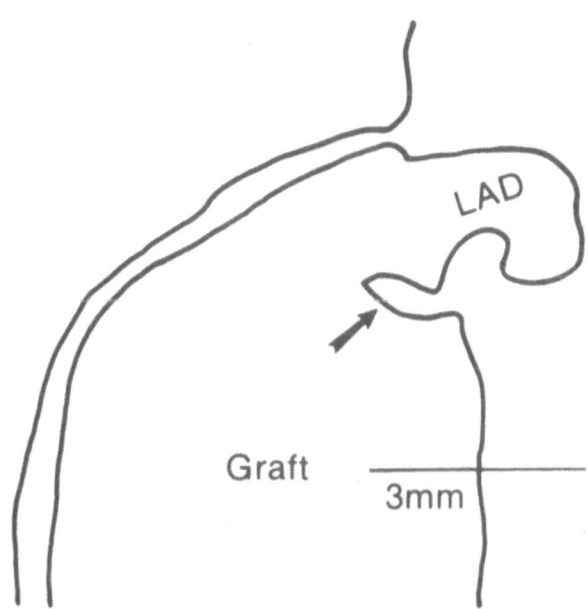

Figure 9. Experimental vein graft-LAD coronary anastomosis in an animal. A deliberate technical error — incorporation of a venous flap into the anastomosis — has been created (arrow). Reproduced from Hiratzka *et al.*, Circulation 73: 1199—1205, 1986, by permission of the American Heart Association, Inc.

110

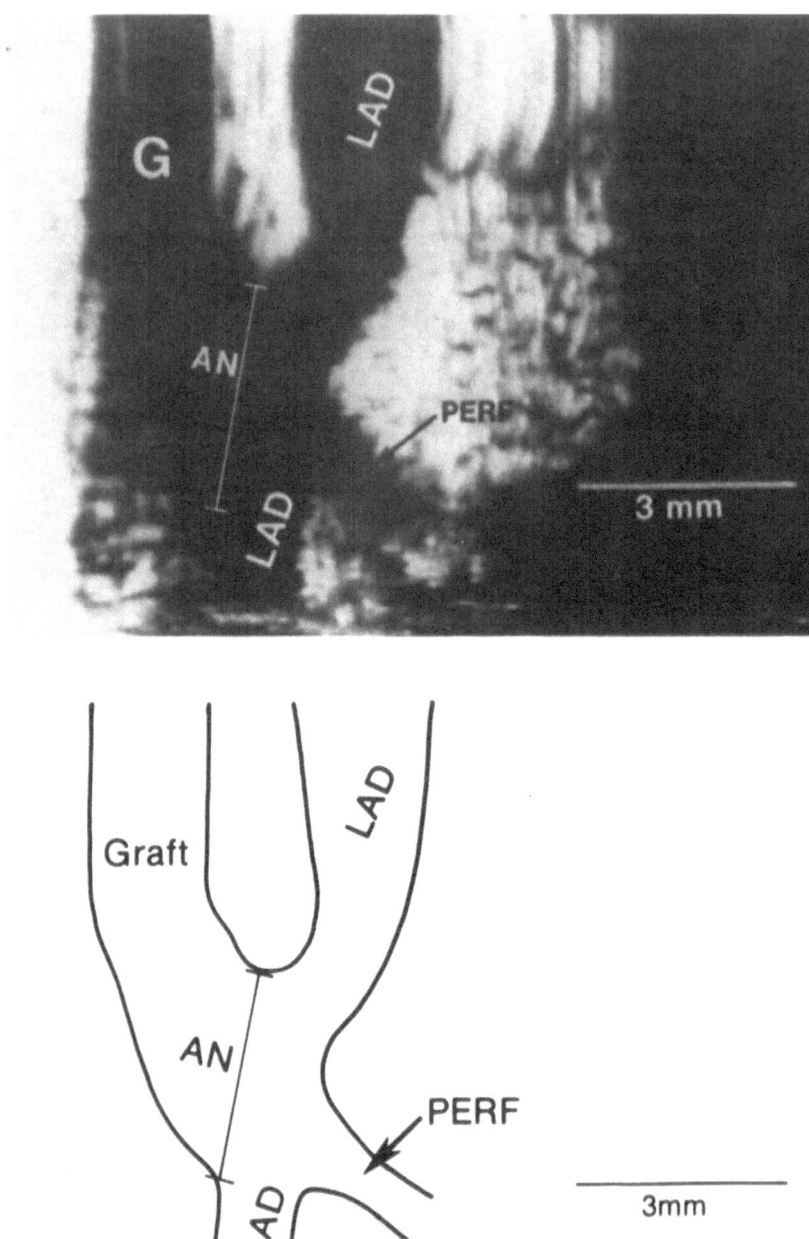

Figure 10. Stop-frame illustration of the vein bypass graft-LAD anastomosis. A technically good anastomosis was achieved with a wide anastomotic opening. G = graft. LAD = left anterior descending coronary artery. AN = anastomosis. PERF = septal perforator. Reproduced from Hiratzka *et al.*, Circulation 73: 1199–1205, 1986, by permission.

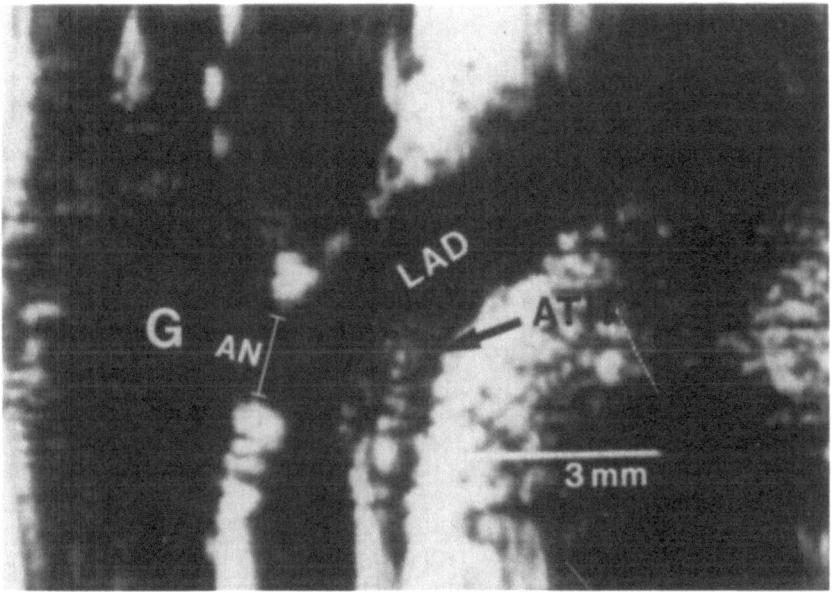

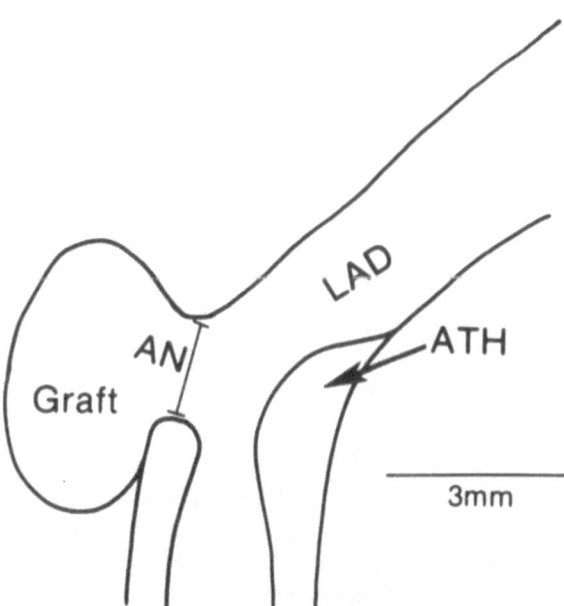

Figure 11. An unsatisfactory vein graft-native vessel anastomosis. The anastomotic opening (AN) is smaller than the diameter of the native left anterior descending coronary artery. In addition, an atherosclerotic plaque (ATH) is present just at the anastomotic site. Reproduced from Hiratzka *et al.*, Circulation 73: 1199—1205, 1986, by permission.

in the high-frequency echo assessment of coronary atherosclerosis. The functional significance of the coronary lesion, of course, is that it interferes with coronary flow. We have developed a unique instrument at the University of Iowa for measuring velocity: a piezoelectric crystal mounted in a suction cup, which uses pulse-Doppler ultrasound at very high transmitted frequency (20 MHz) to measure coronary artery flow velocity. Such probes can be placed on the epicardial coronary vessels without requiring dissection or other trauma to the coronary artery. Phasic and mean coronary velocity is thereby measured during open heart surgery [7].

When coronary arteries are obstructed, myocardial ischemia is produced which immediately induces coronary dilation. When a coronary artery is transiently occluded (10—30 s) while coronary flow velocity is being measured, release of the occlusion and restoration of the normal perfusion pressure causes an immediate and marked increase in coronary flow and velocity. This gradually returns to control levels, usually in less than one minute. Such a vascular response to transient myocardial ischemia is called 'coronary reactive hyperemia'. The Doppler suction probe is an ideal method for the demonstration of such reactive hyperemia. An example is shown in Fig. 12. The ratio of debt area and repayment area can be compared and

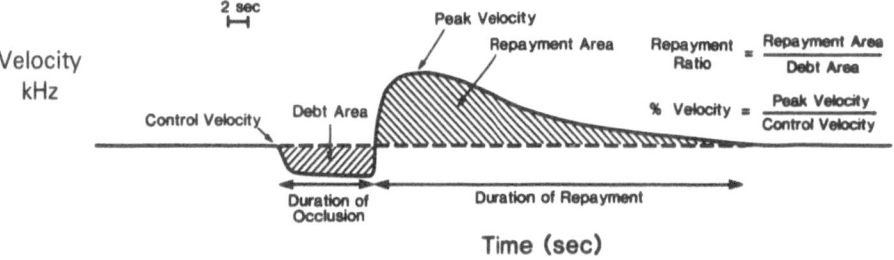

Figure 12. Effect of transient coronary arterial occlusion on coronary artery flow. A marked hyperemia occurs following the brief occlusion resulting in a repayment ratio of 4 : 1. Reproduced from Marcus ML. In: The Coronary Circulation in Health and Disease. McGraw-Hill Book Co., New York, 1983. pg. 75, by permission.

expressed as repayment ratio (repayment area/debt area). The normal dog ratio is about 4. If a coronary stenosis is already present and the artery is partially dilated, the reactive hyperemic response will be blunted or completely abolished. Thus, this technique provides an excellent demonstration of the functional extent of a pre-existing coronary lesion.

We conducted a study where we compared the functional assessment of coronary disease using the Doppler suction probes, to the anatomic assessment permitted by the high-frequency epicardial echocardiographic technique [8]. Cross-sectional coronary artery images were obtained immediately before a 20 second intraoperative coronary occlusion. The artery was then occluded using an atraumatic probe and coronary flow velocity monitored using the suction Doppler technique. Reactive hyperemia was demonstrated after the 20 second coronary occlusion, but this varied depending on the degree of stenosis. We studied 13 patients and divided them into two groups based on the high-frequency echo lumen diameter to wall thickness ratios; a ratio greater than 4.0 was normal and less than 4.0 was considered atherosclerotic. Reactive hyperemia was considered to be normal if the peak and resting flow ratio was greater than $4:1$. We found that reactive hyperemia in the echo-normal group was 5.4 ± 0.7 (range 4.1—6.6), while in the echo-atherosclerotic group, reactive hyperemia was 2.0 ± 3 (range 1.0—4.0, $p < 0.01$ vs. normal). Thus, intraoperative high-frequency echo measurements of coronary arterial wall and lumen were able to identify atherosclerotic lesions which showed a markedly abnormal functional response to brief coronary occlusions [8].

Future applications

The high-frequency echo technique has many potential future applications. We are presently measuring the vasodilating ability of severely atherosclerotic coronary segments by administering intravenous nitroglycerin to patients with coronary atherosclerosis during coronary bypass surgery; initial studies have shown that even severely atherosclerotic segments retain some vasodilating ability [9]. Assessment of coronary arterial shape and the remodeling process induced by coronary atherosclerosis suggests that coronary arteries enlarge in response to developing atherosclerosis in an attempt to preserve lumen size [10]. Tissue characterization techniques to identify subtle changes in coronary arterial walls induced by coronary atherosclerosis are also being employed using this technique.

In conclusion, high-frequency epicardial echocardiography is a valuable tool in assessing the extent, severity and functional significance of coronary disease.

References

1. Rogers EW, Feigenbaum H, Weyman AE, Godley RW, Johnston KW, Eggleton RC: Possible detection of atherosclerotic coronary calcification by two-dimensional echocardiography. Circulation 62: 1046—1053, 1980.
2. Sahn DJ, Barratt-Boyes BG, Graham K, Kerr A, Roche A, Hill D, Brandt PWT, Copeland JG, Mammana R, Temkin LP, Glenn W: Ultrasonic imaging of the coronary arteries in open-chest humans: Evaluation of coronary atherosclerotic lesions during cardiac surgery. Circulation 66: 1034—1044, 1982.

114

3. Sahn DJ, Copeland JG, Temkin LP, Wirt DP, Mammana R, Glenn W: Anatomic-ultrasound correlations for intraoperative open chest imaging of coronary artery atherosclerotic lesions in human beings. J Am Coll Cardiol 3: 1169—1177, 1984.
4. McPherson DD, Armstrong M, Rose E, Kieso RA, Megan M, Hunt M, Hite P, Marcus ML, Kerber RE: High frequency epicardial echocardiography for coronary artery evaluation: In vitro and in vivo validation of arterial lumen and wall thickness measurements. J Am Coll Cardiol 8: 600—606, 1986.
5. McPherson DD, Hiratzka LF, Lamberth WC, Brandt B, Hunt M, Kieso RA, Marcus ML, Kerber RE: Delineation of the extent of coronary atherosclerosis by high-frequency epicardial echocardiography. N Engl J Med 316: 304—309, 1987.
6. Hiratzka LF, McPherson DD, Lamberth WC, Brandt B, Armstrong ML, Schröder E, Hunt M, Kieso R, Megan MD, Tompkins PK, Marcus ML, Kerber RE: Intraoperative evaluation of coronary artery bypass graft anastomoses with high-frequency epicardial echocardiography: Experimental validation and initial patient studies. Circulation 73: 1199—1205, 1986.
7. Marcus M, Wright C, Doty D, Eastham C, Laughin D, Krumm P, Fastenow C, Brody M: Measurement of coronary velocity and reactive hyperemia in the coronary circulation of humans. Circ Res 49: 877—891, 1981.
8. McPherson DD, Hiratzka LF, Brandt B, Lamberth WC, Hunt M, Hartnett J, Clothier J, Eastham C, Kerber RE: Relationship of echo-demonstrated coronary atherosclerosis to reactive hyperemia. (Abstract) Circulation 74: II-85, 1986.
9. McPherson DD, Ross AF, Moyers JR, Hiratzka LF, Brandt B, Hunt M, Kerber RE: Can atherosclerotic coronaries vasodilate? An intraoperative high-frequency epicardial echocardiographic study. (Abstract) Circulation 74: II-468, 1986.
10. McPherson DD, Hunt MM, Hiratzka LF, Brandt B, Lamberth WC, Marcus ML, Kerber RE: Coronary atherosclerosis causes remodeling of arterial geometry: Demonstration by high-frequency epicardial echocardiography. (Abstract) Circulation 74: II-468, 1986.

7. On the accuracy of densitometric measurements of coronary artery stenosis based on Lambert-Beer's absorption law

PIERRE-ANDRÉ DORIOT and W. RUTISHAUSER

SUMMARY. Densitometry of coronary arteries is often thought to be independent of the size and shape of the lumens involved. This belief results from the postulation that Lambert-Beer's absorption law (LB's law) is the appropriate theoretical basis for densitometric measurements on coronary arteries. Experiments with certain phantoms yield, however, results incompatible with the LB-model. For instance, a dependence of the obtained degrees of stenosis on the respective size, shape and rotational orientation (i.e. around the vessel axis and with respect to the incident X-rays) of the lumens can be observed. Since this dependence is not removed by compensation for the nonlinearity introduced by the cinefilm, one must admit that LB's law is not the adequate basis for densitometric measurements of coronary artery stenosis, and that conventional densitometry (i.e. based on LB's law) is likely to produce systematic errors. Using a previously designed, more adequate mathematical-physical model which takes X-ray poly-chromasy and scattered radiation into account, the magnitude of errors of conventionally obtained degrees of stenosis was assessed, as well as the magnitude of errors affecting the residual luminal area, this latter one being obtained from the erroneously assessed degree of stenosis and the area of the intact lumen (determined itself by calibrated diameter measurement).

Introduction

Quantification of coronary artery stenosis by 'diameter' measurements on the intact and stenotic vessel segments is straightforward. However, the accuracy of this morphologic approach is limited, even if different angiographic views are available, because of the irregular shape of the stenotic lumen. A further essential limitation is set by the frequent impossibility of identifying accurately the borders of the lesion in the angiographic images.

Quantification by densitometry is more cumbersome since several conditions must be fulfilled, such as momentary complete filling of the involved arterial segments with contrast medium, no superimposition with other opacified vessels, adequate orientation of the axes of intact and diseased vessel segments with respect to the incident X-rays (more or less perpendicular), etc. The first requirement can be met be injecting the contrast

J. C. Reiber & P. W. Serruys (eds.), New Developments in Quantitative Coronary Arteriography,
115—124.

medium vigorously into the coronary artery. Fulfillment of the two others is still difficult, but could become easier using the procedure for adequate angulation proposed by Wollschläger *et al.* [1], especially if the angiocardiographic unit has an appropriate facility for automatic biplane angulation setting.

Nonetheless, densitometry is often thought to be independent of the size and shape of the involved arterial lumens. This belief results from the assumption that Lambert-Beer's absorption law (LB's law) is the appropriate physical basis for densitometric measurements on coronary arteries. The aim of this contribution is to show why this view is not quite correct and to assess the magnitude of errors resulting from this erroneous concept (Other sources of errors will not be discussed).

A mathematical-physical model for the densitometry of coronary arteries

To assume the applicability of LB's law is equivalent to postulate a linear relationship between the logarithmic transmission 'log T' of an X-ray beam element x_P through a layer of contrast medium, and the thickness t_P of this layer (t_P is measured along the beam element x_P). Denoting the intensity of the beam element x_P by I_{in} when it enters the coronary artery filled with contrast medium, and by $I_{out}(t_P)$ when it leaves it, we have:

$$\log T(t_P) = \log\{I_{out}(t_P)/I_{in}\}$$
$$= \log I_{out}(t_P) - \log I_{in} = -\text{constant} \times t_P.$$

As underlying assumption thereby is, that the (positive) constant is the same for all concerned beam elements in the region of interest. The subsequent assumption that the conversion process in the image intensifier is linear, yields:

$$\log'\{L^*(t_P)/L(t_P)\} = \log L^*(t_P) - \log L(t_P) = -\text{constant} \times t_P,$$

where $L(t_P)$ is the luminance of the vessel pixel P (associated with beam element x_P) on the output screen of the image intensifier before opacification, and $L^*(t_P)$ its luminance during opacification.

If these relations were true, and provided that possible effects resulting from the nonlinear characteristics of the cinefilm can be compensated for, then, densitometry would indeed not depend on the size and shape of the lumens involved, nor on their rotational orientation (i.e. around the axis of the vessel segment) relative to the X-rays (The axes of the two vessel segments are always assumed to be adequately oriented with respect to the incident X-rays).

Experiments with particular phantoms yield, however, results incompatible with the LB-model. For instance, measurements of a 50% stenosis (percentage area reduction) constructed by inserting a plexiglas rod of 'half-moon' cross-section into a cylindrical hole of ˙5 mm diameter drilled in a plexiglass plate and filled with contrast medium, will reveal a clear dependence of the obtained degree of stenosis on the rotational orientation of the 'stenotic' lumen relatively to the incident X-rays (The X-rays are directed perpendicular to the cylinder axis). Since this dependence is not removed by compensation for the nonlinearity introduced by the cinefilm, one must admit that LB's law is not the adequate basis for densitometric measurements of coronary artery stenosis, and that conventional densitometry (i.e. based on LB's law) is likely to produce systematic errors.

In order to better understand the discrepancies between the LB-model and experimental results, we have developed a more adequate mathematical-physical model than the LB-law [2]. Defining the logarithmic ratio as 'luminance $L(t_P)$ of pixel P before opacification of the artery' over 'luminance $L^*(t_P)$ of this pixel during opacification' as the 'luminance contrast' $c_{lum}(t_P)$ of this pixel, and taking X-ray polychromasy and scattered radiation into account, we obtained a second order polynomial relationship between layer thickness t_P of contrast medium inside the coronary artery and resulting 'luminance contrast' $c_{lum}(t_P)$:

$$c_{lum}(t_P) = \log\{L(t_P)/L^*(t_P)\} = \log L(t_P) - \log L^*(t_P)$$
$$= A_{1,P} \cdot t_P + A_{3,P} \cdot t_P^2 + \text{negligible terms of higher order.} \quad (1)$$

(In practice, $L(t_P)$ is replaced by the average luminance of adequately selected background pixels). $A_{1,P}$ being positive and $A_{3,P}$ negative, equation (1) states that the luminance contrast $c_{lum}(t_P)$ does not increase linearly with the thickness t_P of contrast medium, but less strongly. This is mainly due to beam hardening inside the artery and to the presence of scattered radiation. It could be shown, that $A_{1,P}$ and $A_{3,P}$ depend primarily on the actual voltage of the X-ray tube (kV) and on the iodine concentration c_I of the injected, vessel filling contrast medium. This is especially the case when regulation of the delivered dosis is achieved by regulation of the kV only (constant mA and constant exposure times). This results in:

$$c_{lum}(t_P) = A_1(kV, c_I) \cdot t_P + A_3(kV, c_I) \cdot t_P^2. \quad (2)$$

A further additive term $A_2(kV, c_I)m_P t_P$ appears in equation (2), if local variations of the patient's own attenuation, represented by m_P, are also taken into account. This means, in further disagreement with the LB-model, that the luminance contrast of the vessel image depends not only on t_P, but also on the other absorbers/attenuators encountered by the X-ray beam element x_P. In other words, the luminance contrast of a hypothetical contrast medium layer of uniform thickness t would be modulated by local variations of the patient's own X-ray attenuation. However, this secondary effect will be ignored in the following; that means, that we will assume homogeneous patient attenuation along all concerned X-ray beam elements.

One could also have defined coefficients $A_1(kV)$ and $A_3(kV)$ independent of the iodine concentration c_I by using as variable the product 'c_I times thickness t_P':

$$c_{lum}(c_I t_P) = A_1(kV) \cdot c_I t_P + A_3(kV) \cdot (c_I t_P)^2.$$

The functions $A_1(kV, c_I)$ and $A_3(kV, c_I)$ were determined experimentally on our angiocardiographic unit with various iodine concentrations [2]. Different patient attenuations were thereby simulated by different thicknesses of paraffin, yielding kV-values from 55 to 100 kV. It turned out, as expected, that $A_1(kV, c_I)$, $|A_3(kV, c_I)|$ and $|A_3(kV, c_I)/A_1(kV, c_I)|$ decrease with increasing kV and with decreasing iodine concentration. This is mainly due to beam-hardening in the injected artery and in the other absorbing/ attenuating structures, and to the presence of scattered radiation. The values obtained for $A_1(kV, c_I)$ and $A_3(kV, c_I)$ may be somewhat specific for our angiocardiographic unit, but similar angiocardiographic units should produce roughly the same values. It must be pointed out that the mathematical-physical model has been tailored to coronary angiography, and that it is probably not appropriate for densitometric measurements of the left ventricle, for instance.

The experiment demonstrated also that the additional nonlinearity introduced by the 35 mm cinefilm is of secondary importance in comparison with the nonlinearity observed at the output of the image intensifier.

Now that the functions $A_1(kV, c_I)$ and $A_3(kV, c_I)$ have been determined, an algorithm could be designed to correct the native luminance contrast values $c_{lum}(t_P)$ into fictive contrast values $c_{corr}(t_P)$ which are proportional to t_P, according to the following equation obtained from equation (2):

$$c_{corr}(t_P) = A_1(kV, c_I)t_P = \frac{-1 + \sqrt{1 + 4A_3(kV, c_I)/A_1^2(kV, c_I)c_{lum}(t_P)}}{2A_3(kV, c_I)/A_1^2(kV, c_I)}. \quad (3)$$

In this way, the erroneous assumptions of conventional densitometry could be made artificially true.

Domains of error of conventionally measured degrees of stenosis

In densitometry, the cross-sectional area of a vessel lumen is represented by the sum of all contrast values of a slice of unity thickness perpendicular to the vessel axis in the image. Because of equation (2), the cross-sectional area obtained will depend on the kV, on the iodline concentration c_I of the injected contrast medium, on the size of the lumen, and on its shape and rotational orientation relatively to the incident X-rays if the lumen is not circular in shape.

Using equation (2), the densitometric intensity profiles of various hypothetical lumens can be calculated in dependence of the kV, of c_l, and of the respective size, shape and rotational orientation of these lumens. This allows in turn to calculate the error of conventionally measured degree of stenosis. Figure 1 shows for instance the intensity profiles of the intact and stenotic circular lumens of a stenosed artery (75% area reduction). The profiles one would obtain for the LB-model are depicted in plain lines. The intensity profile of the intact lumen (dashed line) is markedly more compressed than the one of the stenotic lumen. Consequently, the true degree of stenosis will be underestimated (71.3%). The underestimation depends on the value of $A_3(kV, c_l)/A_1(kV, c_l)$ and on the respective diameters of the intact and stenotic lumens (and thus on the true degree of stenosis), but of course not on the direction of the incident X-rays.

Calculating the intensity profiles of the intact and stenotic circular lumens as done for Fig. 1, but now from 'no stenosis' to 'total occlusion', and computing the resulting error of the degree of stenosis, yields the curve shown in Fig. 2. This curve represents the error of a conventionally (LB)

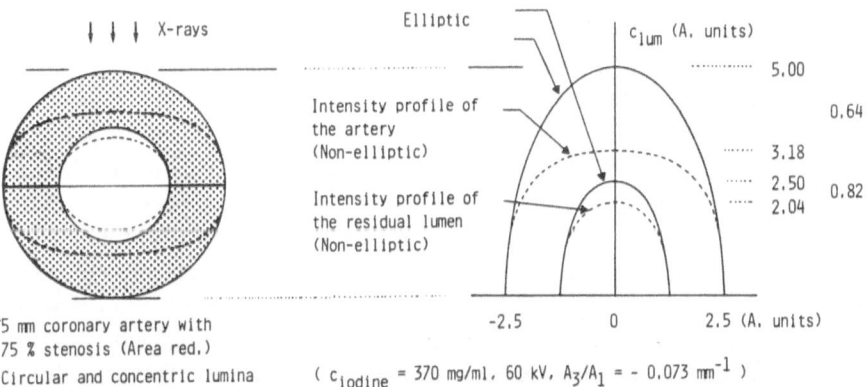

Figure 1. Seventy-five % stenosis (percentage area reduction) on a 5 mm artery with circular intact and stenotic lumens. The corresponding densitometric intensity profiles one would obtain if Lambert-Beer's law (LB) was applicable are depicted at the right in solid lines. The intensity profiles one would obtain in reality are shown in dashed lines. For ease of comparison, the arbitrary units along both axes have been chosen equal to the true vessel dimensions (mm). The ratio of true densitometric arterial diameter to LB arterial diameter is 0.64 (3.18/5 = 0.636); the ratio of true densitometric stenotic diameter to LB stenotic diameter is 0.82 (2.04/2.5 = 0.816). The profile compression is also represented in the left drawing in dashed lines. Since the profile of the intact lumen is more compressed than the one of the stenotic lumen, the degree of stenosis will be underestimated (71.3% instead of 75.0% area reduction).

120

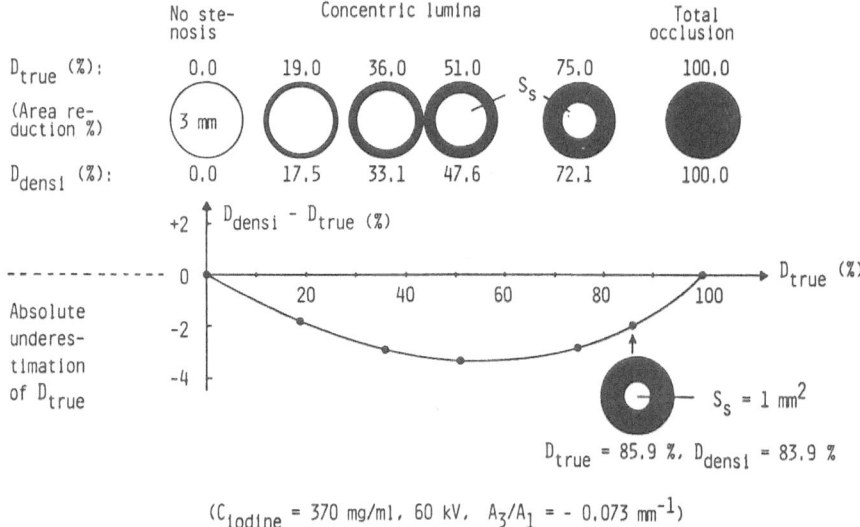

Figure 2. The curve represents the absolute error $E = D_{densi}(\%) - D_{true}(\%)$ in the densitometric degree of stenosis $D_{densi}(\%)$ (percentage area reduction) for a 3 mm artery at 60 kV and 370 mg/ml iodine concentration, under the assumption that intact and stenotic lumens are circular (concentric or not).

measured degree of stenosis for the particular case of circular intact and stenotic lumens, as a function of the true degree of stenosis (0 to 100%), for an arterial diameter of 3 mm, at an X-ray tube voltage of 60 kV, and at an iodine concentration of 370 mg/ml.

The greatest possible over-, respectively underestimation of a particular degree of stenosis can be determined for a given arterial diameter, kV and iodine concentration c_i by replacing in the calculus the previous circular stenotic lumen by the 'slit lumen' depicted in Fig. 3 (top and bottom circles). This particularly shaped lumen will indeed yield the greatest possible overestimation of the true degree of stenosis with regard to all other possible shapes of stenotic lumens with the same cross-sectional area when its long axis is parallel to the incident X-rays (top circles). Inversely, this same lumen will always yield the greatest possible underestimation of the true degree of stenosis when its long axis is perpendicular to the incident X-rays (bottom circles). Thus, calculation of the erroneous degrees of stenosis from 'no stenosis' to 'total occlusion' for the two depicted extreme rotational orientations of the slit lumen yields the boundaries of the domain of errors of conventionally measured degrees of stenosis for a given artery diameter, kV-level and iodine concentration. The error of the "half-moon" stenosis, also depicted in Fig. 3, shows that phantoms presenting such stenoses are more appropriate for test purposes than phantoms presenting circular lumens, since they allow in practice the determination of the maximum error possible.

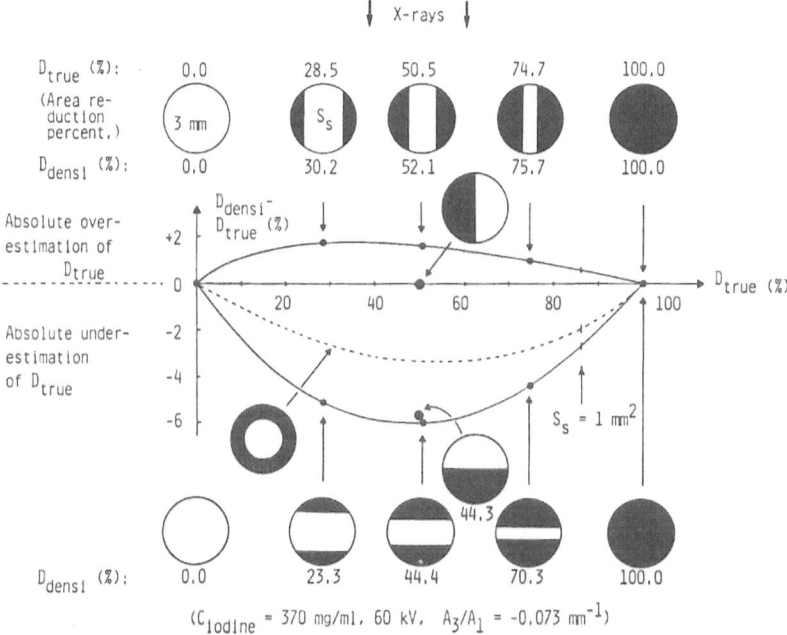

Figure 3. Domain of error of the degree of stenosis for a 3 mm artery at 60 kV and 370 mg/ml iodine concentration. Its upper and lower limits have been determined using the depicted 'slit lumen'. The dashed curve is the error in the degree of stenosis in case of circular intact and stenotic lumens. The also depicted 'half-moon' stenosis demonstrates that phantoms with 'half-moon' stenoses are more appropriate for test purposes than phantoms with circular lumens only, since they reveal in practice the greatest possible error.

Figure 4 shows the domains of error for a 1 mm, 3 mm and 5 mm artery. The errors increase markedly with the arterial diameter and decrease with the X-ray tube voltage (60 and 100 kV). Intermediate stenoses obviously are prone to greater errors than the small or severe ones (As will be demonstrated in the next section, this is not the case if stenosis severity is expressed by the residual cross-sectional area). Although the intact lumen is usually much stronger underestimated by densitometry than the stenotic one, the largest possible errors in the degree of stenosis (expressed in percentage area reduction) remain moderate. The dashed curve in each diagram is the error in the degree of stenosis by a 5 mm artery in case of circular intact and stenotic lumens (concentric or not). If one considers, for a given arterial diameter, a circular stenotic lumen of given cross-sectional area as being the 'average' lumen of all stenotic lumens with the same cross-sectional area (all possible shapes and rotational orientations), then this curve represents the average error of conventionally (LB) measured degrees of stenosis on 5 mm arteries at 60 kV, and 100 kV, respectively, and 370 mg/ml iodine concentration. Thus, conventional densitometry can be expected to underestimate statistically the true degree of stenosis. In our experiments with a phantom

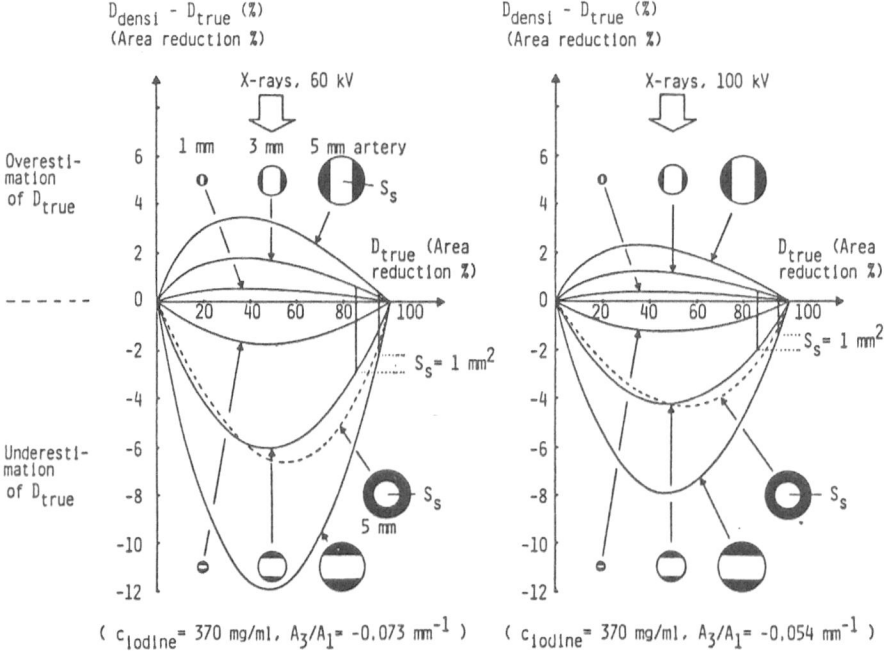

Figure 4. Domains of error in the degree of stenosis of a 1 mm, 3 mm and 5 mm artery at 60 and 100 kV, respectively for an iodine concentration of 370 mg/ml. The dashed curves represent the error in the degree of stenosis for the 3 mm and 5 mm arteries, if the residual lumen is circular. The vertical lines in the right part of the domains of error for the 3 mm and 5 mm arteries represent the possible error in the degree of stenosis when the true residual luminal area S_s is equal to 1 mm².

having circular lumens only, intermediate degrees of stenosis were indeed systematically underestimated [2]. However, since the smallest diameter in this phantom was only 1 mm, further experiments must be performed in order to investigate if other sources of errors may become dominant at still smaller diameters. The smallness of the average error of the degree of stenosis explains why validation studies performed on casts or on phantoms with cylindrical lumens only led to the erroneous conclusion that densitometry is independent of the shape of the stenotic lumen.

Domains of error for lower iodine concentrations would be of course smaller. Lower concentrations have, however, the disadvantage of degrading the signal-to-noise ratio.

Domain of error of the residual area

On the basis of the densitometric data, the cross-sectional area of the stenotic lumen is usually obtained from the measured degree of stenosis and the cross-sectional area of the intact lumen, the last one based on calibrated diameter measurement. The boundaries of the domains of error of residual areas calculated in this way can be determined using the corresponding erroneous degrees of stenosis of the preceding section. Figure 5 shows the domains of error obtained for the 1 mm, 3 mm and 5 mm arteries of Fig. 4, at 60 kV (on the left) and at 100 kV (on the right). As was the case for the degree of stenosis, the domain of error of the residual luminal area increases with increasing artery diameter and with decreasing X-ray tube voltage. Its shape, however, is different: the greatest possible over-, respectively under-estimation of the residual luminal area increase continuously with the true degree of stenosis. Thus, severe stenoses are prone to greater errors in terms of residual luminal area than moderate ones. As the error of the degree of stenosis behaves inversely, the error of the residual cross-sectional area of severe stenoses may be considerable, even if the associated degree of stenosis is accurate to a few percent (This is also the case in the morphologic approach). Since the functionally dominant criterium in coronary artery disease appears to be a residual luminal area of 1 mm², which corresponds to degrees of stenosis of 86 to 95% (percentage area reduction) for arterial

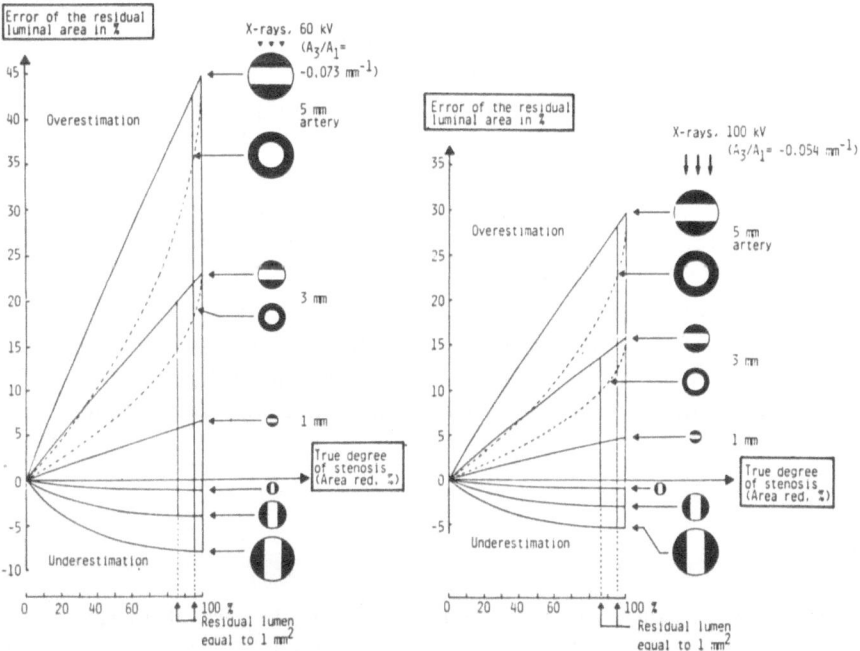

Figure 5. Domains of error in the residual luminal area for the 1 mm, 3 mm and 5 mm arteries, at 60 kV, and 100 kV respectively, and 370 mg/ml iodine concentration.

124

diameters of 3 to 5 mm (vertical lines in Fig. 5), it is important to strive for very high accuracy of the measured degree of stenosis in severe lesions. This means that the native luminance contrast $c(t_P)$ should be corrected pixel by pixel as previously described, or alternatively that the densitometric cross-sectional area of the intact lumen should be corrected by a multiplicative factor (>1), dependent on the arterial diameter, on the kV and on the iodine concentration c_I. This factor can easily be obtained from the ratio function $A_3(kV, c_I)/A_1(kV, c_I)$.

The curves in dashed line in the two diagrams of Fig. 5 represent the error of the residual cross-sectional area if the stenotic lumen of the 3 and 5 mm arteries is circular. These curves show that the residual cross-sectional area can be expected to be statistically overestimated by conventional densitometry, especially in severe stenoses.

Conclusion

Conventional densitometry of coronary arteries is not independent of the shape of the involved lumens as is often claimed, even if one compensates for the nonlinearity introduced by the cinefilm. The computed degrees of stenosis and residual cross-sectional areas depend on the respective size and shape of the intact and stenotic lumens, on their rotational orientation with respect to the incident X-rays, and moreover on the voltage of the X-ray tube (kV) and on the iodine concentration of the injected contrast medium. Although this dependence does not impinge severely on the accuracy of the measured degree of stenosis, a pixel by pixel correction of the native 'luminance contrast' values of the vessel (or some other appropriate correction as suggested) is necessary for accurate measurement of the functionally important residual cross-sectional area.

Measurements on phantoms with circular lumens reveal only average errors. This has often been overlooked and has thus led to too optimistic statements in validation studies. Phantoms presenting 'half-moon' stenoses appear to be much more sensitive in assessing the performances of a measuring system.

References

1. Wollschläger H, Zeiher AM, Lee P, Solzbach U, Bonzel T, Just H: Computed 'triple' orthogonal projections for optimal radiological imaging with biplane X-ray systems. Comput Cardiol, 1986, (in press)
2. Doriot PA, Pochon Y, Rasoamanambelo L, Chatelain P, Welz R, Rutishauser W: Densitometry of coronary arteries — An improved physical model. Comput Cardiol: 91—94, 1985.

8. Morphologic and physiologic validation of quantitative coronary arteriography utilizing digital methods

G. B. JOHN MANCINI

SUMMARY. To assess the *in-vivo* performance of a coronary quantitation program, 16 dogs were instrumented with precision-drilled, plastic cylinders to create intraluminal stenoses ranging from 0.83 mm to 1.83 mm. Biplane, on-line digital coronary angiograms and cine-angiograms were obtained. The on-line digital images were analyzed in nonsubtracted and subtracted modes. Cineangiograms were digitized and quantitated by the same computer program. There was an excellent correlation between known and measured minimal diameter stenoses ($r = 0.87-0.98$, s.e.e. $= 0.09-0.24$ mm). Inter- and intraobserver variability analysis showed high reproducibility ($r = 0.90-0.97$, s.e.e. $= 0.12-0.23$ mm). The best results in both analyses were achieved by nonsubtracted digital imaging and the worst by cineradiography. Measures of percent diameter stenosis, percent area stenosis (geometric and videometric) and absolute minimal cross-sectional area (geometric and videometric) were all highly correlated with independent measures of actual coronary flow reserve. This study provides a direct, *in-vivo*, anatomical and physiological validation of a new and rapid coronary quantitation method suitable for analysis of both digital angiograms and cineangiograms.

Introduction

Quantitative coronary arteriography has been shown to be useful in assessing the extent of coronary disease, its functional significance and its response to therapeutic interventions such as angioplasty, thrombolysis and diet therapy [1]. Most current methods rely either on hand drawn arterial contours or automatic edge-detection algorithms applied to 35 mm cine-angiograms [1, 2]. The purpose of this investigation was to assess the *in-vivo* performance of a new, fully automatic, rapid coronary quantitation program by assessing its accuracy compared to precisely known stenosis dimensions in a range approaching dimensions likely to be encountered clinically, and by comparing the analysis of biplane, on-line digital images to the analysis of cinearteriograms and finally, to determine the relation between morphologic measurements and coronary flow reserve.

J. C. Reiber & P. W. Serruys (eds.), New Developments in Quantitative Coronary Arteriography,
125—141.

Methods

Sixteen mongrel dogs were anesthetized, intubated, and ventilated with a Harvard Ventilator. The proximal left anterior descending and circumflex coronary arteries were dissected free and encircled by appropriately sized and calibrated electromagnetic flow probes, a soft rubber elastic tie and a silk suture. All animals received 12,000 to 15,000 units of heparin in 1000 to 3000 unit intravenous boluses to prevent clot formation.

Baseline measurements of heart rate, systolic blood pressure, left ventricular end-diastolic pressure, peak positive and negative dP/dt, basal epicardial blood flow and reactive hyperemic blood flow after a 20 second coronary occlusion were made. The left main coronary artery was then engaged with a 7F or 8F angiographic catheter under fluoroscopic control. A standard 0.016 mm angioplasty guide wire was passed through the catheter and advanced into one of the main coronary arteries. The angiographic catheter was then removed, leaving the wire in place. Precision drilled, radiolucent, Nylon cylinders were advanced into either or both of the proximal coronary arteries. The distal 2 mm of the cylinders were precision drilled to produce lumen diameters ranging from 0.71 mm to 1.83 mm. The cylinders were positioned by inserting them over the tip of the appropriately sized catheter which was then advanced over the guide wire and into position in the proximal coronary arteries. Once in a suitable position, the cylinders were sutured into place by rapidly tying the silk suture around the segment of coronary artery containing the intraluminal cylinder while the advancing catheter and guide wire were quickly removed to reestablish antegrade flow.

After reattainment of hemodynamic stability, all pressure and flow measurements were repeated, instruments were then removed, ribs were reapproximated and the chest wound was closed.

Biplane digital coronary angiograms were then obtained in projections that optimized separation of the stenotic area from surrounding vessels. Angiograms were acquired on a digital angiographic computer (DPS-4100C, ADAC Laboratories, Edenvale, CA) interfaced to a standard cineangiographic system (Philips Optimus M200, Eindhoven, the Netherlands). The radiographic input signal was kept constant (fixed kVp, mA and pulse width X-ray exposure). A 12.5 cm field of view and a small focal spot size (0.6 mm, nominal) were used. Images were acquired at 10 frames per second in a 512×512 matrix with 256 gray levels. Images underwent logarithmic lookup transformation to account for Lambert-Beer exponential X-ray absorption. Cineangiograms in the identical views were also acquired using the same radiographic technique. The frame rate for these images was 30 per second. Care was taken to ensure that both the stenotic area and the angiographic catheter were within the central portion of the radiographic field in order to minimize any possible effects of pincushion distortion. Care was also taken to ensure that the optical densities of interest were on the linear portion of the sensitometric curve of the film (Kodak CFR) by routinely analyzing a density step-wedge.

In order to analyze the cinefilm, orthogonal images which showed the lesions optimally were projected on a Vanguard Viewer (Model XR-15, Melville, NY) which was optically coupled to a video camera identical to the one in the on-line digital system. Using 2.4 : 1 optical magnification, the resulting video signal corresponding to a sub-region of the 35 mm frame was digitized at $512 \times 512 \times 8$ bit resolution onto the same digital angiographic computer system. The video noise of this method of film digitization was reduced by averaging four video frames prior to storage.

The digital images were processed both with and without mask subtraction. The single mask frame and the image best demonstrating the stenosis were selected so as to minimize any misregistration artifacts in the region of the stenosis. Subtracted and non-subtracted digital images underwent gray-scale inversion to produce white-on-black pictures comparable to the gray-scale of negative film images. All images were subjected to a gray-scale modification to linearly expand their individual scene dynamic range to fill the full 8-bit dynamic range of the digital radiographic system. This pre-processing step is fully automated. All directly acquired digital images were then subjected to digital magnification by a factor of four and the digitized film images were digitally magnified by a factor of two. This was achieved by bilinear pixel interpolation using the system's array processor. Although this digital magnification does not improve the density of the spatial sampling of the electronic imaging methods, it does provide additional precision in the analysis techniques of the quantitation program. The final overall magnifications of the digital images and the digitized film images were ×4 and ×4.8, respectively. These magnifications were experimentally determined to optimize the quantitative analyses of both film and digital images. The analyzed effective pixel resolution was thus 2048×2048 for the on-line digital images and 2458×2458 for the digitized film images.

All images were analyzed using a previously described automatic coronary quantitation program [3]. The centerline of the arterial segment within the analysis region is determined by analyzing circular pixel density profiles of decreasing radii using simple signal processing techniques to locate the angular positions of the proximal and distal portions of the arterial segment at each radius. Linear density profiles perpendicular to the arterial centerline are extracted over the entire length of the arterial segment. Initial edge points are found by noting the density of points at the first and second derivatives of each perpendicular density profile and then determining the location of the points which fall at a value of 75% of the difference between the densities at these derivative extrema (i.e. weighted toward the first derivative extrema). This method was found to give best accuracy and precision of measurement of radiographic phantoms in the 0.5–5 mm diameter range [3]. These initial gradient-determined edge points are then examined for spatial continuity and outliers are discarded. The gray-scale densities of initial edge points are then used to determine final edge points using local thresholding. The set of accepted threshold densities for either edge (independently) is smoothed and any threshold values discarded during the first pass are replaced by linear interpolation from neighboring valid edge points. Each perpendicular profile is reanalyzed and the location of final edge points are determined using this locally adaptive threshold method. The geometric diameter at any point along the centerline is the distance along each perpendicular profile between edge points on opposite sides of the artery. Calibration is achieved by measuring a magnification factor based on the known size of the angiographic catheter. Calibrations were obtained from the nonsubtracted images and film images. The catheter in the sub-tracted images was not used for calibration because of the routine occur-rence of spatial misregistration. The computer program determines video-densitometric cross-sectional area at each point along the centerline by integrating the densities across the perpendicular profile from edge to edge. These areas are corrected for background by subtracting a linearly inter-polated background determined by the density values at the edge points. The final computer output consists of the arterial image with arterial edges and centerline and plots of geometric diameter (calibrated with reference to the known diameter of the angiographic catheter), densitometric relative cross-sectional area, maximal percent diameter stenosis and maximal area (densitometric) percent stenosis (Fig. 1). Approximately one minute is required to complete the analysis of each view of a single lesion.

This process was repeated for the digitally acquired images after applying a geometric image transformation which removes pincushion distortion following a previously described method [4]. Film images were not corrected for pincushion distortion.

Of the 16 animals studied, three fibrillated immediately after placement of the stenotic cylinder and postmortem examination revealed thrombosis of the lumena. Three animals fibrillated during contrast injection and one animal died secondary to coronary dissection. In the nine remaining dogs there were 8 cylinders in circumflex arteries and 5 cylinders in left anterior descending arteries. One stenosis was excluded from analysis because it had slipped from its suture and contrast streaming around the cylinder could not be excluded. One stenosis could not be optimally separated from small, adjacent, perforating branches. Two stenoses could not be analyzed because calibration of the angiographic catheter was not reproducible due to poor contrast density between it and the background. One stenosis required editing of the automatically determined edges to preclude spurious tracking

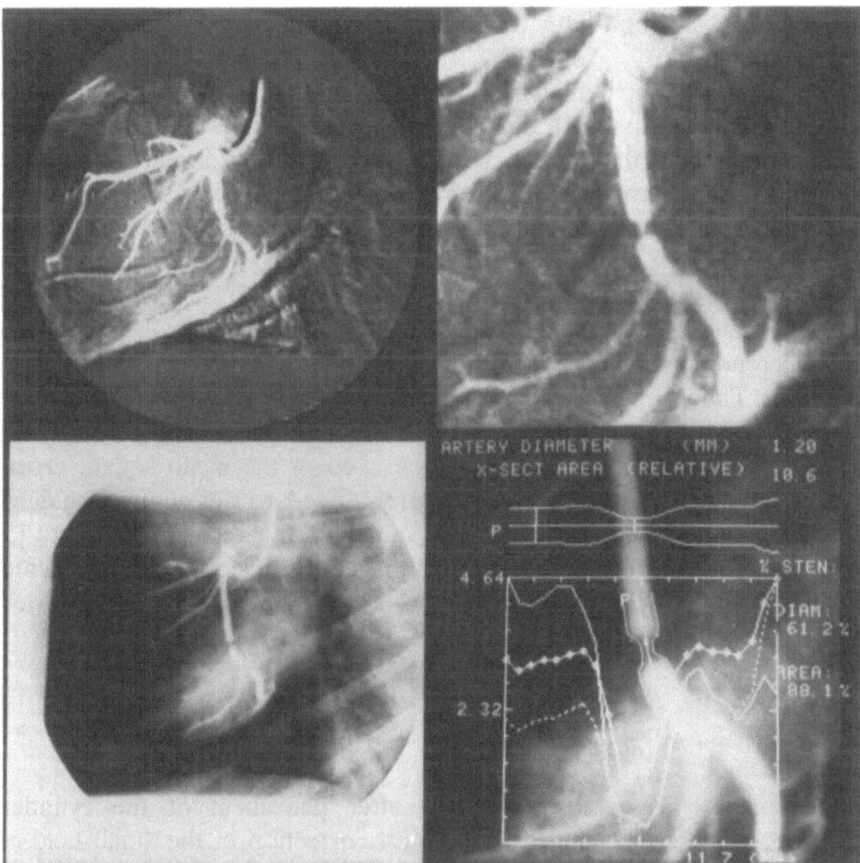

Figure 1. Images from a study with a stenosing cylinder in the circumflex artery of a dog. The left hand upper and lower panels show the subtracted and nonsubtracted images, respectively. The right hand panels show the magnified views. The lower right hand panel shows the screen overlay with the quantitative parameters, stylized arterial segment and the plots of geometric diameter (diamonds), densitometric relative cross-sectional area (solid line) and the approximation of cross-sectional area as calculated from the geometric diameter data, assuming circular cross-section (dashed line). The automatically determined edge is shown on this image. (Reproduced from Mancini *et al.*, Circulation 75: 452–460, 1987 with permission from the American Heart Association Inc.)

of adjacent rib and soft-tissue shadows in the nonsubtracted image and, therefore, was excluded from analysis. Finally, one dog died during the final contrast injection and images could not be analyzed in the subtracted mode. Thus, eight nonsubtracted and eight subtracted on-line digital images and nine film images could be analyzed and these ranged in minimal diameter between 0.83 and 1.83 mm. In one of these regions, the corresponding reactive hyperemia could not be determined accurately because of instability of the electromagnetic flow probe after insertion of the cylinder. Postmortem examination in all dogs from which data was analyzed showed absence of any intraluminal clot.

Each image set was analyzed by an independent observer to obtain minimum diameter, percent diameter stenosis and relative area stenosis. Results from each orthogonal view were averaged. Intraobserver and inter-observer variability were established by a repeated analysis performed at least three weeks later by the original observer and by a second, independent observer.

Results were analyzed by standard linear, polynomial and logarithmic regression analyses; however, no statistically significant improvements were noted when polynomial and logarithmic regressions were compared to linear regressions. Thus, all regression results referred to below represent the linear regression results. Standard errors of the estimate (s.e.e.) were tested using the standard F statistic derived from the ratio of the mean square errors. Subsequently, an analysis of covariance was used to determine significant differences in the slope and intercept values of the regression results [5]. Correlation coefficients were tested by a Fisher Z transformation [6]. Hemo-dynamic data were compared with a paired Student's t-test. Results were considered significant when $p < 0.05$.

Results

Hemodynamics measured before and after placement of the cylinders showed no significant changes. Pincushion correction of the small field-of-view images with centrally located stenoses and catheters did not affect the results and therefore only uncorrected data are presented. Figure 2 shows the results of the measured minimum diameter as assessed by the automated technique compared to the known lumen diameters. A high correlation was obtained for both the subtracted and nonsubtracted on-line digital acquisi-tions. Automated analysis of film acquisitions showed a poorer overall correlation and almost a tripling of the standard error of the estimate. Table 1 summarizes the full regression results. Statistical analyses showed no significant differences amongst modalities with regard to slope, intercept and r values. The standard error of the estimate was significantly greater with the use of film ($p < 0.03$ compared to subtracted and unsubtracted images).

Figures 3 and 4 show the relations between percent diameter stenosis and reactive hyperemia, and percent area (videodensitometric) stenosis and reac-tive hyperemia, respectively. All image modalities were highly correlated with the measured reactive hyperemia and no significant differences were noted amongst the different image modalities. Moreover, no significant differences in the precision of correlation with reactive hyperemia was found

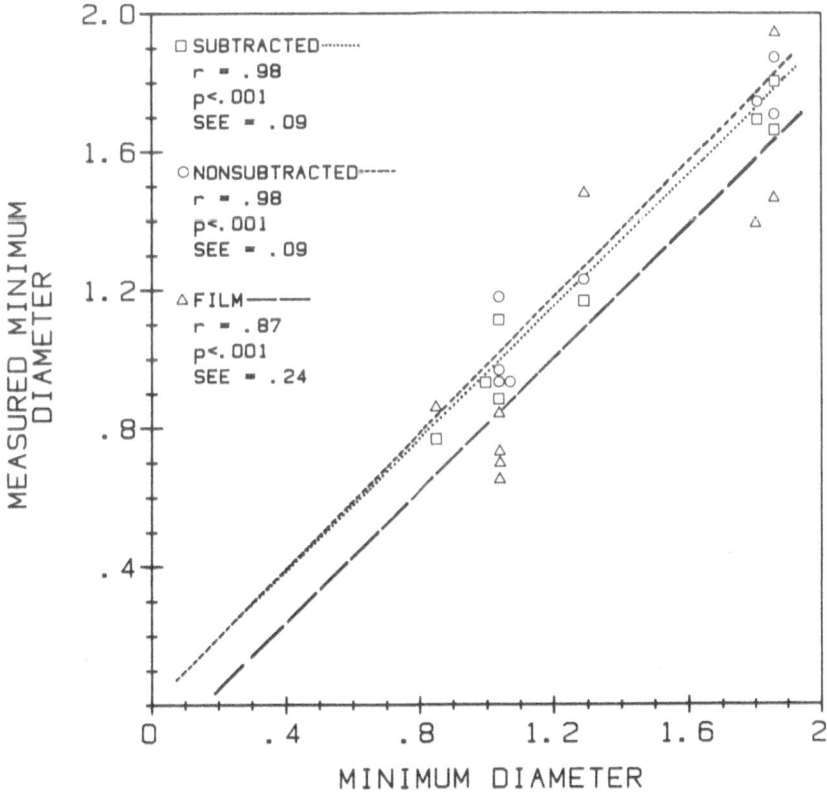

Figure 2. Regression analyses between known and measured stenosis diameters (in milli-meters) from the subtracted (squares), nonsubtracted (circles) and film (diamonds) images. The lines represent the regression lines for each image modality. SEE = standard error of the estimate in millimeters. (Reproduced from Mancini *et al.*, Circulation 75: 452–460, 1987 with permission from the American Heart Association Inc.)

Table 1. Regression results for analyses of different image modalities in determining minimum diameter.

Image	*r* value	slope	*y* intercept	s.e.e. (mm)	*p* value
Nonsubtracted	0.98	0.98	−0.02	0.09[a]	0.001
Subtracted	0.98	0.95	−0.01	0.09[a]	0.001
Film	0.87	0.97	−0.13	0.24	0.001

s.e.e. = standard error of the estimate in millimeters, [a] *p* < 0.03 vs s.e.e. of film analysis. (Reproduced from Mancini *et al.*, Circulation 75: 452–460, 1987 with permission from the American Heart Association Inc.)

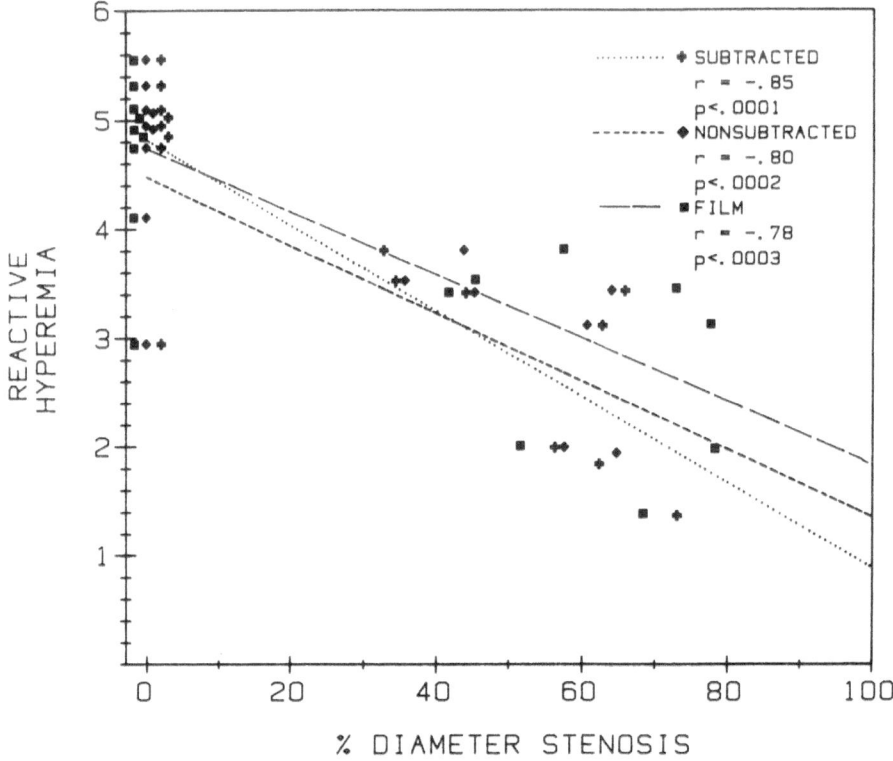

Figure 3. Regression analysis between quantitative percent diameter stenosis determined from each image type and reactive hyperemia. Regression lines are shown. No significant differences amongst these analyses was found. (Reproduced from Mancini *et al.*, Circulation 75: 452—460, 1987 with permission from the American Heart Association Inc.)

between percent area and percent diameter measurements. All methods showed *r* values between 0.78 and 0.85.

Figures 5 and 6 show the relation between stenotic segment area, measured both geometrically and videodensitometrically, versus reactive hyperemia. As in the prior analyses, all image modalities yielded quantitative parameters that were highly correlated with reactive hyperemia ($r = 0.77-0.83$) and no statistical differences amongst modalities was noted.

Table 2 shows the results of inter- and intraobserver variability for measurement of the minimum stenosis diameter and geometric cross-sectional areas. All *r* values ranged from 0.90 to 0.97 with the best results occurring in nonsubtracted, on-line digital images ($r = 0.97$, s.e.e. $= 0.12$ mm). No statistical differences were noted amongst *r* values, slopes, intercepts or standard errors of the diameter measurements. However, in both the intra- and interobserver analyses, the standard error of the estimate for cross-

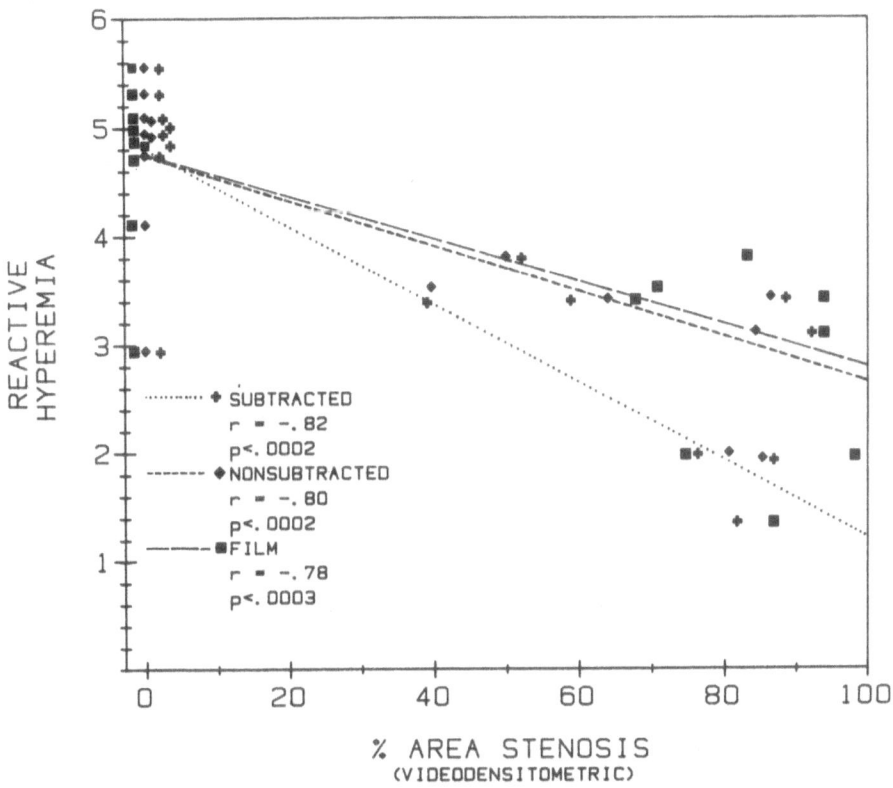

Figure 4. The relation between reactive hyperemia and videometrically determined percent area stenosis. No statistically significant differences in these regressions were found. (Reproduced from Mancini *et al.*, Circulation 75: 452—460, 1987 with permission from the American Heart Association Inc.)

sectional area measurements was greater for the film analyses than the nonsubtracted on-line digital image results (intraobserver variability: 0.56 mm^2 for film vs. 0.02 mm^2 for nonsubtracted images, $p < 0.02$; interobserver results: 0.50 mm^2 for film vs. 0.15 mm^2 for nonsubtracted images, $p < 0.005$). Although the standard error of the estimate for cross-sectional area was smaller for the subtracted compared to film images, this difference was not statistically significant.

Discussion

This study represents the first time that any fully automated, coronary

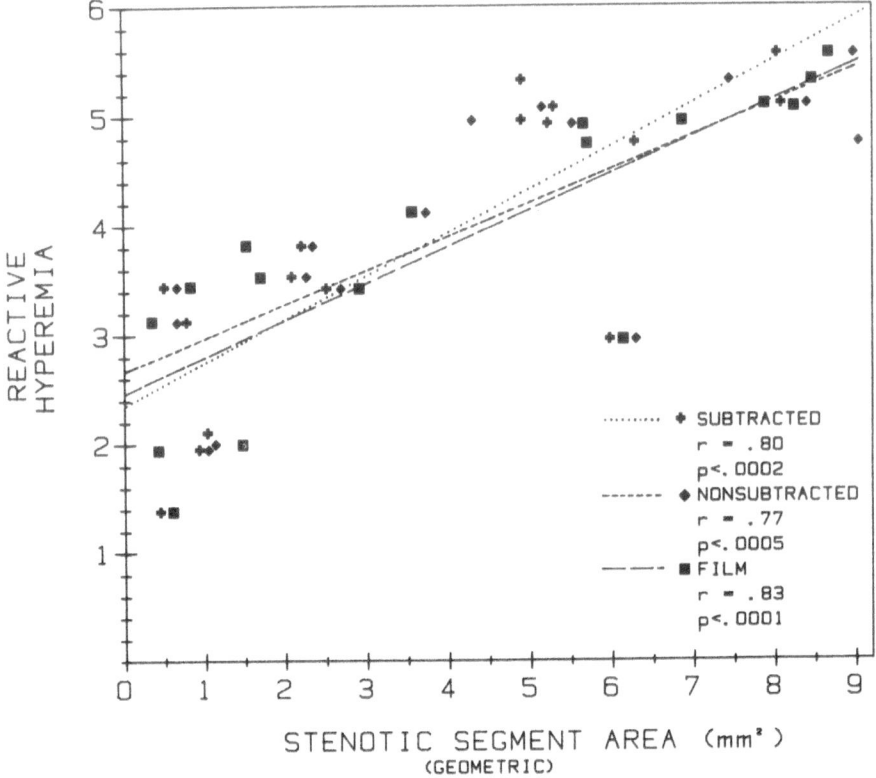

Figure 5. The relation between reactive hyperemia and geometrically determined stenotic segment area is shown. No statistically significant differences were noted amongst results from different image modalities. (Reproduced from Mancini *et al.*, Circulation 75: 452–460, 1987 with permission from the American Heart Association Inc.)

quantification algorithm has been validated on both morphologic and physiological grounds in an *in-vivo* model. The study demonstrates that minimal luminal diameter can be rapidly and accurately measured with this technique and that on-line digital images allow greater morphological precision than routinely processed cineangiograms. The study demonstrates that the clinically used indexes of coronary stenosis assessed by the current technique bear significant relations to reactive hyperemia, a physiological measure of the importance of a coronary stenosis.

Morphometric precision

Numerous methods have been proposed for the quantitation of coronary

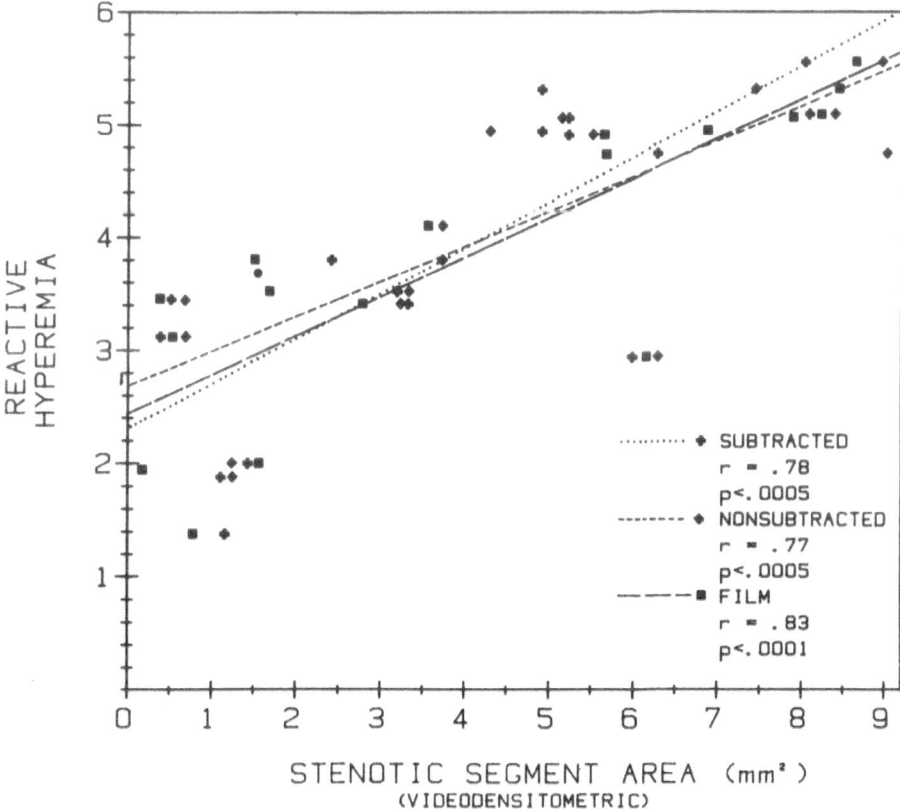

Figure 6. The relation between reactive hyperemia (RH) and stenotic segment area determined from a combination of the videodensitometric data and the catheter calibration is shown. No statistical differences among the regressions was noted. (Reproduced from Mancini *et al.*, Circulation 75: 452—460, 1987 with permission from the American Heart Association Inc.)

lesions and the precision of most of these methods has been determined either in radiographic phantom models, in arterial strips harvested from cadavers or in non-cardiac, *in-vivo* models [1, 2, 3, 7—16]. No prior method has been validated in an *in-vivo* cardiac model. The proposed methodology demonstrates very accurate measurements of precision-drilled stenosis cylinders that were imaged in a closed-chest preparation in the coronary arteries of a beating heart. This model very closely mimics the conditions to be anticipated clinically. The results suggest that clinical implementation should provide a highly accurate method for morphological quantitation of coronary stenoses. Several conditions, however, must be met. First, adequate separation of the lesion from adjacent structures is required to minimize the likelihood of inaccurate edge detection. Although the program has been

Table 2. Results of intra- and interobserver variability analyses.

		Nonsubtracted	Subtracted	Film
		($n = 8$)	($n = 8$)	($n = 9$)
Intraobserver	r	0.97	0.90	0.92
	s.e.e.	0.12 mm	0.21 mm	0.23 mm
		0.20 mm^2	0.29 mm^2	0.56 mm^2 [a]
	p	<0.0001	<0.003	<0.0005
Interobserver	r	0.97	0.90	0.92
	s.e.e.	0.12 mm	0.19 mm	0.21 mm
		0.15 mm^2	0.25 mm^2	0.50 mm^2 [b]
	p	<0.0001	<0.003	<0.0006

s.e.e. = standard error of the estimate. [a] $p < 0.02$, [b] $p < 0.005$ for film versus nonsubtracted results. (Reproduced from Mancini *et al.*, Circulation 75: 452—460, 1987 with permission from the American Heart Association Inc.)

designed to allow operator editing of edges, this procedure may increase inter- and intraobserver variability. One stenosis in this study required such editing and was, therefore, excluded from analysis. It is anticipated that diverse clinical conditions and variations in imaging characteristics of different X-ray systems will mandate use of such editing features, particularly in designation of 'normal' segments and in analyzing stenoses at branch points. Secondly, the accuracy of the absolute measurements is heavily dependent on the reliability of the calibration system used. The angiographic catheter was used for this purpose in preference to more elaborate methods that might be more difficult to implement clinically. Inaccuracies of this approach have been shown to arise from several factors including catheter material, manufacturing variabilities in lumen size and the differential magnification that occurs when the stenosis and the catheter tip are at different distances from the X-ray source [1, 2, 17]. Nevertheless, this remains the most convenient approach and the results from this study and others suggest that it yields values of sufficient accuracy. The importance of the calibration is underscored by the occurrence of two instances in this study that precluded accurate calibration due to poor image contrast between the catheter and background. Under such circumstances only relative measures of stenosis severity are feasible. Finally, calibration of the nonsubtracted digital images were used for the analysis of the subtracted digital images as well because of the frequent occurrence of spatial misregistration, which often resulted in spurious edges in the area of the catheter shaft.

Overestimation of diameters less than 1 mm has been previously reported for several automated techniques [1, 3, 12, 18]. The diameters studied in this investigation ranged from 0.71—1.83 mm and the smallest diameter imaged successfully was 0.83 mm. The regression analyses do not suggest over-estimation of sizes within this range. Figure 2 and Table 1 show regression slopes that were actually less than unity. It is postulated that this is due to measurement of only the minimal stenosis diameter, not average diameters over the entire length of the stenosis [3]. Phenomena such as motion un-sharpness, limited spatial resolution, oblique orientation of the vessel with respect to the X-ray beam, and geometric magnification would all lead to over- not underestimation, thus, providing the rationale for using this approach. It is unknown whether lumena of smaller caliber could also be measured as accurately *in-vivo* but physical limitations in maintaining patency and antegrade flow precluded a direct assessment of much smaller lumena in the dog model.

Digital versus film images

Few direct comparisons of digital coronary arteriography and film based arteriography are available. Tobis and coworkers [19] compared hand-held caliper determinations of coronary stenoses from standard cineangiograms and digital angiograms obtained with fluoroscopic and radiographic exposure levels which were processed by either a blurred mask or a single mask frame. In addition, the latter digital images were assessed from edge-enhanced and magnified images. No significant difference in mean percent diameter stenosis measurements or in variability of measurements from any of the three different images were reported. Vas and coworkers [20] assessed visual estimation from both cinefilm and digital caliper measurements from magni-fied digital images and concluded that no differences exist between the two methods and that the use of digital calipers can substantially reduce inter- and intraobserver variability. Bray *et al.* [21] compared cineangiograms to digital angiograms processed by the high-pass temporal filtration technique. Using hand-held caliper methods, this group showed a modest correlation between percent stenosis measurements from the two image types and no difference in interobserver variability. Absolute diameters and their accuracy could not be evaluated in these studies nor were automated approaches used.

In contrast, the current study allows a direct comparison of digital and cine images for absolute quantifiability using a fully automated approach. The results showed some deterioration in accuracy and reproducibility when film is used for quantitative coronary arteriography. In addition, the results suggest that analysis of subtracted images yields results of equivalent precision but with slightly higher inter- and intraobserver variability. This increased inter- and intraobserver variability was not significantly different from the higher variability seen in the film analyses. This increase is felt to be due to increased image noise and the potential presence of subtraction artifacts.

Factors limiting precise stenosis measurement have been recently reviewed [1, 2]. Although film-based radiography has a very high theoretical resolution, numerous factors prevent attainment of this maximal resolution in clinical circumstances. The difference in attenuation coefficients between iodinated contrast medium and tissues is not great and may perturb edge-detection in areas with significant variations in background density. The usual measurement of the resolving power of a system by using tungsten wires or lead strips does not truly reflect this much poorer object contrast in coronary angiograms. Moreover, the usable spatial resolution of film, considering the physical properties of cesium iodide image intensifiers, the effects of the main objective lens in the image distributor and the cine camera optics, is markedly deteriorated from the theoretical intrinsic resolution of cinefilm and is approached by that of a high quality video imaging tube [20]. A second major factor is that the automated edge-detection scheme used in this investigation was optimized for the noise frequency of digital images. Finally, this investigation was performed on a routinely used clinical imaging system with only one film type and one processing method. Different processing systems and film types may show a different relative accuracy when compared to digital images. Thus, the small differences shown in this study may not apply under all circumstances and in all laboratories. Moreover, in spite of these differences, the relation between commonly measured parameters of coronary stenosis and reactive hyperemia could not be shown to be significantly different amongst modalities suggesting that no major clinical differences are present.

The slight improvement in accuracy of nonsubtracted over subtracted images is likely related to small degrees of misregistration artifact and increased noise of subtracted images in the region of the stenosis that affected the edge-detection algorithm. Such problems might be improved with the use of blurred masks or EKG-gated masks. Of practical importance, however, is that the acquisition of nonsubtracted images is faster and less technically demanding than the acquisition of subtracted images because patient and cardiac motion will not affect the images as severely. Despite great advances in other aspects of digital imaging, misregistration artifact due to patient motion remains one of the commonest causes of image degradation and, therefore, the demonstrated accuracy of nonsubtracted quantitative digital angiography should enhance clinical implementation and acceptability of the proposed techniques.

Comparison to flow reserve measurements

Very accurate coronary quantitation has been shown to be useful in both reflecting and predicting coronary flow reserve [23]. Thus, it was important to substantiate that the proposed computer-generated results bore some relation to the physiological importance of the resultant stenoses. As demonstrated in Figures 3—6, this was indeed the case. This establishes the potential usefulness of this specific automatic program for studies designed to assess the relation between morphological parameters and physiological aspects of coronary flow. It should be emphasized, however, that in this dog model there were no ambiguities in designation of the normal segment and the model was relatively uniform with regard to hemodynamics and other factors that might significantly affect flow reserve measurements. Despite this, only moderate correlations with flow reserve were obtained with all indexes and this is in keeping with the finding that such relationships in heterogeneous patients with more diverse clinical circumstances are even less well correlated [23, 24].

Clinical importance

Quantitative coronary arteriography by previously proposed methods has been shown to give a marked reduction in the variability of stenosis measurements and increase the precision with which interventions can be assessed. Despite this, most methods still require tedious post-processing and hand-drawn outlines of cinearteriograms. Moreover, the time required to process film carefully also severely limits the ability and suitability of these approaches to provide information during patient studies. Rapidly available coronary quantitation is of immediate potential clinical value in the setting of coronary angioplasty, thrombolytic therapy and unstable angina [25—29]. Despite the growing body of literature suggesting that morphological criteria have an important role in predicting potential outcome under these circumstances, no other method is available to provide this information conveniently during the course of a procedure. The immediate availability of digital images, the ease of acquiring nonsubtracted images even in ill patients and the availability of the proposed program that requires only a short time for analysis of a single view is expected to overcome the major impasses to routine clinical application of coronary quantitation. The routine availability of precise, physiologically meaningful and prognostically important information at the time of coronary arteriography and intervention studies will be useful in both refining the therapy of patients and in understanding the complex anatomical-physiological relationships that determine their prognosis.

Acknowledgement

This study was supported by the Veterans Administration, Washington D.C. and the American Heart Association of Michigan, Lathrup Village, Michigan.

140

References

1. Brown BG, Bolson EL, Dodge HT: Quantitative computer techniques for analyzing coronary arteriograms. Prog Cardiovasc Dis 28: 403—418, 1986.
2. Reiber JHC, Kooijman CJ, Slager CJ, Gerbrands JJ, Schuurbiers JCH, Boer A den, Wijns W, Serruys PW: Computer assisted analysis of the severity of obstructions from coronary cineangiograms: A methodological review. Automedica 5: 219—238, 1984.
3. LeFree MT, Simon SB, Mancini GBJ, Vogel RA: Digital radiographic assessment of coronary arterial geometric diameter and videodensitometric cross-sectional area. Proc SPIE 626: 334—341, 1986.
4. LeFree MT, Mulvaney JA, Vogel RA: Image corrections for digital radiographic geometric and videodensitometric distortions. Radiology 157P: 36, 1985 (Abstract).
5. Neter J, Wasserman W: Applied linear statistical models, Irwin RD, Inc., Homewood, Illinois, 1974, pp 702—703.
6. Snedecor GW, Cochran WG: Statistical Methods, The Iowa State University Press, Ames, Iowa, 1972, pp 185—186.
7. Brown BG, Bolson E, Frimer M, Dodge HT: Quantitative coronary arteriography: Estimation of dimensions, hemodynamic resistance, and atheroma mass of coronary artery lesions using the arteriogram and digital computation. Circulation 55: 329—337, 1977.
8. Kishon Y, Yerushalmi S, Deutsch V, Neufeld HN, Koprak A: Measurement of coronary arterial lumen by densitometric analysis of angiograms. Angiology 30: 304—312, 1979.
9. Sandor T, Als AV, Paulin S: Cine-densitometric measurement of coronary arterial stenoses. Cathet Cardiovasc Diagn 5: 229—245, 1979.
10. Spears JR: Rotating step-wedge technique for extraction of luminal cross-sectional area information from single plane coronary cineangiograms. Acta Radiol Diagn 22: 217—225, 1981.
11. Kruger RA: Estimation of the diameter of an iodine concentration within blood vessels using digital radiography devices. Med Phys 8: 652—658, 1981.
12. Spears JR, Sandor T, Als AV, Malagold M, Markis JE, Grossman W, Serur JR, Paulin S: Computerized image analysis for quantitative measurement of vessel diameter from cineangiograms. Circulation 68: 453—461, 1983.
13. Jaques P, DiBianca F, Pizer S, Kohout F, Lifshitz L, Delany D: Quantitative digital fluorography. Computer vs. human estimation of vascular stenoses. Invest Radiol 20: 45—52, 1985.
14. Nichols AB, Gabrieli CFO, Fenoglio Jr JJ, Esser PD: Quantification of relative coronary arterial stenosis by cinevideodensitometric analysis of coronary arteriograms. Circulation 69: 512—522, 1984.
15. Wright GA, Taylor KW, Rowlands JA: Noise in stenosis measurement using digital subtraction angiography. Med Phys 12: 705—712, 1985.
16. Simons MA, Kruger RA: Vessel diameter measurement using digital subtraction radiography. Invest Radiol 20: 510—516, 1985.
17. Reiber JHC, Kooijman CJ, Boer A den, Serruys PW: Assessment of dimensions and image quality of coronary contrast catheters from cineangiograms. Cathet Cardiovasc Diagn 11: 521—531, 1985.
18. Kirkeeide RL, Fung P, Smalling RW, Gould KL: Automated evaluation of vessel diameter from arteriograms. Comput Cardiol: 215—218, 1982.
19. Tobis J, Nalcioglu O, Iseri L, Johnston WD, Roeck W, Castleman E, Bauer B, Montelli S, Henry WL: Detection and quantitation of coronary artery stenoses from digital subtraction angiograms compared with 35-millimeter film cineangiograms. Am J Cardiol 54: 489—496, 1984.

20. Vas R, Eigler N, Miyazono C, Pfaff JM, Resser KJ, Wiess M, Nivatpumin T, Whiting J, Forrester J: Digital quantification eliminates intraobserver and interobserver variability in the evaluation of coronary artery stenosis. Am J Cardiol 56: 718—723, 1985.

21. Bray BE, Anderson FL, Hardin CW, Kruger RA, Sutton RB, Nelson JA: Digital subtraction coronary angiography using high-pass temporal filtration: A comparison with cineangiography. Cathet Cardiovasc Diagn 11: 17—24, 1985.

22. Mistretta CA: X-ray image intensifiers. In: Haus AG, (ed): The physics of medical imaging: recording system measurements and techniques. American Institute of Physics, New York 1979, pp 182—205.

23. Harrison DG, White CW, Hiratzka LF, Doty DB, Barnes DH, Eastham CL, Marcus ML: The value of lesion cross-sectional area determined by quantitative coronary angiography in assessing the physiologic significance of proximal left anterior descending coronary arterial stenoses. Circulation 69: 1111—1119, 1984.

24. Legrand V, Mancini GBJ, Bates ER, Hodgson JMcB, Gross MD, Vogel RA: Comparative study of coronary flow reserve, coronary anatomy and the results of radionuclide exercise tests in patients with coronary artery disease. J Am Coll Cardiol 8: 1022—1032, 1986.

25. Harrison DG, Ferguson DW, Collins SM, Skorton DJ, Ericksen EE, Kioschos JM, Marcus ML, White CW: Rethrombosis after reperfusion with streptokinase: importance of geometry of residual lesions. Circulation 69: 991—999, 1984.

26. Serruys PW, Reiber JHC, Wijns W, Brand M vd, Kooijman CJ, Katen H ten, Hugenholtz PG: Assessment of percutaneous transluminal coronary angioplasty by quantitative coronary angiography: diameter versus densitometric area measurements. Am J Cardiol 54: 482—488, 1984.

27. Wilson RF, Holida MD, White CW: Quantitative angiographic morphology of coronary stenoses leading to myocardial infarction or unstable angina. Circulation 73: 286—293, 1986.

28. Johnson MR, Brayden GP, Ericksen EE, Collins SM, Skorton DJ, Harrison DG, Marcus ML, White CW: Changes in cross-sectional area of the coronary lumen in the six months after angioplasty: a quantitative analysis of the variable response to percutaneous transluminal angioplasty. Circulation 73: 467—475, 1986.

29. Brown BG, Gallery CA, Badger RS, Kennedy JW, Mathey D, Bolson EL, Dodge HT: Incomplete lysis of thrombus in the moderate underlying atherosclerotic lesion during intracoronary infusion of streptokinase for acute myocardial infarction: quantitative angiographic observations. Circulation 73: 653—661, 1986.

9. Comparison of automated edge detection and videodensitometric quantitative coronary arteriography

ROBERT A. VOGEL, M. SANZ, and G. B. J. MANCINI

SUMMARY. To increase the precision of the evaluation of coronary artery stenosis severity, we have implemented a digital radiographically based computer program which measures absolute and relative coronary artery dimensions using automated edge detection and relative coronary cross-sectional area using videodensitometry. We have compared automated edge detection and densitometric data for, (1) dimensional accuracy using *in-vitro* arterial phantoms, (2) independence from arteriographic projection in patients undergoing coronary angioplasty and, (3) correlation with coronary flow reserve and stress scintigraphic data in patients undergoing diagnostic catheterization. Both the diameter measurements assessed by automated edge detection and the videodensitometric cross-sectional area measurements were found to correlate closely ($r > 0.98$) with known dimensions of an arterial phantom containing contrast-filled cylindrical chambers ranging from 0.5—5.0 mm diameter. Although both methods were statistically equivalently accurate, automated edge detection tended to overestimate diameters less than 1.0 mm. Dependence of stenosis severity estimation on the arteriographic projection was evaluated in 13 patients undergoing coronary angioplasty. Comparison of arterial diameter and videodensitometric cross-sectional area estimations in the RAO- and LAO-views demonstrated greater independence from projection for the absolute diameter data. We have also compared quantitative arteriographic data with stress thallium scintigraphy, radionuclide ventriculography and digitally assessed coronary flow reserve information in 19 patients without prior myocardial infarction or coronary collaterals. Of all quantitative parameters of coronary stenosis severity, percent diameter stenosis best predicted functional impairment. Videodensitometric cross-sectional area predicted functional impairment least well. These data suggest that although *in-vitro* estimations of automated edge detection and videodensitometric methodologies are both highly accurate, absolute and relative diameter assessments are to be preferred over videodensitometric data, because of greater independence from arteriographic projection and closer correspondence to coronary flow reserve and exercise physiological data.

Introduction

During the last ten years, in an attempt to improve the assessment of coronary artery stenosis severity, several quantitative arteriographic methods have been developed which have been shown to reduce interobserver variability [1—3]. These initial efforts tended to be time consuming and did not take into consideration the distortions of spatial dimensions caused by

J. C. Reiber & P. W. Serruys (eds.), New Developments in Quantitative Coronary Arteriography,
143—152.

pincushion and differential magnification effects. Brown *et al.* described a cinefilm based method which incorporated pincushion and magnification distortion correction and utilized operator-interactive coronary edge definition [4]. This geometric approach can be applied to orthogonal views of a single coronary lesion with a resultant analysis of absolute cross-sectional area having been reported to be both reproducible and accurate. Spears *et al.* have, however, pointed out that errors in analyzing elliptical stenoses can occur even using geometric analysis of orthogonal views [5]. Although crescentic lesions are uncommon in coronary atherosclerosis, concentric and eccentric elliptical lesions are commonly encountered. An alternative approach to geometric analysis is that of videodensitometry which has usually been applied to the estimation of relative cross-sectional area. This approach has limitations as well. It can be affected by contrast streaming, overlap of contrast containing and non-contrast containing structures, and vessel foreshortening due to lack of orthogonality of the arteriographic projection. Videodensitometric approaches described by several groups may be improved using digital coronary arteriography because of the greater density resolution of the digital methodology compared to that of cinefilm imaging [6—10]. Advances in digital computers have enabled the implementation of automated approaches to coronary artery edge detection and densitometric cross-sectional area evaluation [11]. The question then arises whether absolute or relative arterial dimensions or densitometric cross-sectional area is optimum for the evaluation of coronary artery stenosis from a clinical viewpoint. This manuscript describes data relevant to this question obtained from *in-vitro* and *in-vivo* studies.

Quantitative arteriographic methodology

Our laboratory has recently implemented an automated edge detection method which analyzes both geometric (absolute diameter) and videodensitometric (relative area) parameters of digitally acquired and stored selective coronary arteriograms. This method can be used to evaluate coronary stenoses during interventional procedures as it requires neither film development nor subjective operator edge tracing. Pincushion distortion is corrected on the original arteriogram using a vectorial pixel shifting algorithm. Regional vectors are determined using data derived from imaging an orthogonal ball bearing phantom. Image matrices of either 512 × 512 or 1024 × 1024 pixels with 8 bit gray levels can be analyzed using this program, which requires minimal operator interaction and approximately five seconds running time.

The digital arteriographic frames are stored with the ECG-signal facilitating selection of end-diastolic images. The initial step is magnification calibration which uses the catheter as a reference. The operator identifies the catheter using a light pen, following which the computer magnifies that region of the arteriogram four-fold for 512 × 512 images. The operator then identifies an acceptable point along the catheter. An automated edge detection algorithm identical to that used for the stenosis quantification (see below) determines the catheter diameter over an approximate one cm length. With knowledge of the catheter size, the image magnification can then be calibrated.

The operator then identifies the stenosis under investigation which is then magnified and subjected to automated analysis using the following scheme. A polar coordinate search algorithm is used to identify the central line of the artery following operator assignment of the approximate center of the lesion and the length of the artery to be evaluated. Orthogonal lines at 0.25 mm intervals are then identified which lie perpendicular to the arterial centerline. The first and second derivatives of the contrast medium density are analyzed along these lines. The arterial edge is determined at an arbitrary spacing between the maximum first and second derivatives and the arterial density is determined at this point. Using continuity criteria, a threshold-based contour is determined which best passes through these derivative determined 'edges'. Finally, the cumulative arterial contrast density is summed between the opposite edges of each perpendicular segment from which is subtracted a linearly interpolated background.

Color-coded data are presented superimposed on both the original and schematized arterial segment including absolute diameter, percent diameter narrowing, and relative cross-sectional (densitometric) area. This technique has been validated in arterial phantoms as well in a canine model using transarterially placed stenoses of known dimension and standard selective coronary arteriography. Excellent correlations with known phantom and stenosis dimensions have been found [12—14].

Phantom validation

In order to determine the accuracy of this quantitative arteriographic approach, we initially designed and constructed a radiographic arterial phantom containing seven arterial models, each with different proximal, lesional and distal diameters. Stenosis diameters ranged from 0.5—4.0 mm diameters and proximal and distal regions varied from 1.0—5.0 mm diameters. Fourteen different degrees of stenosis severity were thus available for measurement with ranges from 17 to 87 percent diameter stenosis. The phantom was filled with 100 percent concentration of iodine contrast medium and imaged using a standard angiographic X-ray system interfaced to a commercially available digital radiographic system. Clinical imaging conditions were approximated through the use of 15 cm scattering medium, 0.6 mm focal spot, 70—80 kVp X-ray energy, and 25 microroentgen per frame X-ray intensity. Images were obtained in the 12.5 cm field-of-view, with coupling of a pulse progressive readout high signal-to-noise ratio video camera directly through a 10 bit analogue-to-digital converter to 512 × 512 8 bit gray scale computer disk memory.

Correlations of the phantom arterial diameter determined by automated edge detection and videodensitometrically assessed phantom cross-sectional area were made with known dimensions. Very high correlations were noted in both instances ($r = 0.99$). Standard errors of 0.1 mm and 2 percent were found for absolute diameter and relative area estimates, respectively. As described by other investigators, the arterial diameter of the 0.5 mm chamber was overestimated at a value of approximately 0.8 mm. It is likely that this is due to the focal spot size and the image intensifier modulation transfer function, as this overestimation was not subsequently reduced by the use of 1024 × 1024 pixel matrix digital resolution. Overestimation of small diameters was not found, however, for videodensitometric estimations. Subsequent validation studies, however, performed in canine models using transarterially placed stenoses of known dimension have failed to reveal overestimations of diameters less than 1 mm using either absolute diameter or videodensitometric relative area methods [14]. The latter finding is likely attributable to the use of minimal diameter data employed in the *in-vivo* study in contrast to mean data employed in the *in-vitro* study. These validation data suggest that both the automated edge detection, absolute diameter, and videodensitometric relative cross-sectional area approaches are both highly and equally accurate in assessing arterial size when freed from the problems of arterial projection encountered in clinical imaging.

Clinical effects of arteriographic projection

Videodensitometric relative cross-sectional area analysis has been suggested as a means of assessing asymmetric lesions as the technique is theoretically unaffected by radiographic projection as long as the view is perpendicular to the arterial axis. Clinical factors contributing to the inaccuracy of videodensitometry, however, include beam hardening, X-ray scatter, veiling glare, image intensifier nonuniformity and nonlinearity, video camera and A-D converter nonlinearity, contrast media screening, vessel and contrast density overlap, and foreshortening due to lack of orthogonality between projection and vessel orientation. An initial clinical study performed by Nichols *et al.* [14], reported a very high correlation between right and left anterior oblique projection analyses of 10 coronary artery stenoses. However, only selected non-post angioplasty arteries were employed, the inclusion being determined upon lack of foreshortening in both projections. We have chosen to study the dependence of videodensitometry on projection in a prospective manner including arteriograms obtained both before and after coronary angioplasty. It is in the latter instance that videodensitometry would have its greatest theoretical benefit due to the great eccentricity of post-dilatation lesions.

Using the programs described above, we have analyzed 42 pairs of right and left anterior oblique arteriograms acquired before and after coronary angioplasty in 13 consecutive patients [15—16]. Electrocardiographically-gated digital subtraction was employed to minimize retrovessel contrast density. Relative and absolute arterial dimensions based on automated edge detection and videodensitometric cross-sectional areas were determined using the program described above. Analysis of intra- and inter-observer variability demonstrated that minimal arterial diameter was the most reproducible quantitative arteriographic parameter. The finding of poorer reproducibility for percent diameter stenosis suggests that identification of the 'normal' segment is a significant source of inter-observer variability. Videodensitometric cross-sectional area determined in the right and left anterior oblique projections showed poor correlation ($r = 0.46$), which was less than the value found for comparison of minimal vessel diameter in the two projections ($r = 0.59$) (Fig. 1). These data which were recently confirmed [17], do not support the independence of videodensitometric cross-sectional area from the arteriographic projection in nonselected patients. Moreover, this approach provides neither absolute diameter nor absolute cross-sectional area data.

Quantitative arteriography vs flow physiology

Recent developments in Doppler velocity probes and catheters, and digital radiographic parametric flow imaging now allow the assessment of coronary flow reserve to be performed in clinical situations. Initial clinical studies comparing visually assessed coronary percent diameter stenosis and intra-operatively measured coronary flow reserve have demonstrated poor correlations [18]. A closer correlation between minimal cross-sectional area determined by quantitative coronary arteriography and coronary flow reserve was found in selected groups of patients with coronary stenoses limited to specific sites [19]. Exclusion of patients with prior myocardial infarction, coronary collaterals, and multi-vessel disease has also been found to improve the correlation between quantitative arteriography and digital radiographically assessed coronary flow reserve [20]. Recent analysis of such selected patients also suggests that quantitatively assessed percent diameter stenosis also correlates closely with flow reserve data [21]. Previous studies, however, have not determined which of the many parameters assessable by

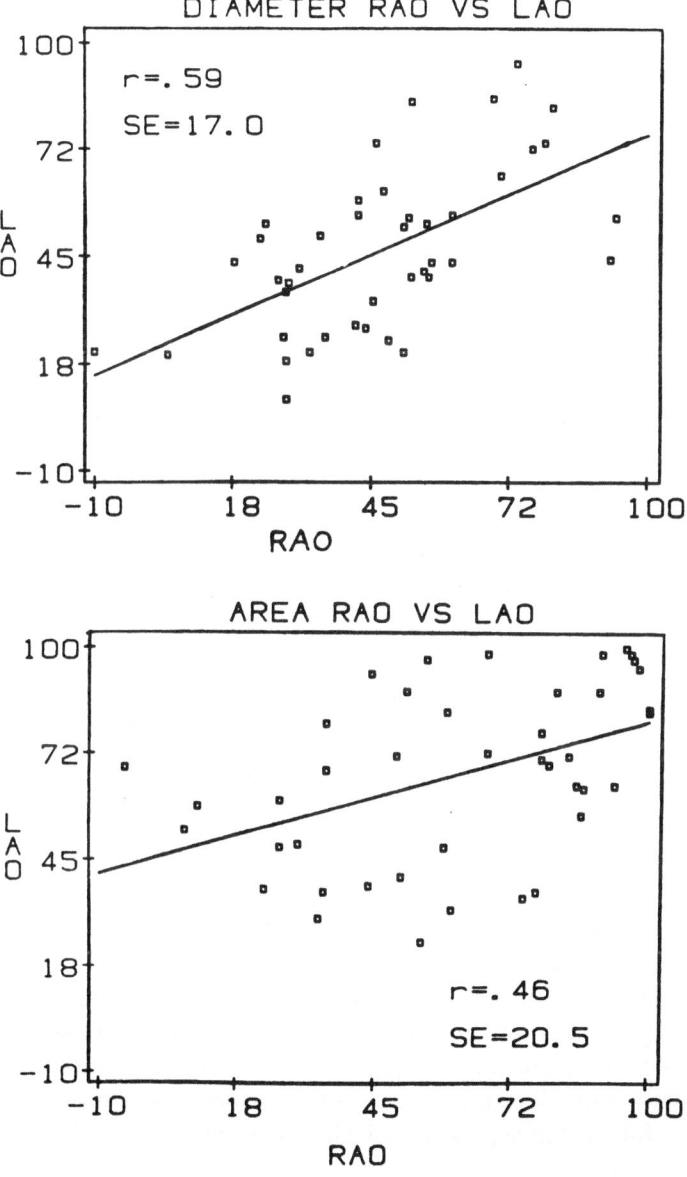

Figure 1. Top Panel — Comparison of quantitative coronary arteriographic percent diameter stenosis measurements of arteriograms obtained in the left anterior oblique (LAO)- and right anterior oblique (RAO)-projections. Bottom Panel — Comparison of videodensitometric relative percent cross-sectional area measurements obtained in the LAO- and RAO-projections.

quantitative arteriography best correlate with coronary flow reserve and stress scintigraphy in the clinical situation.

To determine which parameter of coronary artery stenosis best correlates with flow physiology, we compared quantitative arteriographic data obtained on 45 coronary artery distributions in 19 prospective patients found to have coronary artery disease during diagnostic studies. Quantitatively assessed percent diameter stenosis, minimal stenosis diameter, orthogonal projection absolute cross-sectional area, and videodensitometric relative cross-sectional area were compared with digital radiographically assessed coronary flow reserve and stress thallium myocardial perfusion imaging and stress radionuclide ventriculography. No patients had evidence of prior myocardial infarction or coronary collaterals, and lesions were approximately equally distributed between the three major perfusion beds. Thirty-seven of 43 regional distributions showed concordance of normal flow reserve and stress scintigraphic data, or abnormal flow reserve and stress scintigraphic data. Six distributions were found to have low coronary flow reserve values with normal stress scintigraphy. All occurred in patients who had lower flow reserve values and abnormal scintigraphy found in other distributions. It was judged that the patients terminated exercise on symptomatic appreciation of this ischemia and could not exercise further. These latter distributions were considered to be abnormal for this study.

Of the parameters analyzed, percent diameter stenosis best separated the normal from the abnormal flow physiology groups, followed in order by minimal absolute diameter, minimal cross-sectional area determined by biplane diameter analysis, and videodensitometric cross-sectional area. Respective values used to differentiate normal from abnormal segments for the four parameters include: 50 percent diameter stenosis (Fig. 2), 1.1 mm minimal diameter (Fig. 3), 1.0 mm^2 minimal cross sectional area (Fig. 4), and 75 percent videodensitometric cross-sectional area reduction (Fig. 5). Moreover, only two of 36 lesions less than 47 percent stenosis or greater than 52 percent stenosis were found to have discordance between their quantitative arteriography and flow physiology. Three times as many distributions were incorrectly diagnosed using a 5 percent wide videodensitometric ambiguous zone dividing normal and abnormal distributions. These data suggest that in situations without prior myocardial infarction or collaterals, quantitative arteriographic estimation of percent diameter stenosis is the parameter most clinically useful for the separation of physiologically normal from abnormal distributions.

Conclusions

We have found that automated quantitative arteriography can be performed quickly and successfully on almost all coronary arteriograms. Observer variability is substantially reduced by the use of absolute diameter measurements. This type of analysis would therefore be especially applicable to

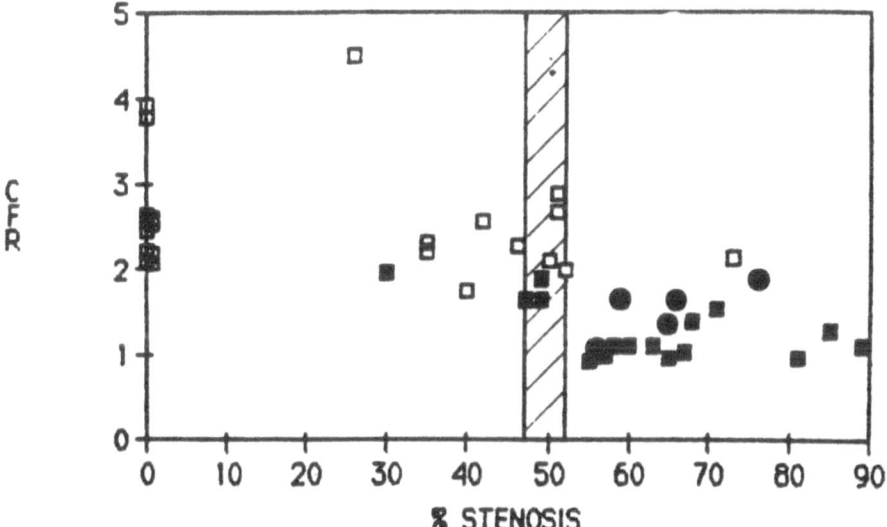

Figure 2. Coronary flow reserve (CFR) values are plotted against percent diameter stenosis obtained by quantitative coronary arteriography. Open squares values denote regional measurements obtained on distributions associated with normal stress scintigraphy. Closed squares represent data obtained from distributions with abnormal stress scintigraphy. Closed circles denote data obtained from regions with abnormal CFR values and normal stress scintigraphy in patients with other distributions associated with lower CFR values and abnormal scintigraphy. The hatched region represents a five percent wide border zone, which best separates physiologically normal from physiologically abnormal distributions.

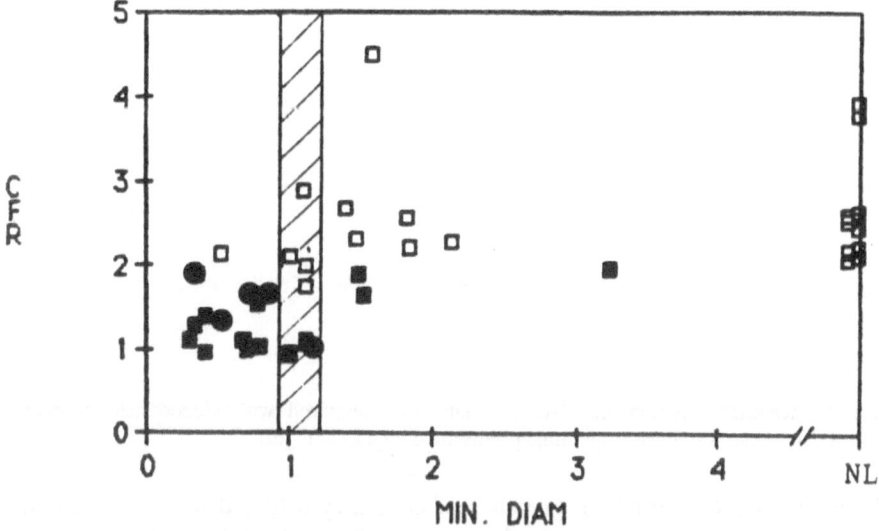

Figure 3. Segmental coronary flow reserve data are compared with quantitative coronary arteriographically measured arterial minimum diameter. Individual data points are coded as described in Figure 2.

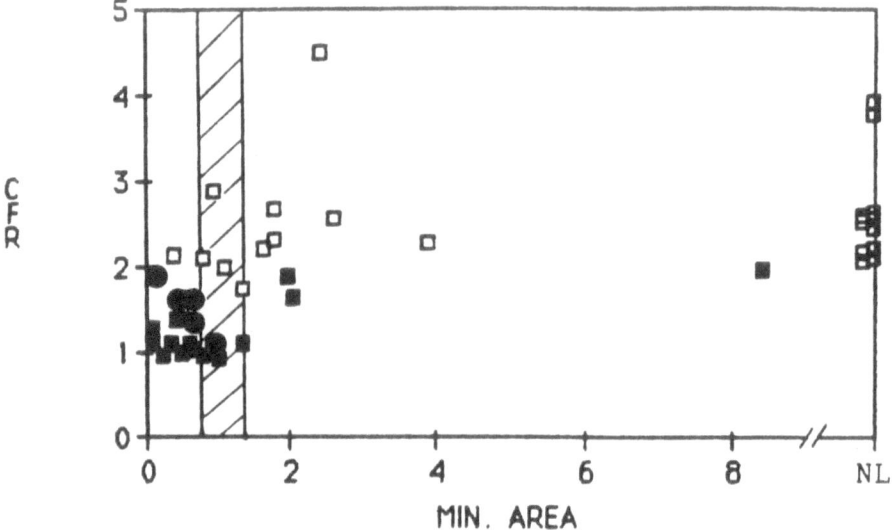

Figure 4. Regional coronary flow reserve data are compared with quantitative coronary arteriographically assessed minimal lesional cross-sectional area obtained from two orthogonal projections. Individual data points are coded as in Figure 2.

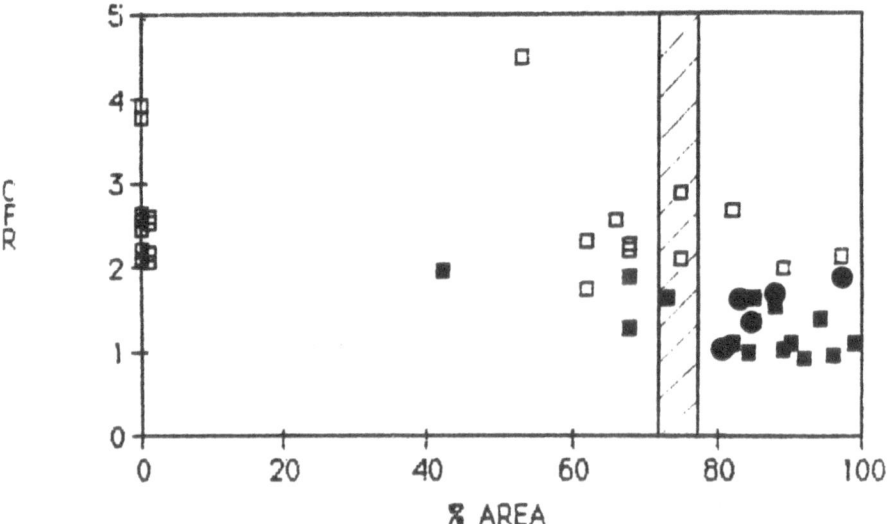

Figure 5. Regional coronary flow reserve data are compared with videodensitometrically assessed percent area stenosis. Individual points are coded as in Figure 2.

studies of progression and regression of coronary artery disease. In patients without substantial alterations of coronary flow physiology due to prior infarction, or collateralized vessels, good correlations between quantitative parameters and coronary flow reserve and stress scintigraphic findings are likely to occur. Of those parameters currently measurable, percent diameter stenosis and minimal diameter both assessed by automated edge detection techniques, best determine the clinical consequences of individual coronary stenoses. Videodensitometric relative cross-sectional area does not appear to be independent of radiographic projection nor highly predictive of flow physiology.

References

1. Gensini GG, Kelly AE, DaCosta BCB, Huntington PP: Quantitative angiography: The measurement of coronary vasomobility in the intact animal and man. Chest 60: 522—530, 1971.
2. Feldman RL, Pepine CJ, Curry RC, Conti CR: Quantitative coronary arteriography using 105-mm photospot angiography and an optical magnifying device. Cathet Cardiovasc Diagn: 5: 195—201, 1979.
3. Rafflenbeul W, Smith LR, Rogers WJ, Mantle JA, Rackley CE, Russell Jr RO: Quantitative coronary arteriography: Coronary anatomy of patients with unstable angina pectoris reexamined 1 year after optimal medical therapy. Am J Cardiol 43: 699—707, 1979.
4. Brown BG, Bolson E, Frimer M, Dodge HT: Quantitative coronary arteriography: Estimation of dimensions, hemodynamic resistance, and atheroma mass of coronary artery lesions using the arteriogram and digital computation. Circulation 55: 329—337, 1977.
5. Spears JR, Sandor T, Baim DS, Paulin S: The minimum error in estimating coronary luminal cross-sectional area from cineangiographic diameter measurements. Cathet Cardiovasc Diagn 9: 119—128, 1983.
6. Sandor T, Als AV, Paulin S: Cine-densitometric measurement of coronary arterial stenoses. Cathet Cardiovasc Diagn 5: 229—245, 1979.
7. Crawford DW, Brooks SH, Barndt Jr R, Blankenhorn DH: Measurement of atherosclerotic luminal irregularity and obstruction by radiographic densitometry. Invest Radiol 12: 307—313, 1977.
8. Kishon Y, Yerushalmi S, Deutsch V, Neufeld HN: Measurement of coronary arterial lumen by densitometric analysis of angiograms. Angiology 39: 304—312, 1979.
9. Hoornstra K, Hanselman JMH, Holland WPJ, Wey Peters GW de, Zwamborn AW: Videodensitometry for measuring blood vessel diameter. Acta Radiol Diagn 21: 155—164, 1980.
10. Nichols AB, Gabrieli CFO, Fenoglio JJ, Esser PD: Quantification of relative coronary arterial stenosis by cinevideodensitometric analysis of coronary arteriograms. Circulation 69: 512—522, 1984.
11. Reiber JHC, Serruys PW, Kooijman CJ, Wijns W, Slager CJ, Gerbrands JJ, Schuurbiers JCH, Boer A den, Hugenholtz PG: Assessment of short-, medium-, and long-term variations in arterial dimensions from computer-assisted quantitation of coronary cineangiograms. Circulation 71: 280—288, 1985.
12. LeFree MT, Simon SB, Lewis RJ, Bates ER, Vogel RA: Digital radiographic coronary artery quantification. Comput Cardiol: 99—102, 1985.
13. LeFree MT, Simon SB, Mancini GBJ, Vogel RA: Digital radiographic assessment of coronary arterial geometric diameter and videodensitometric cross-sectional area. SPIE 626: 334—341, 1986.
14. Mancini GBJ, Simon SB, McGillem MJ, LeFree MT, Friedman HZ, Vogel RA: Auto-

mated quantitative coronary arteriography: Morphologic and physiologic validation in vivo of a rapid digital angiographic method. Circulation 75: 452—460, 1987.

15. Sanz M, LeFree MT, Mancini GBJ, Mickelson JK, Starling M, Topol E, Vogel RA: Inter-observer and orthogonal view variability of automated quantitative analysis of digital subtraction coronary angiograms. Comput Cardiol: 189—192, 1986.

16. Sanz ML, Mancini GBJ, LeFree MT, Mickelson JK, Starling MR, Vogel RA, Topol EJ: Variability of quantitative digital subtraction coronary angiography before and after percutaneous transluminal coronary angioplasty. Amer J Cardiol 60: 55—60, 1987.

17. Tobis J, Nalcioglu O, Johnston WD, Qu L, Reese T, Sato D, Roeck W, Montelli S, Henry WL: Videodensitometric determination of minimum coronary artery luminal diameter before and after angioplasty. Amer J Cardiol 59: 38—44, 1987.

18. White CW, Wright CB, Doty DB, Hiratzka LF, Eastham CL, Harrison DG, Marcus ML: Does visual interpretation of the coronary arteriogram predict the physiologic importance of a coronary stenosis? N Engl J Med 310: 819—824, 1984.

19. Harrison DG, White CW, Hiratzka LF, Doty DB, Barnes DH, Eastham CL, Marcus ML: The value of lesion cross-sectional area determined by quantitative coronary angiography in assessing the physiologic significance of proximal left anterior descending coronary arterial stenoses. Circulation 69: 1111—1119, 1984.

20. LeGrand V, Mancini GBJ, Bates ER, Hodgson JMcB, Gross MD, Vogel RA: Comparative study of coronary flow reserve, coronary anatomy and results of radionuclide exercise tests in patients with coronary artery disease. J Am Coll Cardiol 8: 1022—1032, 1986.

21. Zijlstra F, Ommeren J. van Reiber JHC, Serruys PW: Does the quantitative assessment of coronary artery dimensions predict the physiologic significance of a coronary stenosis? Circulation 75: 1154—1161, 1987.

10. Issues of validation in quantitative coronary angiography

DAVID M. HERRINGTON, G. A. WALFORD, and T. A. PEARSON

SUMMARY. Quantitative coronary angiography (QCA) is an important new tool in the study of coronary artery disease. Validation of these techniques is crucial for their ongoing development and refinement, identification of appropriate applications, planning for their use in clinical studies, and comparing results of these studies. Validation of these techniques is difficult for a number of reasons. These include numerous potential sources of error, heterogeneity of goals, designs, and analysis of previously conducted QCA validation studies, and the lack of a true gold standard against which to compare the results of QCA techniques. Principles concerning the design and analysis of future QCA validation studies are described in detail. Recent work using more sophisticated phantoms or independent measures of luminal dimensions to validate QCA techniques are also mentioned.

Introduction

Quantitative coronary angiography (QCA) is rapidly becoming an important tool in the study of coronary anatomy, function and disease. It offers enormous potential advantages through more accurate assessment of coronary pathology. Thanks to diligent efforts by several investigators these advantages have begun to be realized [1—3]. However, despite the progress that has been made, there remain several issues that could limit the successful future application of these techniques to the study of coronary disease. The validation and standardization of these techniques is one such issue. The following material is a presentation of some of the issues and problems concerning the validation and standardization of QCA techniques. The first part is a description of the importance of validation and standardization. The second part is a discussion of some of the problems encountered by those attempting to validate QCA techniques, and some guidelines for future validation studies. Some newer approaches to QCA validation will also be presented.

J. C. Reiber & P. W. Serruys (eds.), New Developments in Quantitative Coronary Arteriography,
153—166.

Importance of validation and standardization

There are four reasons why validation and standardization are important for the future of QCA techniques. First, validation is important for ongoing development and refinement of QCA techniques. New approaches to edge detection, image enhancement, and estimating luminal dimensions are continually being developed and incorporated into QCA techniques. Careful validity testing identifies additions or modifications that are truly advantageous.

Second, good validation tests alert investigators to conditions where the technical performance is inadequate, such as at the extremes of stenosis values or when the lumen is asymmetric. This information may modify the types of clinical studies a technique could be used for. For example, a QCA technique may perform well when evaluating vessels with circular lumen, but not when evaluating asymmetric ones. It would be inappropriate to use this technique to study lesions after PTCA. Without a clear understanding of a technique's strengths and weaknesses through careful validation studies, it is impossible to identify appropriate applications of the technique.

Third, a validation study is required to determine the variability of a technique. This information is needed to calculate sample sizes for clinical studies. Table 1 shows the relationship between the variability of a QCA measure of stenosis and the sample size required to determine a 20% difference in progression of disease. Small errors in the estimated variability of a technique from inadequate validation leads to major differences in predicted number of study subjects required. The time and monetary implications of such errors would not be trivial.

Table 1. Effect of QCA technique variability on sample size required to detect a 20% reduction in % diameter stenosis.

Standard Deviation of QCA Measure of % Diameter Stenosis	Sample Size* (total)
3%	35
4%	62
5%	97
6%	140
7%	191

* Includes 20% increase to account for dropouts.

Finally, without uniform approaches to validation using standardized measures of disease it is impossible to compare results from different institutions. This limits the potential collective benefit of a number of investigators studying the same or related topics using different QCA techniques. Table 2 shows the results of two published studies that illustrate this problem [4, 5]. In study A, 24 people underwent successful streptokinase reperfusion and the residual lumen were evaluated using a QCA technique. Seven out of 13 with a residual minimum cross-sectional area less than $0.4 \ mm^2$ went on to suffer restenosis compared to 0 out of 7 with a residual minimum cross-sectional area greater than $0.4 \ mm^2$. In study B, 57 subjects underwent successful streptokinase reperfusion and the residual stenoses were also evaluated with a QCA technique. All seven of those with restenosis had a residual percent diameter stenosis greater than 58%. Both studies addressed the exact same issue, but because different measures of stenosis were used the results can not be compared. Using the same measures would have been helpful for those trying to synthesize an understanding of the relationship between residual lumen dimensions and subsequent restenosis. However, even if both studies used the same measure of luminal dimensions, comparisons would be difficult unless they were also validated in similar ways.

Table 2. Two Studies [4, 5] of restenosis after successful streptokinase reperfusion.

Study A — 24 patients
- 7/13 with residual *cross-sectional area*
  < 0.4 mm² developed restenosis
- 0/11 with residual *cross-sectional area*
  > 0.4 mm² developed restenosis

Study B — 57 patients
- 7/7 with restenosis had a residual
  % diameter stenosis > 58%

The magnitude of this problem is amplified by the fact that there are several large clinical trials underway that will use QCA measures of disease as the primary or secondary endpoint. Furthermore, virtually all future clinical trials concerning arteriographically defined coronary disease will use some form of QCA as a primary or secondary endpoint. Unless a uniform approach to validation and standardized measures of disease are used it will be difficult to generalize the results from one QCA based clinical trial to other centers that use different QCA techniques. This would be unfortunate given the enormous time and expense involved in conducting these clinical trials. Thus, validation and standardization of QCA techniques are important not only for those developing new techniques, but also for those applying these techniques in clinical studies, those interpreting the results of these clinical studies, and those providing funds for such clinical investigations.

QCA validation: problems

Even if an investigator believes the importance of good validation studies for QCA techniques, there are a number of problems that make it difficult to actually carry out these studies. The first problem is the enormous number of variables encountered in standard clinical coronary angiography that could lead to spurious estimates of luminal dimensions by even the most advanced QCA technique. These variables include radiographic variables such as kV, focal spot, quantum mottle, scatter, veiling glare, and pincushion and magnification distortion; angiographic variables such as the concentration of intraluminal contrast, projection angles, and overlying stuctures; patient related variables such as vasomotor tone, and cardiac and respiratory motion; and operator variability. These factors undoubtedly influence the results of QCA measures of coronary disease. Ideally, when developing a QCA technique the effect of each of these factors on the results should be determined while all other parameters remain constant. This allows for specific changes in the technique or in image acquisition to minimize effects of those variables with the greatest impact. In practice, this is an arduous task, and no single investigator has isolated and measured the effect of every potential source of error. Fortunately, it appears that with new, larger image intensifiers, good angiographic technique, and use of standardized protocols in the catherization laboratory (e.g. routine use of coronary vasodilators), some of these problems will be overcome. Establishment of common procedural standards in all catheterization laboratories would reduce the importance of these factors when comparing results from different institutions. More work needs to be done to determine the strategy for frame selection that is the most reliable for the purposes of comparison (e.g. best diastolic view, average of several views through the cardiac cycle, average of several views from different projections).

The second difficulty in QCA validation is that no standards exist for the design of an adequate QCA validation study and the description of the results. To illustrate this fact, data from validation studies of seven different QCA techniques are presented in Table 3 [6—15]. The phantoms or lesions used to evaluate these techniques ranged from brass rods and drilled holes in plexiglass to human coronary lesions imaged during routine coronary angiography. There was diversity in the numbers of phantoms or lesions used. The range was 1 to 38 with a median value of 8. The range of repeated evaluations of the same phantom or lesion was 1 to 12 with a median value of 3. There were also a wide variety of strategies adopted with respect to the repeated evaluations of lesions or phantoms (Table 4). This heterogeneity of validation strategies was so extensive that, in fact, no two techniques were validated in precisely the same manner. There was a similar lack of consensus on how to describe results of these validation studies (Table 3).

Table 3. Reported bias and precision of seven different film based QCA techniques.

Author	Ref	Type of Images Used	# of phantoms or lesions	# of reps	Bias %DS	Bias Dmin	Precision %DS	Precision Dmin	Comments
Alderman et al.	6	clinical angiograms	23	3				pooled SD 0.06 mm; coef. var. 3.5%	same frame × 3
	6	clinical angiograms	23	2				pooled SD 0.19 mm; coef. var. 9.5%	2 different injections
Brown et al.	7	brass phantom with stenosis	1	NS		within 0.08 mm			
	7	clinical angiograms	8	9			avg. SD of estimate 3%	avg. SD of estimate 0.10 mm	3 trained operators × 3 different frames
Cashin et al.	8	clinical angiograms	8	3			resid. var. (ANOVA) 6.8%		similar QCA technique to Siebes et al. 3 adjacent frames
Harrison et al.	9	brass phantom with stenosis	1	NS		within 3%			same QCA technique as Brown et al.
	9	clinical angiograms	18	3				Mean ± SD of % diff. 7 ± 1%	" 3 projections of same lesion
Mancini et al.	10*	canine angiograms with intracoronary prostheses	8	2		mean error −0.18 mm		SD of error 0.20 mm	better results reported using on-line digital images

Table 3 (continued)

Author	Ref	Type of Images Used	# of phantoms or lesions	# of reps	Bias %DS	Bias Dmin	Precision %DS	Precision Dmin	Comments
Nichols et al.	11	plastic phantoms eccentric stenoses contrast filled	9	3	corr. coef. 0.99 SEE 3.9%				
	11	clinical angiograms	19	6		corr. coef. 0.96 SEE 6%			avg. results from: same frame × 2 (same operator), and same frame × 2 (different operators)
Reiber et al.	12	plastic lumen filled with contrast	9	6—12	mean error 2%	mean error −0.03	overall precision 2.68%	overall precision 0.09 mm	avg. results from phantoms with 50%, and 100% contrast
	13	clinical angiograms	38	2			SD of error 2.74%	SD of error 0.1 mm	13 stenotic segments and 25 normal segments
Seibes et al.	14	plastic phantoms with stenosis contrast filled	3	NS	% error (range) −2 to 13%	% error (range) −8 to 15%			
Spears et al.	15	plastic phantoms (over live human chest)	14	1	Mean absolute error 0.06 mm (Mean absolute error 0.11 mm)				avg. results using different edge detectors, contrast concentration, focal spot size, position in *x-y* plane, magnification, motion, kV, and thickness of scattering media

ANOVA = analysis of variance; avg. = average; corr. coef. = correlation coefficient; coef. var. = coefficient of variation; Dmin = minimum diameter; DS = diameter stenosis; kV = kilovoltage; NS = not stated; resid. var. = residual variance; S.D. = standard deviation; SEE = standard error of the estimate; * = mean and S.D. of the error provided via personal communication with Dr. Mancini.

Table 4. Strategies used for repeated evaluations of lesions or phantoms in 10 QCA validation studies.

- same cineframe
- adjacent cineframes
- adjacent cardiac cycles
- different injections of the same vessel segment
- different projections of the same vessel segment
- different catheterizations separated by: days, weeks, months

---

The heterogeneity of validation study designs and methods of describing results is a serious impediment for those attempting to thoughtfully compare the results of these validation studies, or the results of clinical studies using these different QCA techniques. A more standardized approach to validation testing and reporting results would be helpful for the scientific community involved with the development and application of QCA techniques. With this in mind, there are some general principles of validation testing that would be helpful for future QCA validation studies. First, the goals of the validation test should be clearly stated at the outset, and the design of the test should be specifically tailored for those goals. Validation tests performed during the development and refinement of a technique should not be confused with tests intended to determine the variability of a technique in preparation for a clinical study.

Second, the full range of disease expected in the planned clinical application should be represented in the validation study. This is especially challenging when attempting to create phantoms that adequately represent severe stenoses. It is generally difficult to create phantoms with minimal luminal dimensions less than 0.5 mm in diameter, yet many patients with severe coronary disease have stenotic lumens at least that small. Several investigators have resorted to highly specialized, industrial techniques to produce phantoms with diameters in the 0.5 mm range.

Third, it is better to validate a technique using many different phantoms or lesions with only a few repeated measures than only a few phantoms or lesions with lots of repeated measures. This will allow one to more fully characterize the performance of a technique in the range of expected values in real clinical applications, and at the same time provide the needed information about the variability of the test.

Finally, lesions or phantoms should be evaluated in random order by operators who are unaware of the true dimensions or the results of previous evaluations. Investigators that have already performed QCA validation studies will realize that these principles are not always entirely feasible, but they should be adhered to as closely as possible.

The results of validation studies should be separated into measures of bias and measures of variability (Fig. 1). Bias is a estimate of how close, on the average, a measured value is from the truth. Precision or variability are estimates of how close repeated measures are to each other; or put another way, they are measures of the spread in the data. When describing bias there are several options. The most straight forward is the mean error (Fig. 2). The

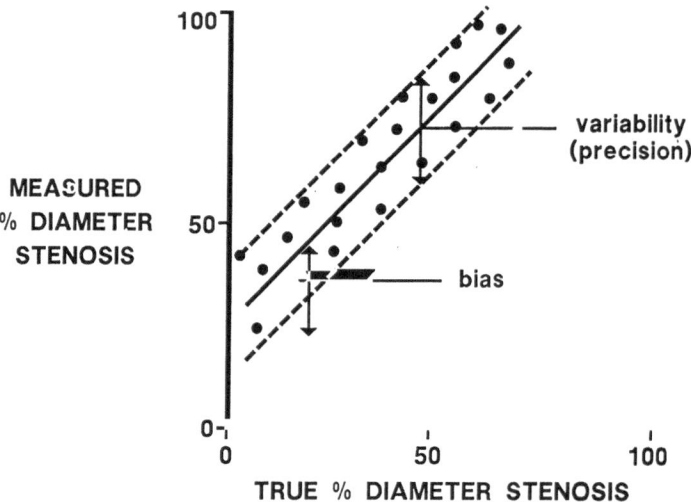

Figure 1. Results of a hypothetical QCA validation study. Arrows indicate the two essential features of a validation study, bias and precision.

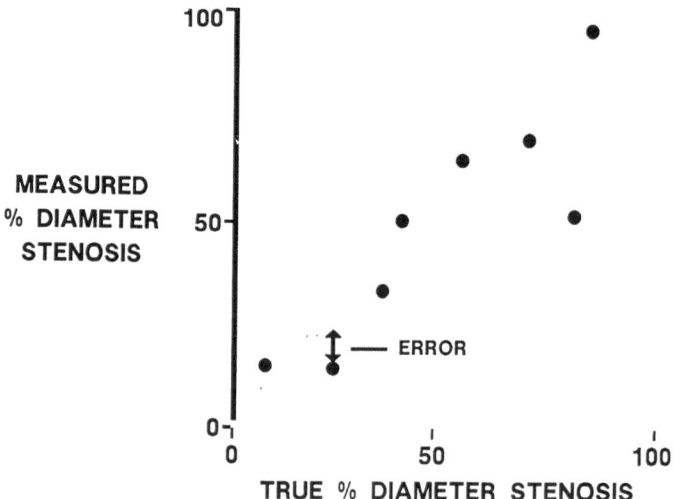

Figure 2. Arrow indicates the error of a single measurement in a QCA validation study. Bias can be expressed as the mean of the errors of multiple measurements.

advantage of the mean error is that it is simple, uniformly understood, and easy to compare from study to study. Its disadvantage is that it is greatly affected by extreme values. The median error is less affected by extreme values, but statistical theory for comparing median values is not well understood. The mean absolute error suffers the same problem with extreme values, and in addition it hides the direction of the bias and is statistically less convenient than the simple mean error. The slope and intercept using simple linear regression may be useful for those familiar with interpreting the results; however, far too many investigators are guilty of plugging numbers into a computerized statistical package without a good understanding of the assumptions involved in using regression techniques. The correlation coefficient is a measure of how well the data is estimated by a straight line. It does not measure how close that line is to the line of identity and it is an inappropriate measure of bias (Fig. 3).

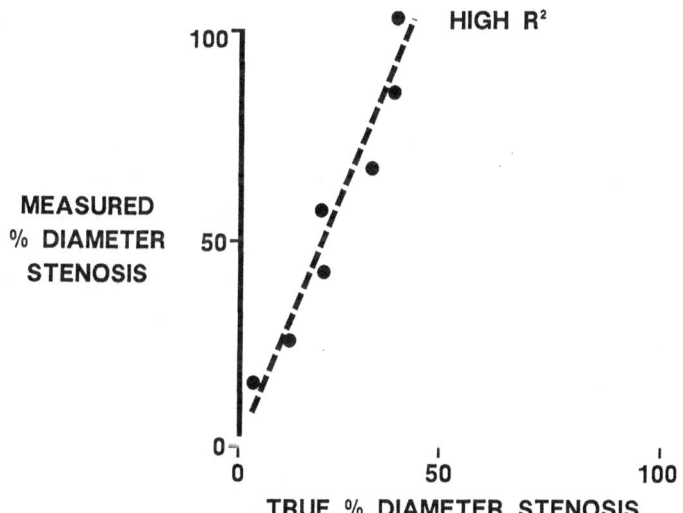

Figure 3. Validation data with a high correlation coefficient (R^2) from a severely biased QCA technique.

When describing the variability of a QCA technique the standard deviation of the errors can be used. When repeated evaluations of several phantoms or lesions are performed the pooled standard deviation can be used (Fig. 4). Like the mean error, the standard deviation is simple, uniformly understood, and easy to compare. Simple linear regression, correlation coefficients, or analysis of variance can also be helpful in some circumstances to those who are familiar with these techniques.

There are two special situations to keep in mind when analyzing the results of a validation test. The first situation occurs when the bias or

162

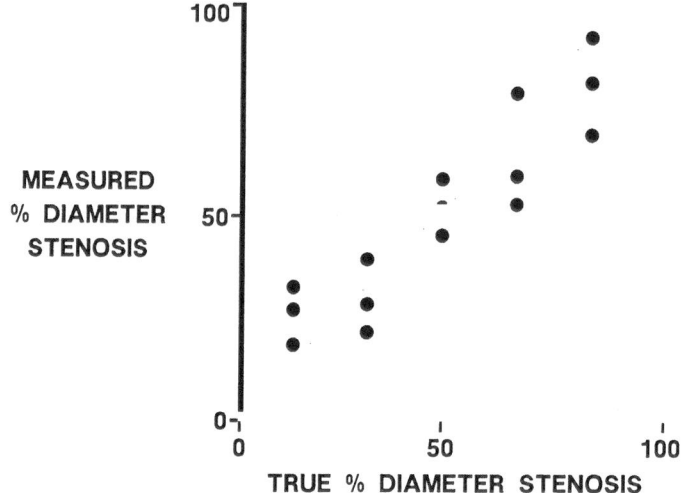

Figure 4. Multiple measurements of five lesions or phantoms. Precision of the QCA technique can be expressed as the pooled standard deviation of these values.

precision of a test is linearly dependent on the size of the vessel being measured (Fig. 5). In this case the measures of bias can be expressed as a percent of the size of the vessel. When describing variability, the coefficient of variation should be used. The second situation occurs when the bias or precision of a test is dependent on the size of the vessel being measured, but not in a simple linear fashion (Fig. 6). In this situation simple descriptive

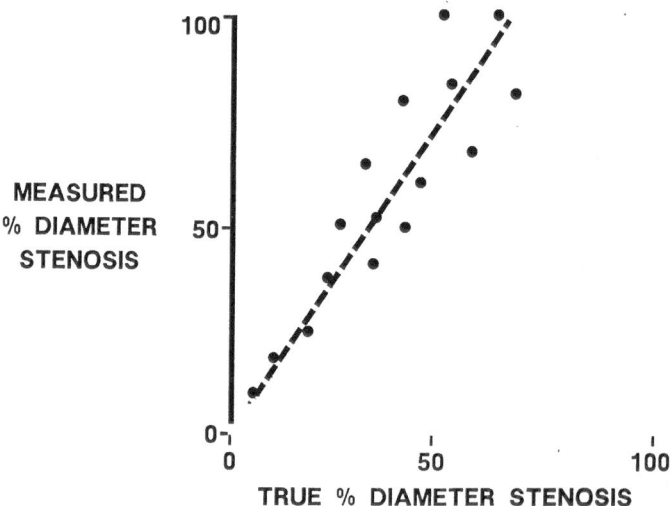

Figure 5. Example of bias and precision linearly related to the size of the vessel being measured. Percent error and coefficient of variation can be used to describe this data.

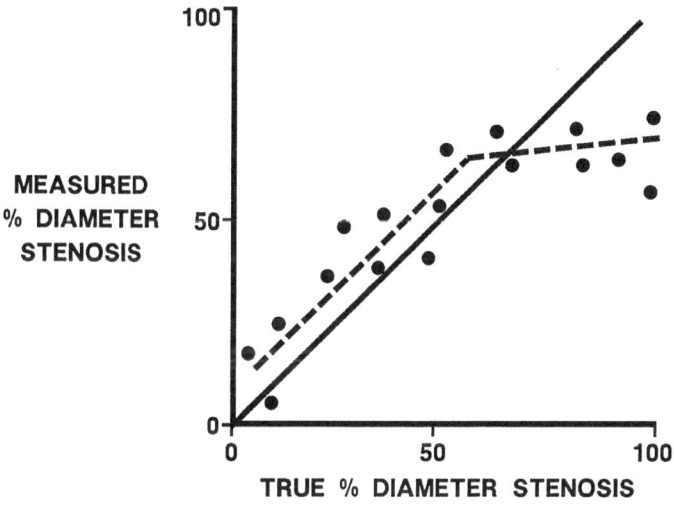

Figure 6. Example of bias and precision nonlinearly related to the size of the measured vessel.

statistics and a graphical description of the data are the best way to present the results.

Finally, no analysis of QCA validation tests or results of studies using QCA measures is complete without a careful examination of the plotted data. It allows you to identify extreme values, and check for linearity and constant variance in the data. The simple descriptive statistics including the mean and standard deviation of the error should always be included to facilitate comparison of results from other institutions. Regression techniques and coefficient of variation may also be helpful in some instances.

The third difficulty with QCA validation is that there is no independent measure of *in-vivo* coronary luminal dimensions to serve as a gold standard to compare with the results of a QCA technique. Thus it is impossible to determine technique bias using standard clinical coronary angiograms. Images of phantoms may be used to estimate the bias (as well as the precision), but one should be careful about extrapolating those results to the use of the technique in clinical studies. Realistic estimates of technique bias is especially important when QCA measures are used to predict coronary flow because of the fourth power of the radius in models predicting coronary flow from anatomy [16]. Several investigators have made special efforts to arrive at more realistic estimates of the bias of QCA techniques. Johnson *et al.* have used high-frequency epicardial ultrasound to measure the luminal dimensions of vessels at coronary bypass surgery to compare with QCA measures of the same vessels from a previously acquired angiogram [17]. This has the advantage of using real human coronary atherosclerotic pathology. However, it is difficult to know to what extent changes in vasomotor

164

tone, pulse pressure, and other metabolic parameters may have altered the luminal dimensions between the time of the angiogram and the time of surgery.

Mancini and Vogel *et al.* have developed a canine model for coronary stenoses where cylindrical plastic prostheses with known luminal dimensions are inserted into coronaries of live dogs [10]. This provides the opportunity for validation studies in the face of sources of variability that have been difficult to replicate in more conventional phantom models such as cardiac motion and inhomogeneity of intraluminal contrast.

We have been working on a third approach for validating QCA techniques using postmortem hearts. A radiopaque polymer is injected into the coronary vessel segment of interest. This is allowed to cure as the heart is fixed. The heart is then placed into the pericardial space of an embalmed human chest and taken to the catherization laboratory where standard angiographic images are acquired (Fig. 7). After the film is reviewed, the

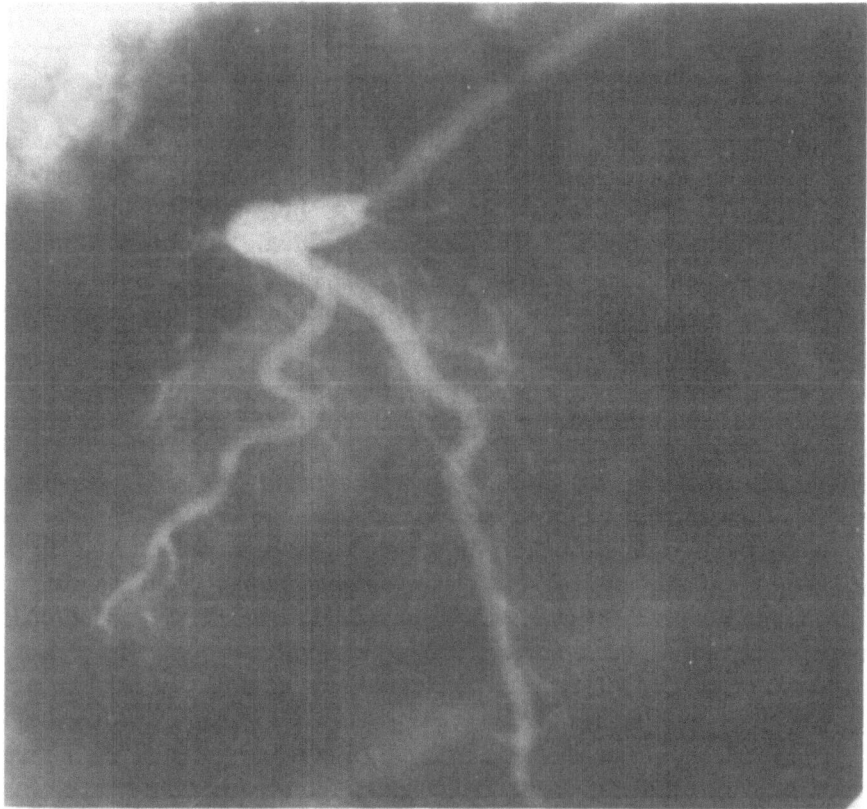

Figure 7. Angiographic image of a postmortem human heart injected with a radiopaque plastic polymer.

vessel segment of interest is dissected from the myocardium and sectioned in 0.5 mm increments perpendicular to the long axis of the vessel. The cross-sectional area profile can then be determined by computer assisted histoplanimetry. This approach results in images that closely resemble human coronary angiography and at the same time provides accurate estimates of the true luminal dimensions, however, it does not include factors such as motion artifact or inhomogeneity of intraluminal contrast.

In summary, QCA is an exciting and powerful tool in the study of coronary disease. Validation and standardization of these techniques will be crucial for the successful future application of these techniques. Unfortunately, because of the current heterogeneity in approaches to validation and to describing results, it is very difficult to compare published data from validation studies or clinical investigations using QCA measures. Future validation studies should have clearly specified goals and designs tailored to achieve those goals. Multiple phantoms that span the range of stenosis severity to be studied and that resemble clinical coronary angiography should be evaluated in a random and blinded fashion. The analysis of validation studies should always include a plot of the data and the mean and standard deviation of the error to allow for meaningful comparison to results from other institutions. Efforts to create more realistic phantoms, and develop other independent measures of coronary dimensions will provide additional information about the performance of QCA techniques. In the future, cooperative interlaboratory efforts to uniformly compare different QCA techniques and establish standardized approaches to validation will clearly enhance the utility of quantitative coronary angiography.

Acknowledgements

This work has been supported in part by the Andrew Mellon Foundation, New York, N.Y. and the National Heart, Lung, and Blood Institute Research Grant in Preventative Cardiology, # T32 HL 07642.

References

1. Brown BG, Bolson EL, Dodge HT: Arteriographic assessment of coronary atherosclerosis. Review of current methods, their limitations, and clinical applications. Arteriosclerosis 2: 2—15, 1982.
2. Reiber JHC, Kooijman CJ, Slager CJ, Gerbrands JJ, Schuurbiers JCH, Boer A den, Wijns W, Serruys PW: Computer assisted analysis of the severity of obstructions from coronary cineangiograms: A methodological review. Automedica 5: 219—238, 1984.
3. Brown BG, Bolson EL, Dodge HT: Quantitative computer techniques for analyzing coronary arteriograms. Prog Cardiovasc Dis 28(6): 403—418, 1986.

4. Harrison DG, Ferguson DW, Collins SM, Skorton DJ, Ericksen EE, Kioschos JM, Marcus ML, White CW: Rethrombosis after reperfusion with streptokinase: Importance of geometry of residual lesions. Circulation 69: 991—999, 1984.

5. Serruys PW, Wijns W, Brand M van den, Ribeiro V, Fioretti P, Simoons ML, Kooijman CJ, Reiber JHC, Hugenholtz PG: Is transluminal coronary angioplasty mandatory after successful thrombolysis? Quantitative coronary angiographic study. Br Heart J 50: 257—265, 1983.

6. Alderman EL, Berte LE, Harrison DC, Sanders W: Quantitation of coronary artery dimensions using digital image processing. Digital Radiography 314: 273—278, 1981.

7. Brown BG, Bolson E, Frimer M, Dodge HT: Quantitative coronary arteriography. Estimation of dimensions, hemodynamic resistance, and atheroma mass of coronary artery lesions using the arteriogram and digital computation. Circulation 55: 329—337, 1977.

8. Cashin WL, Brooks SH, Blankenhorn DH, Selzer RH, Sanmarco ME, Benjauthrit B: Computerized edge tracking and lesion measurement in coronary angiograms: A pilot study comparing smokers with non-smokers. Atherosclerosis 52: 295—300, 1984.

9. Harrison DG, White CW, Hiratzka LF, Doty DB, Barnes DH, Eastham CL, Marcus ML: The value of lesion cross-sectional area determined by quantitative coronary angiography in assessing the physiologic significance of proximal left anterior descending coronary arterial stenoses. Circulation 69: 1111—1119, 1984.

10. Mancini GBJ, Simon SB, McGillem MJ, LeFree MT, Friedman HZ, Vogel RA: Auto-mated quantitative coronary arteriography: Morphologic and physiologic validation in vivo of a rapid digital angiographic method. Circulation 75(2): 452—460, 1987.

11. Nichols AB, Gabrieli CFO, Fenoglio JJ, Esser PD: Quantification of relative coronary arterial stenosis by cinevideodensitometric analysis of coronary arteriograms. Circulation 69: 512—522, 1984.

12. Reiber JHC, Kooijman CJ, Slager CJ, Gerbrands JJ, Schuurbiers JCH, Boer A den, Wijns W, Serruys PW, Hugenholtz PG: Coronary artery dimensions from cineangiograms — Methodology and validation of a computer-assisted analysis procedure. IEEE Transactions on Medical Imaging MI3: 131—141, 1984.

13. Reiber JHC, Serruys PW, Kooijman CJ, Wijns W, Slager CJ, Gerbrands JJ, Schuurbiers JCH, Boer A den, Hugenholtz PG: Assessment of short-, medium-, and long-term variations in arterial dimensions from computer-assisted quantitation of coronary cine-angiograms. Circulation 71: 280—288, 1985.

14. Siebes M, D'Argenio DZ, Selzer RH: Computer assessment of hemodynamic severity of coronary artery stenosis from angiograms. Comput Methods Programs Biomed 21: 143—152, 1985.

15. Spears JR, Sandor T, Als AV, Malagold M, Markis JE, Grossman W, Serur JR, Paulin S: Computerized image analysis for quantitative measurement of vessel diameter from cine-angiograms. Circulation 68: 453—461, 1983.

16. Gould KL: Quantification of coronary artery stenosis in vivo. Circ Res 57: 341—353, 1985.

17. Johnson MR, McPherson DD, Fleagle SR, Hunt M, Hiratzka L, Skorton DJ, Kerber R, Collins SM: Videodensitometric analysis of coronary stenoses: Validation using high-frequency epicardial echocardiography. Circulation 72(III): III-261, 1985.

11. Early regression and late progression in coronary artery lesions in the first 3 months following coronary angioplasty

KEVIN J. BEATT, H. E. LUIJTEN, J. H. C. REIBER and
P. W. SERRUYS

SUMMARY. In order to determine the changes in stenotic lesions following coronary angioplasty, detailed quantitative angiographic measurements were performed in 254 patients (292
lesions) immediately post-angioplasty and then at one of three predetermined follow-up times,
at 30, 60 or 90 days. The absolute changes in mm of the minimal lumen diameter were
compared for the three groups, and a relatively high follow-up rate of 88% was achieved. In
the groups of patients followed-up at 30 and 60 days, the response was variable with 6% of the
lesions showing a significant improvement in both groups and 1% and 12% respectively,
showing a deterioration. At 90 days no lesions were seen to improve with 23% deteriorating.

Early following angioplasty lesions exhibit a variable response with more improving than
deteriorating. At 60 days the restenosis process is evident, with the number of lesions
deteriorating almost doubling between 60 days and 90 days.

Introduction

The incidence of restenosis following PTCA has become an important index
for defining the longterm success rate of the procedure. However, despite a
number of studies, some involving relatively large numbers of patients, the
incidence of restenosis in the overall PTCA population remains poorly
defined. This is due to a number of factors, which alone or in combination
may lead to distortion of the data. The first of these is the failure to use a
reproducible quantitative angiographic measurement system for defining the
vessel diameter. Visual estimation of stenosis severity alone yields unaccept-
able errors in the assessment of changes in the coronary lesion [1—4], and an
automated edge detection system will further enhance the accuracy of a
quantitative system [5].

Secondly, the rate of restenosis varies considerably according to the
definition used. Restenosis rates are conventionally based on the change in
percentage diameter stenosis; the criteria used are arbitrary and may not
reflect the true changes occurring in the vessel.

Thirdly, follow-up studies addressing restenosis should be performed
prospectively, with all or as many patients as possible undergoing repeat
angiography at preset follow-up times. Reinvestigation determined predomi-

J. C. Reiber & P. W. Serruys (eds.), New Developments in Quantitative Coronary Arteriography,
167—180.

nantly by the recurrence of symptoms, will bias the results so that they do not reflect the outcome of the PTCA population as a whole.

In order to better define the true incidence of restenosis, and to determine the change of lesion characteristics with time, we performed an angiographic study in patients who had undergone a successful PTCA. Patients were reinvestigated at 30, 60 and 90 days (following the dilatation procedure) and measurements were performed using a computer based quantitative angiographic system (CAAS).

Study population

Initially 290 patients were entered into the study having undergone successful coronary angioplasty, defined as: (1) less than 50 percent diameter stenosis on visual inspection of the post-angioplasty coronary angiogram performed in multiple views; (2) no in-hospital complications, namely recurrence of angina, coronary bypass grafting, repeat percutaneous transluminal coronary angioplasty (PTCA), acute myocardial infarction, or death.

Both patients with stable and unstable angina pectoris, as defined previously [6], were included. Patients with acute myocardial infarction receiving a thrombolytic agent who subsequently had immediate coronary angioplasty were excluded.

Allocation of patients to one of three predetermined times for follow-up angiography was made sequentially according to the study period in which the dilatation was performed; those falling in the first study period being reinvestigated at 30 days, the second at 60 days, the third at 90 days. Of the 290 patients who met the inclusion criteria, 254 patients had repeat angiography suitable for quantitative analysis. The reasons for failure to complete the study are detailed in Fig. 1.

Recatheterization was considered to be contra-indicated for the following reasons: severe concomitant disease (e.g. renal failure, lung cancer), peripheral vascular disease, or multiple (> 4) prior angiographic investigations.

Of the total study group of 254 patients (292 lesions), 93 patients were recatheterized at 30 days (110 lesions), 79 patients at 60 days (89 lesions) and 82 patients at 90 days (93 lesions).

The baseline clinical characteristics in the three groups were comparable for the variables shown in Table I. The mean time from PTCA to follow-up angiography in the three study groups was 40 days, 58 days and 102 days, respectively.

Where clinically indicated (early recurrence of symptoms), patients were re-investigated before their preset time, but in order not to adversely bias the earlier groups and so allow valid statistical comparison of the individual groups, analysis was performed according to their original allocation group.

**PATIENTS WITH SUCCESSFUL PTCA
(< 50% DSTEN POST-PTCA)**

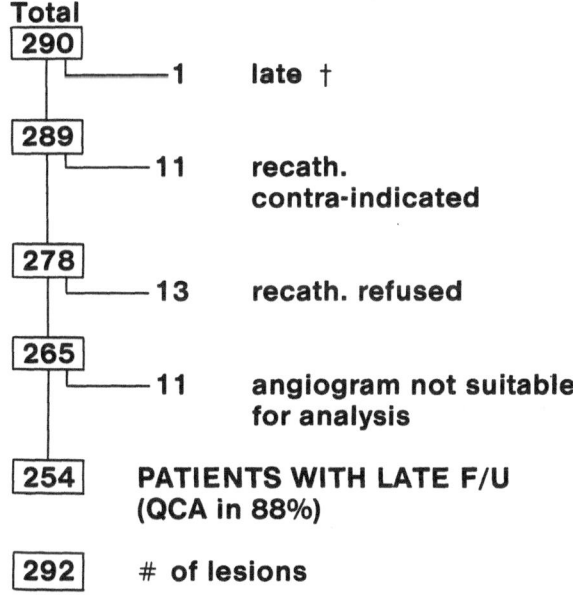

Figure 1. Flow chart of the total number of patients who met the inclusion criteria, and the reasons for failure to complete the study. F/U = follow-up; QCA = quantitative coronary angiography; Recath. = recatheterization.

Prior myocardial infarction was defined according to the Minnesota code, [7] and in the case of an electrocardiographic conduction abnormality making interpretation difficult, the presence of regional akinesia or dyskinesia on the left ventriculogram was used as the criterion for a previous infarction. In Table II are shown for each study group the type of vessel dilated, the number of patients with tandem lesions, and the number of patients with more than one lesion dilated.

Methods

Coronary angioplasty was performed with a steerable, movable guide-wire system via the femoral route. Details regarding the procedure used in our laboratory have previously been described [6]. At the beginning of the angioplasty procedure all patients received 10,000 I.U. of heparin i.v., 500 mg of acetylsalicylic acid i.v., and a continuous infusion of Rheomacrodex® (low molecular weight dextran) was started. After dilatation 10 mg of nifedipine

Table I. Clinical characteristics of 290 patients with successful percutaneous transluminal coronary angioplasty entered into the study.

Characteristics	Follow-up period			
	30 Days No. (%)	60 Days No. (%)	90 Days No. (%)	overall No. (%)
No. of patients	93	79	82	254
No. of lesions	110	89	93	292
Mean no. of lesions dilated/pt.	1.18	1.13	1.13	1.15
Age (mean ± s.d.)	57±9 (range, 35—75)	57±9 (range, 31—75)	56±9 (range, 32—74)	57±9 (range, 31—75)
Sex ratio (M/F)	5.6 (79/14)	5.1 (66/13)	3.3 (63/19)	4.5 (208/46)
Time from PTCA to F/U (days)	40±7 (range, 18—62)	61±12 (range, 11—80)	102±18 (range, 33—164)	80±38 (range, 11—164)
Extent of C.A.D. (No. of vessels) 1	63 (68)	55 (70)	59 (72)	177 (70)
2	25 (27)	20 (25)	18 (22)	63 (25)
3	5 (5)	4 (5)	5 (6)	14 (6)
Previous coronary bypass grafting	8 (9)	4 (5)	3 (4)	15 (6)
Previous myocardial infarction	25 (27)	24 (30)	20 (24)	69 (27)
Previous coronary angioplasty	10 (11)	2 (3)	11 (13)	23 (9)

C.A.D. = coronary artery disease; F = female sex; F/U = follow-up angiography; M = male sex; s.d. = standard deviation.

was given orally every two hours for the first twelve hours after PTCA, and then three to six times a day together with 500 mg of acetylsalicylic acid orally once a day until repeat angiography. Beta-blockers were withdrawn unless hypertension was present.

Quantitative coronary angiography

The quantitative analysis of the stenotic coronary segments was carried out with the computer-assisted Cardiovascular Angiography Analysis System (CAAS), which has been described in detail [8, 9]. In summary, to analyze a coronary arterial segment in a selected frame of 35 mm cinefilm, an optically magnified (magnification factor 2) portion of the image encompassing that segment is converted into video format by means of a cine-video converter. The contours of the vessel are detected automatically on the basis of the weighted sum of first- and second-derivative functions applied to the digitized brightness information. Calibration of the diameter data of the vessels in absolute values (mm) is achieved by using the contrast catheter as a scaling device. To this end, the contours of a user-defined portion of the optically magnified catheter (optical magnification factor $2\sqrt{2}$) are detected automatically. Both the arterial segment and catheter contours are corrected for pincushion distortion caused by the image intensifier. From the arterial contours, the vessel diameter function, in millimeters, is determined by computing the shortest distances between the two contour sides. A representative analysis, with the detected contours and the diameter function superimposed on the digitized video image, is shown in Fig. 2.

The reference diameter or the normal diameter of the coronary artery at the site of obstruction is difficult to standardize and is usually defined visually using the nearest coronary artery segment that appears normal. A number of errors may be produced in this way: firstly, there is a large individual variation in the choice of the segment used, and secondly, because of the variation in the vessel diameter, typical of atherosclerotic vessels, adjacent segments will not always represent the normal diameter of the vessel at the site of the obstruction. To avoid these potential errors we have used an 'interpolated' reference diameter measurement. The principle behind this technique is the computer estimation of the original diameter within the obstructed region assuming that no local coronary disease is present. This is calculated from the computed reference diameters of the proximal and distal segments, and after the vessel has been reconstructed the interpolated reference diameter is taken as the value coincident with the site of maximal narrowing [10—11]. The precision of the contour detection process has previously been validated using plexiglass phantoms filled with contrast medium [12]. We have found that using our measurement system, the overall accuracy (average difference between true and measured values) and the precision (pooled standard deviation of the differences) of the obstruction diameter is minus 30 and plus 90 microns, respectively [8].

In order to standardize the method of analysis of the PTCA and follow-up angiograms, the following four measures were undertaken: first, multiple matched views, orthogonal if possible, were analyzed for each patient and the results averaged; second, the X-ray system was repositioned in the settings corresponding as much as possible to the projections used during the previous angiographies. For this purpose, the angular settings of the X-ray gantry and the various height levels were readjusted according to the values previously documented with the on-line registration system. Third, for all studies cineframes to be analyzed were selected at end-diastole to minimize any possible foreshortening effect. Fourth, the user-determined

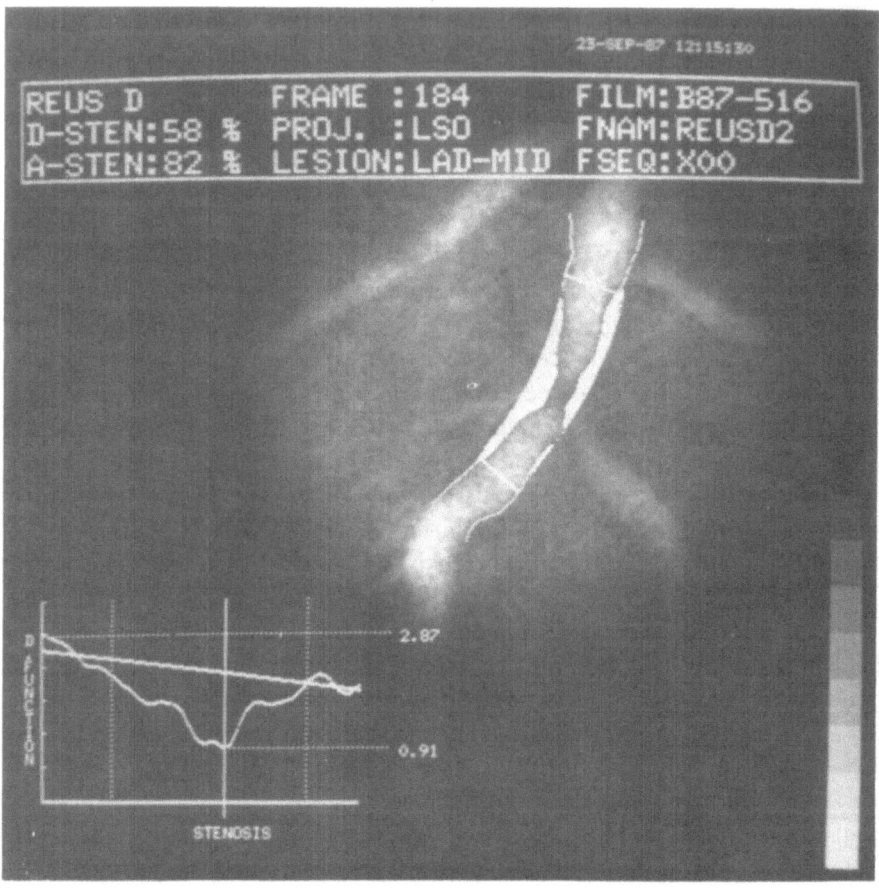

Figure 2. A single frame angiogram of a left coronary artery with superimposition of the automated contours at the coronary artery segment of interest. Beneath this is shown the diameter function of the detected contours of the left anterior descending coronary artery. The minimal lumen diameter (0.91 mm) and the interpolated diameter function line (i) from which the reference diameter is derived, are shown on the diameter function plot.

beginning and end-points of the major coronary segments between side branches, where possible, were identified according to the definitions of the American Heart Association. Finally, Polaroid pictures were taken of the video image with the detected contours superimposed, to ensure that the analyses were performed on the same coronary segment in the consecutive angiograms.

Absolute measurements of the reference diameter and minimal obstruction diameter were recorded in millimeters. A change of greater than 0.72 mm was taken to represent a significant change. This is based on twice the variability of the obstruction diameter (0.36 mm) when coronary angiography is repeated over an interval of 90 days [8].

Statistical analysis

To compare the three follow-up groups with respect to baseline characteristics (Tables I and II), univariate analysis of variance was performed for the continuous variables, and chi-square analysis for discrete variables. Univariate analysis (BMDP statistical software, University of California Press, Berkeley, California 1985) was performed on the quantitative angiographic data.

Table II. Type of vessel dilated, number of patients with tandem lesions, and number of patients with more than one lesion dilated for each of the four study groups.

	30 Days No. (%)	60 Days No. (%)	90 Days No. (%)	overall No. (%)
Vessel dilated				
LAD	61 (56)	61 (69)	55 (59)	177 (61)
LCX	18 (16)	16 (18)	19 (20)	53 (18)
RCA	26 (24)	11 (12)	16 (17)	53 (18)
Bypass	4 (4)	0 (0)	2 (2)	6 (2)
LMCA	1 (1)	1 (1)	1 (1)	3 (1)
No. of patients with tandem lesion	6 (6)	2 (3)	2 (2)	10 (4)
No. of patients with more than 1 lesion dilated	15 (16)	10 (13)	10 (12)	35 (14)

Bypass = aortocoronary bypass graft; LAD = left anterior descending artery; LCX = left circumflex artery; LMCA = left main coronary artery; RCA = right coronary artery.

Results

In the three follow-up groups 254 patients completed angiographic follow-up. As a result of PTCA there was an expected significant improvement in the minimal lumen diameter and diameter stenosis in each of the 3 groups ($p < 0.0001$). The changes in the mean minimal lumen diameter and the mean reference diameter occurring between post-PTCA and follow-up are shown in Fig. 3. In the groups that had follow-up angiography performed at 30 and 60 days, there were small nonsignificant changes in both these values. However, at 90 days there was a highly significant decrease in not only the minimal lumen diameter, but also in the reference diameter.

The changes in the individual minimal lumen diameters (mm) of all the lesions divided into the 3 follow-up groups are represented in Fig. 4. Individual lesions that have undergone a change greater or equal to 0.36 mm are distinguished by a closed circle. Regression is defined as an increase, and

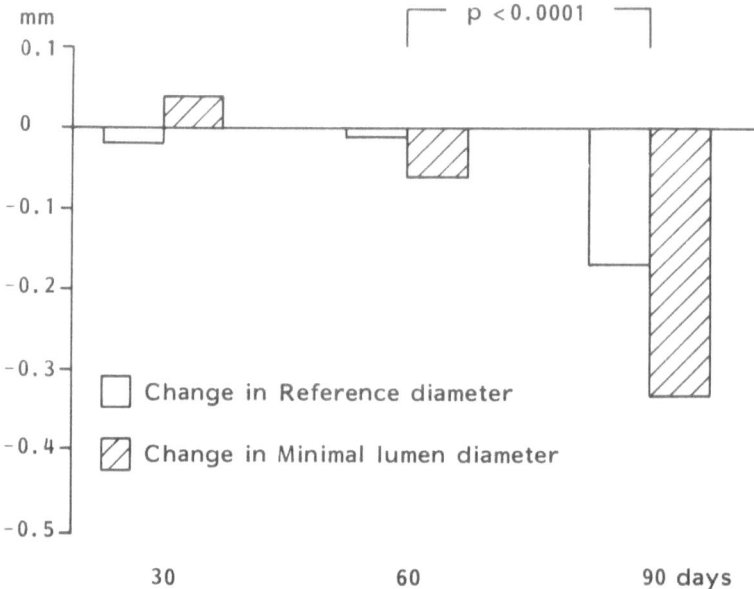

Figure 3. Change in reference diameter and minimal lumen diameter for the three follow-up groups. For the 90 days group both these changes are significantly greater than in the two previous follow-up groups (*p* < 0.0001).

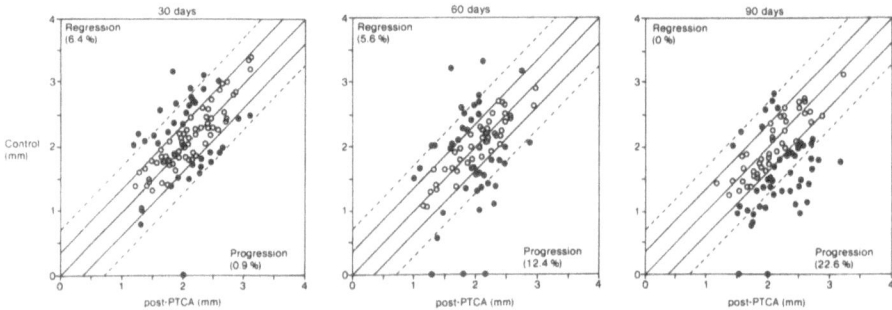

Figure 4. Individual minimal lumen diameter (mm) post-PTCA compared with that at control angiography for the three groups. The two solid lines on either side of the identity line correspond to the long-term variability (0.36 mm) of repeated measurements for this para-meter. This variability is one standard deviation of the differences of the duplicate angio-graphic measurements. Here two standard deviations were used (2 × 0.36 = 0.72 mm; dashed lines) as a criterion for lesion progression or regression. Based on this criterion the percentage of lesions showing progression or regression (outside of dashed lines) are shown within the relevant brackets.

progression as a decrease of at least 0.72 mm (twice the variability) and these values fall outside the dotted lines. It can be seen that the mean change for each group does not reflect the number of individual lesions undergoing a significant change. In the group followed up at 30 days there were a greater number of lesions undergoing regression than progression. At 60 days the percentage of patients showing progression was twice that of regression and at 90 days this percentage had doubled with virtually no lesions exhibiting regression.

Figure 5 illustrates the incidence of restenosis according to a number of commonly used criteria, and to the criterion for a change of greater than 0.72 mm. There is a wide variation in the incidence according to the criteria used, although the incidence of restenosis increases progressively up to at least 90 days, irrespective of the criteria chosen.

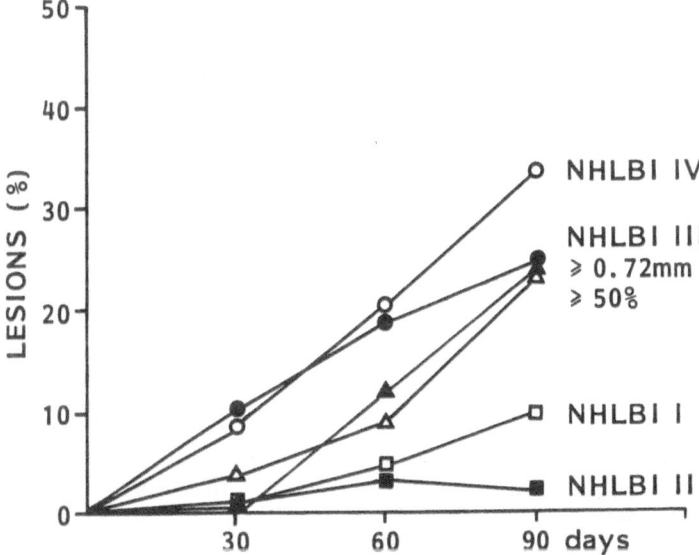

Figure 5. Shown are the percentages of lesions that fulfil three of the restenosis criteria: NHLBI IV, defined by a loss of greater than 50% of the gain achieved at PTCA; ⩾0.72 mm, defined by a change of ⩾0.72 mm between post-PTCA and follow-up; and thirdly, ⩾50% stenosis at follow-up. Using these three criteria the incidence of restenosis increases up to at least 90 days.

Discussion

Method of assessment

Percutaneous transluminal coronary angioplasty has developed into a well accepted method of revascularization. Although the immediate benefits of the procedure are well established and often striking, the longterm outcome is less well defined; undoubtedly, the feature that most limits the usefulness of this procedure is the incidence in restenosis of the dilated lesion in the months following the procedure [14—17]. Various methods of assessing the results of angioplasty have been addressed by Serruys and others [10, 18]. The absolute measurement of a coronary stenosis based on a series of single frame angiograms remains the most direct method of assessing the degree of coronary artery obstruction. Accurate measurement of any change in the coronary artery stenosis must be based on reproducible quantitative measurements. The use of computer assisted automatic edge detection of the lesion contours is also important, particularly in the situation post-angioplasty when the contours of the dilated lesions tend to be irregular and are subject to a greater inter- and intra-observer variability [5]. Using an automatic edge detection measurement system in combination with a strict protocol, both for the timing of repeat follow-up measurements and for the angiographic projections studied, will allow a high degree of accuracy to be obtained. The variability of the mean minimal lumen diameter for repeat short (5 min.), medium (60 min.), and long term (90 days) observations was found to be 0.34 mm, 0.22 mm and 0.36 mm, respectively. We have taken the long term variability, the value for the least well controlled group, as the basis of our criteria for lesions that undergo a significant change. The variability represents one standard deviation of the differences between the paired measurements from the first and second angiograms, and would result in a 16% false positive rate, while the use of two standard deviations as a criterion (0.72 mm) results in a false positive rate of 2.5%. It provides an index of restenosis based on the absolute change in the lesion rather than a change relative to the reference diameter; by using this value we are able to obtain a better insight into the changes in coronary anatomy that occur following PTCA.

Early remodeling of dilated lesion

The data of patients followed up at 30 days suggest that the early response following PTCA is extremely variable with more patients exhibiting a regression of the stenosis than those exhibiting progression. This is well shown in Fig. 4. The lack of uniformity in response following PTCA has been documented in the past [16, 17], but no factor has been identified that can predict with any reliability or consistency the lesions that will show either progression or regression.

Lesion regression rates of 30% have previously been described following angioplasty, but in a small group of patients, using different criteria and without specific reference to time following angioplasty of the selected subgroups. Spontaneous lesion regression may occur as part of the atherosclerotic process [19—22] in undilated coronary artery lesions; however, we cannot exclude further changes following our last observation point at 90 days. It may be that the irregular nature of the lesion post-angioplasty does not allow accurate baseline measurement, particularly if a dissection has occurred, but our system using automatic detection of the vessel contours will minimize the variability of this measurement. Distortion of the baseline value will mean that any consequent measurement based on this will be inaccurate.

An alternative explanation for the early variable response is that of platelet deposition or dissolution. Thrombus may be present at the site of the stenosis prior to dilatation, or alternatively deposition may occur early after dilatation as has been demonstrated in animal models [23]. Therefore, behavior of platelets at the site of dilatation following angioplasty may account for the early variable response seen.

Late progression

In the group of patients followed up at 60 days the variability in response is again exhibited, but at 90 days there is a distinct change in the pattern. There are fewer patients exhibiting a regression in the minimal lumen diameter, with many more patients showing a deterioration. This general trend towards deterioration is responsible for the relatively large change in the mean minimal lumen diameter and the highly statistical difference between this group and the 2 groups followed up earlier at 30 and 60 days ($p < 0.0001$).

This progression of the minimal lumen diameter reflects the well known deterioration in percent diameter stenosis in studies where the mean follow-up time post-angioplasty was greater than two months [14—17]. Animal studies have shown that following angioplasty of normal arteries there is initially significant platelet deposition, particularly if an intimal tear has occurred, and subsequently proliferation of smooth muscle cells. In the pig model [23] it has been shown that intimal proliferation occurs between 7 and 14 days and this same process has been identified in at least 7 postmortem hearts that were examined over a similar time period to that involved in our study (17—150 days) [24—28]. These reports comment on this difference between the dilated segments and nondilated segments, but do not differentiate between changes within stenotic segments and those without. More recently, Wallar *et al.* [29] has reported fribrocellular proliferation in the left main stem coronary artery which was not targeted for angioplasty, but may have been traumatized by either the balloon dilatation or guiding catheters. However, the former seemed the more likely as there was evidence of the restenosis process along the entire segment occupied by the dilating balloon. The histological evidence suggests that the restenosis process found in animals is the same as that responsible for the deterioration in the minimal lumen diameter and the reference diameter shown in our study. Kaltenbach *et al.* [13] in one of the few studies with a high percentage follow-up rate showed, that almost all patients who develop restenosis do so within the first three months. We are able to show that a restenosis process takes place predominantly between two and three months, but at this time we are unable to comment on the possibility of the process continuing beyond this period.

There is very little data concerning the change in the reference diameter following angioplasty, which is perhaps surprising as animal studies would suggest that coronary artery segments involved in the dilatation procedure would also expect to be involved in the intimal proliferation process [23]. The fact that, in our study, the acceleration of deterioration in the reference diameter occurs at the same time as that in the minimal lumen diameter suggests that the underlying process is the same. The change has an important effect on the percentage diameter stenosis measurement and will tend to underestimate the restenosis process. It further reinforces the importance of using an accurate measurement system in this type of study.

Conclusion

The use of an accurate computer-assisted system for the measurement of coronary artery lesions has enabled a more accurate determination of the changes that occur in coronary artery lesions following dilatation. Early following the procedure there is a variable response with both improvement and deterioration of the minimal lumen diameter, whereas by 90 days the response is more uniform with a significant deterioration being evident. The change in reference diameter follows a similar pattern to that of the mean minimal' lumen diameter, presumably because it is also involved in the dilatation process, and will lead to an underestimation of changes that occur if percentage diameter stenosis is used as the sole measurement.

References

1. DeRouen TA, Murray JA, Owen W: Variability in the analysis of coronary arteriograms. Circulation 55: 324–328, 1977.
2. Detre KM, Wright E, Murphy ML, Takaro T: Observer agreement in evaluating coronary angiograms. Circulation 52: 979–986, 1975.
3. Zir LM, Miller SW, Dinsmore RE, Gilbert JP, Harthorne JW: Interobserver variability in coronary angiography. Circulation 53: 627–632, 1976.

4. Scoblionko DP, Brown BG, Mitten S, Caldwell JH, Kennedy JW, Bolson EL, Dodge HT: A new digital electronic caliper for measurement of coronary arterial stenosis: comparison with visual estimates and computer-assisted measurements. Am J Cardiol 53: 689—693, 1984.

5. Sanz ML, Mancini GBJ, LeFree MT, Mickelson JK, Starling MR, Vogel RA, Topol EJ: Variability of quantitative digital subtraction coronary angiography before and after percutaneous transluminal coronary angioplasty. Am J Cardiol 60: 55—60, 1987.

6. Feyter PJ de, Serruys PW, Brand M van den, Balakumaran K, Mochtar B, Soward AL, Arnold AER, Hugenholtz PG: Emergency coronary angioplasty in refractory unstable angina. N Engl J Med 313: 342—346, 1985.

7. Blackburn H: Electrocardiographic classification for population comparisons. The Minnesota code. J Electrocardiol 2: 5—10, 1969.

8. Reiber JHC, Serruys PW, Kooijman CJ, Wijns W, Slager CJ, Gerbrands JJ, Schuurbiers JCH, Boer A den, Hugenholtz PG: Assessment of short-, medium-, and long-term variations in arterial dimensions from computer-assisted quantitation of coronary cineangiograms. Circulation 71: 280—288, 1985.

9. Reiber JHC, Serruys PW, Kooijman CJ, Slager CJ, Schuurbiers JCH, Boer A den: Approaches toward standardization in acquisition and quantitation of arterial dimensions from cineangiograms. In: Reiber JHC, Serruys PW, (eds.). State of the art in quantitative coronary arteriography. Martinus Nijhoff Publishers, Dordrecht/Boston/Lancaster, 1986: 145—172.

10. Wijns W, Serruys PW, Reiber JHC, Brand M van den, Simoons ML, Kooijman CJ, Balakumaran K, Hugenholtz PG: Quantitative angiography of the left anterior descending coronary artery: correlations with pressure gradient and results of exercise thallium scintigraphy. Circulation 71: 273—279, 1985.

11. Kooijman CJ, Reiber JHC, Gerbrands JJ, Schuurbiers JCH, Slager CJ, Boer A den, Serruys PW: Computer-aided quantitation of the severity of coronary obstructions from single view cineangiograms. First IEEE Comp Soc Int Symp on Medical Imaging and Image Interpretation, IEEE Cat No. 82 CH 1804-4, 1982, pp 59—64.

12. Reiber JHC, Serruys PW, Slager CJ: Quantitative coronary and left ventricular cineangiography; methodology and clinical applications. Martinus Nijhoff Publishers, Boston/Dordrecht/Lancaster, 1986.

13. Kaltenbach M, Kober G, Scherer D, Vallbracht C: Recurrence rate after successful coronary angioplasty. Eur Heart J 6: 276—281, 1985.

14. Leimgruber PP, Roubin GS, Hollman J, Cotsonls GA, Meier B, Douglas JS, King III SB, Gruentzig AR: Restenosis after successful coronary angioplasty in patients with single-vessel disease. Circulation 73: 710—717, 1986.

15. Holmes Jr DR, Vlietstra RE, Smith HC, Vetrovec GW, Kent KM, Cowley MJ, Faxon DP, Gruentzig AR, Kelsey SF, Detre KM, Raden MJ van, Mock MB: Restenosis after percutaneous transluminal coronary angioplasty (PTCA): A report from the PTCA Registry of the National Heart, Lung, and Blood Institute. Am J Cardiol 53: 77C—81C, 1984.

16. Johnson MR, Brayden GP, Ericksen EE, Collins SM, Skorton DJ, Harrison DG, Marcus ML, White CW: Changes in cross-sectional area of the coronary lumen in the six months after angioplasty: a quantitative analysis of the variable response to percutaneous transluminal angioplasty. Circulation 73: 467—475, 1986.

17. Levine S, Ewels CJ, Rosing DR, Kent KM: Coronary angioplasty: clinical and angiographic follow-up. Am J Cardiol 55: 673—676, 1985.

18. Legrand V, Aueron FM, Bates ER, O'Neill WW, Hodgson JMcB, Mancini GBJ, Vogel RA: Value of exercise radionuclide ventriculography and thallium—201 scintigraphy in evaluating successful coronary angioplasty: comparison with coronary flow reserve, translesional gradient and percent diameter stenosis. Eur Heart J 8: 329—339, 1987.

19. Kramer JR, Kitazuma H, Proudfit WL, Matsucha Y, Williams GW, Sones FM: Progession and regression of coronary atherosclerosis: Relation to risk factors. Am Heart J 105: 134—144, 1983.
20. Bruschke AVG, Wijers TS, Kolsters W, Landmann J: The anatomic evolution of coronary artery disease demonstrated by coronary arteriography in 256 nonoperated patients. Circulation 63: 527—536, 1981.
21. Kramer JR, Matsuda Y, Mulligan JC, Aronow M, Proudfit WL: Progression of coronary atherosclerosis. Circulation 63: 519—526, 1981.
22. Shub C, Vlietstra RE, Smith HC, Fulton RE, Elveback LR. The unpredictable progression of symptomatic coronary artery disease. A serial clinical-angiographic analysis. Mayo Clin Proc 56: 155—160, 1981.
23. Steele PM, Chesebro JH, Stanson AW, Holmes Jr DR, Dewanjee MK, Badimon L, Fuster V: Balloon angioplasty. Natural history of the pathophysiological response to injury in a pig model. Circ Res 57: 105—112, 1985.
24. Essed CE, Brand M van den, Becker AE: Transluminal coronary angioplasty and early restenosis: fibrocellular occlusion after wall laceration. Br Heart J 49: 393—396, 1983.
25. Waller BF, McManus BM, Gorfinkel HJ, Kishel JC, Schmidt ECH, Kent KM, Roberts WC: Status of the major epicardial coronary arteries 80 to 150 days after percutaneous transluminal coronary angioplasty. Analysis of 3 necropsy patients. Am J Cardiol 51: 81—84, 1983.
26. Austin GE, Ratliff NB, Hollman J, Tabei S, Philips DF: Intimal proliferation of smooth muscle cells as an explanation for recurrent coronary artery stenosis after percutaneous transluminal coronary angioplasty. J Am Coll Cardiol 6: 369—375, 1985.
27. Hollman J, Austin GE, Gruentzig AR, Douglas Jr JS, King III SB: Coronary artery spasm at the site of angioplasty in the first 2 months after successful percutaneous transluminal coronary angioplasty. J Am Coll Cardiol 2: 1039—1045, 1983.
28. Waller BF, Rothbaum DA, Gorfinkel HJ, Ulbright TM, Linnemeier TJ, Berger SM: Morphologic observations after percutaneous transluminal balloon angioplasty of early and late aortocoronary saphenous vein bypass grafts. J Am Coll Cardiol 4: 784—792, 1984.
29. Waller BF, Pinkerton CA, Foster LN: Morphologic evidence of accelerated left main coronary artery stenosis: a late complication of percutaneous transluminal balloon angioplasty of the proximal left anterior descending coronary artery. J Am Coll Cardiol 9: 1019—1023, 1987.

12. How to assess the immediate results of PTCA. Should we use pressure gradient, flow reserve or minimal luminal cross-sectional area?

PATRICK W. SERRUYS, F. ZIJLSTRA, Y. JUILLIÈRE,
P. J. DE FEYTER, M. VD BRAND, H. SURYAPRANATA, and
J. H. C. REIBER

SUMMARY. Intracoronary blood flow velocity measurements with a Doppler probe, and the radiographic assessment of myocardial perfusion with contrast media have previously been used to investigate regional coronary flow reserve. We have applied both techniques in the same patients to measure the immediate improvement in coronary flow reserve as a result of angioplasty. In a group of 13 consecutive patients with a single proximal stenosis, coronary flow reserve was measured pre- and post-angioplasty by digital subtraction cineangiography, while Doppler measurements before and after papaverine were obtained pre- and post-angioplasty in the proximal part of the stenotic vessel. As a result of the angioplasty, coronary flow reserve measured with the radiographic technique (mean ± s.d.) increased from 1.1. ± 0.4 to 2.2 ± 0.4 ($p < 0.001$), while coronary flow reserve measured with the Doppler probe (mean ± s.d.) increased from 1.2 ± 0.3 to 2.4 ± 0.4 ($p < 0.001$). Pharmacologically induced hyperemia measured with the radiographic technique and with the Doppler probe were linearly related ($r = 0.91$ with an SEE = 0.3); this excellent relation confirmed the reliability of the intracoronary measurements. Using these two independent techniques coronary flow reserve immediately after angioplasty was found to be substantially improved but still abnormal. In a more recent study, we selected 18 patients without angina and with normal exercise thallium scintigraphy 5 months after successful percutaneous transluminal coronary angioplasty. We compared their coronary flow reserve with the flow reserve of 24 patients with angiographically normal coronary arteries, to establish whether angioplasty can restore coronary flow reserve of atherosclerotic coronary arteries to a normal level. We studied the quantitative cineangiographic changes and the concomitant alterations in coronary flow reserve resulting from angioplasty, as well as the subsequent changes 5 months later. Coronary flow reserve was measured with digital subtraction cineangiography. Angioplasty resulted in an increase in minimal obstruction area (mean ± s.d.) from 1.0 ± 0.5 to 3.6 ± 0.8 mm² and in coronary flow reserve (mean ± s.d.) from 1.0 ± 0.3 to 2.5 ± 0.6 immediately following angioplasty. Five months later, a substantial and significant ($p < 0.05$) late increase in obstruction area (4.3 ± 1.4 mm²) and flow reserve (3.8 ± 1.1) had occurred. In 72% of our patients coronary flow reserve was restored to normal, 5 months after angioplasty.

It is concluded that changes in stenosis geometry are likely to be one of the major determinants of this late normalization of coronary flow reserve.

Introduction

Since the introduction of coronary angioplasty in 1977 [1], this procedure has

J. C. Reiber & P. W. Serruys (eds.), New Developments in Quantitative Coronary Arteriography,
181—206.

gained increasing importance in the treatment of coronary artery obstructions. So far, the immediate results of the procedure have been assessed by coronary angiography and on the basis of the residual pressure gradient. However, the change in luminal size of an artery following the mechanical disruption of its internal wall cannot be assessed accurately from the detected angiographic contours [2, 3]. Also, while the measured residual pressure gradient may have long-term prognostic value, it reflects only the hemodynamic state at rest [4, 5]. Recently, the assessment of coronary flow reserve have been proposed as a better method to evaluate the functional consequences of a coronary artery obstruction [6, 7].

Papaverine is currently regarded as the ideal vasodilator for the induction of maximal hyperemia, since its intracoronary administration results in a potent and short-lasting hyperemia [8, 9].

Intracoronary blood flow velocity measurements with a Doppler probe, and the radiographic assessment of myocardial perfusion with contrast media have previously been used to investigate regional coronary flow reserve [10—16]. In the present study we applied both techniques to measure the immediate improvement in coronary flow reserve as a result of PTCA. Although coronary angioplasty has been shown to result in symptomatic, hemodynamic and functional improvement [17—19], doubt has remained whether this procedure can restore coronary flow reserve of atherosclerotic coronary arteries to a normal level [20—22]. Therefore, we selected 18 patients that were free of angina and had a normal exercise thallium scintigram 5 months after angioplasty, and compared their radiographically measured coronary flow reserve with the flow reserve of 24 patients with angiographically normal coronary arteries. We describe the quantitative cineangiographic changes and the concomitant alterations in coronary flow reserve resulting from the acute intervention, as well as the subsequent changes as observed 5 months after coronary angioplasty.

Patients and methods

The first study group consisted of thirteen patients who underwent an elective PTCA for angina pectoris. All patients had evidence of myocardial ischemia as indicated either by ECG changes at rest or at exercise, and/or during exercise thallium scintigraphy. Informed consent was obtained for the additional investigations. All patients were studied without premedication, but their medical treatment (nitrates, calcium antagonists and beta-blockers) was continued on the day of the procedure.

The second study population consisted of 24 patients with angiographically normal coronary arteries (12 have been published previously) [14] and 18 patients with single vessel coronary artery disease. These 18 patients had undergone successful angioplasty for disabling angina refractory to intensive pharmacological treatment. They were selected on the basis of a normal exercise thallium scintigram and complete relief of chest pain 5 months after angioplasty, when coronary angiography and left ventriculography were performed as part of an ongoing study on restenosis after angioplasty. Informed consent was obtained for all investigations. Before angioplasty pharmacological treatment consisted of nitrates, calcium antagonists and beta-blockers, and during the 5 months after angioplasty the patients were treated with aspirin 500 mg/day and nifedipine 60 mg/day. All 42 patients had normal systolic and diastolic wall motion and an ejection fraction of more than 55%. Patients with left ventricular hypertrophy, valvular heart disease, angiographic evidence of collateral circulation, anemia, polycythemia or hypertension were excluded because these conditions may influence coronary flow reserve [23—25].

Protocol of the investigational procedure in the first study group

1. Coronary cineangiography was performed in at least two, preferably orthogonal, projections for quantitative analysis of the coronary artery stenosis.
2. Coronary flow reserve was assessed by digital subtraction cineangiography (DSC), following the induction of pharmacological hyperemia (PH) by 12.5 mg papaverine injected through the guiding catheter, (8 Fr, Angiomedics®).
3. A long guide wire (length: 315 cm, diameter: 0.014 inch) was passed through the coronary artery stenosis.
4. A balloon catheter with a Doppler probe (DOP) at the tip was advanced over the guide wire into the coronary artery to measure coronary blood flow velocity. The precise location of the tip of the balloon catheter with respect to the stenotic lesion — immediately proximal to the lesion and beyond any major side branches — was determined by injection of contrast medium. After recording of the baseline intracoronary blood flow velocity, PH was induced by injecting 12.5 mg papaverine through the guiding catheter. The ratio of peak mean intracoronary blood flow velocity to the baseline value (PH-DOP) was then determined.
5. Thereafter, the balloon was advanced across the stenosis and 3 to 6 inflations up to 12 atmospheres were used to dilate the stenosis until repeat cineangiography showed a good result (< 50% diameter stenosis). The mean total inflation time was 172 s/patient (range: 148—352 s).
6. During and following each balloon inflation coronary blood flow velocity was recorded continuously with the Doppler probe situated across the stenotic lesion (Fig. 1a). Reactive hyperemia immediately after the final balloon deflation (RH) was calculated as the ratio of maximal mean intra-

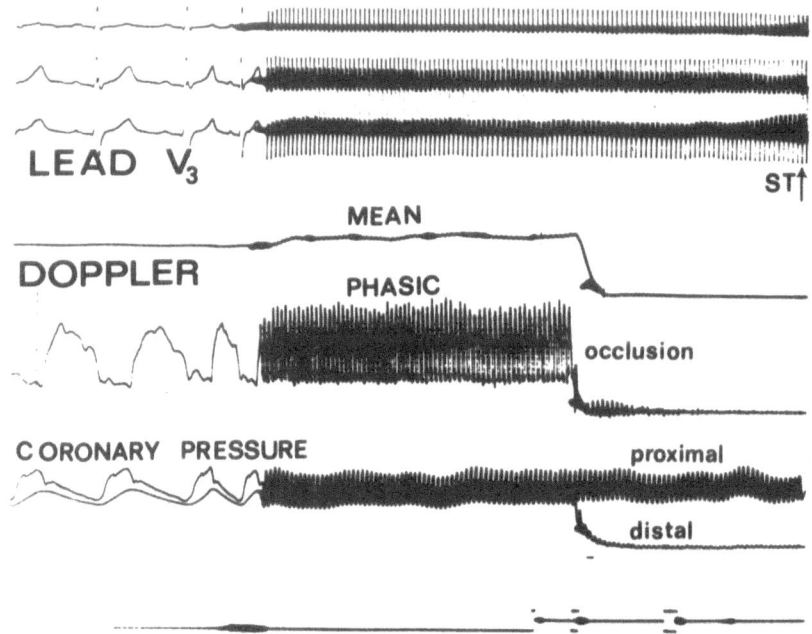

LEAD V₃   ST↑

MEAN

DOPPLER

PHASIC

occlusion

CORONARY PRESSURE   proximal

distal

Fig. 1a.

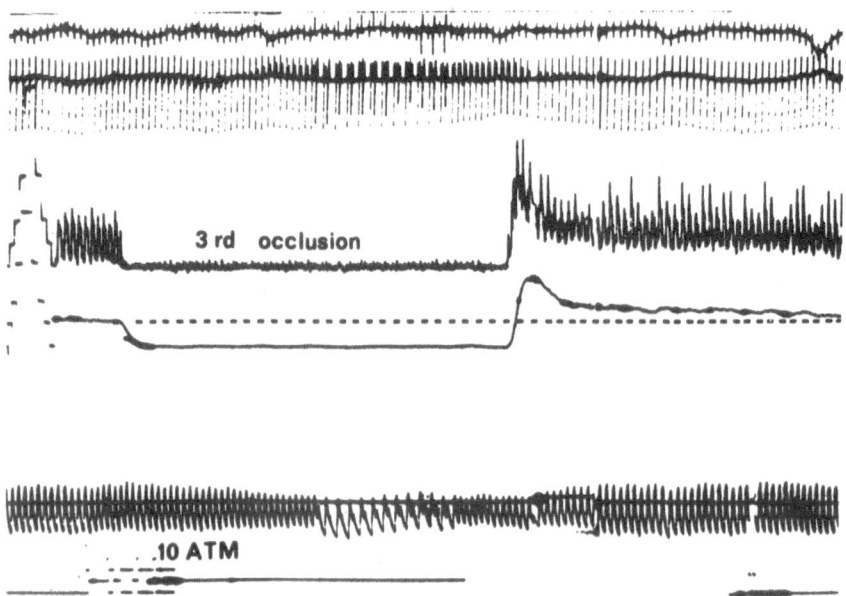

3rd occlusion

.10 ATM

Fig. 1b.

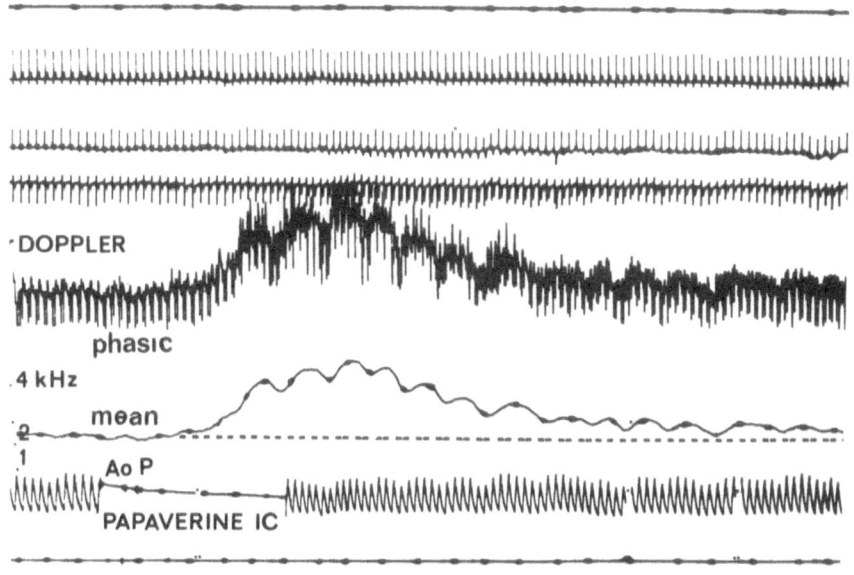

Fig. 1c.

Figure 1. (a) ECG-leads, mean and phasic Doppler signal, translesional pressure-gradient before and during a balloon inflation. The precordial lead V3 shows ST-segment elevation. (b) Example of reactive hyperemia after a third transluminal occlusion using a balloon inflating pressure of 10 atmosphere (ATM). (c) Example of hyperemia pharmacologically induced with intracoronary (i.c) papaverine and measured with the Doppler probe in the prestenotic segment of the dilated vessel. From top to bottom: ECG-leads, phasic and mean Doppler signal and aortic pressure (AoP).

coronary blood flow velocity to stabilized blood flow velocity, observed after the hyperemia had subsided (Fig. 1b).
7. With the Doppler tip pulled back into the proximal part of the coronary artery, PH-DOP was assessed again (Fig. 1c).
8. After removal of the balloon catheter and the guide wire, coronary flow reserve was measured with digital subtraction cineangiography, (PH-DSC, as in 2).
9. Coronary cineangiography was repeated post-PTCA in the same projections as used at the start of the procedure (see 1), for quantitative analysis of the coronary artery stenosis.

Intracoronary blood flow velocity measurements

A 20 MHz ultrasonic crystal mounted on the tip of the angioplasty catheter was used in all patients. Recently, Sibley *et al.* [16] validated clinically and experimentally the ability of a similar catheter with an end-mounted piezo-electric crystal to provide accurate continuous on-line measurements of coronary blood flow velocity and vasodilator reserve [16]. A balloon diameter size of 3.0 mm was used in 10 patients, and 3.4 mm in 3 patients. The cross-sectional area of the catheter with the balloon deflated was 1.5 mm^2.

The Doppler crystal is a 1.0 mm diameter annulus with a 0.5 mm central hole (see Fig. 2). Two leads are soldered to the crystal and pass through the

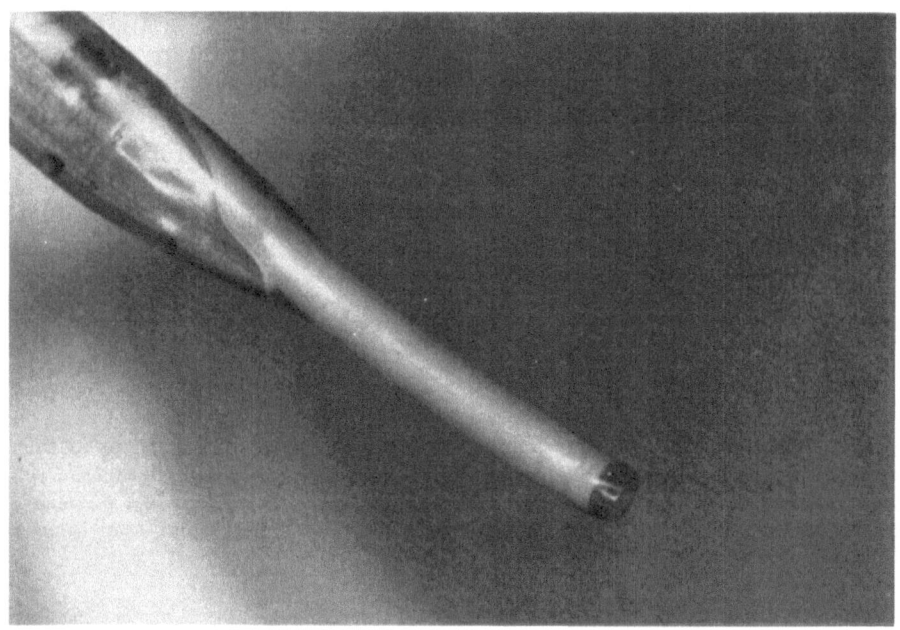

(a)

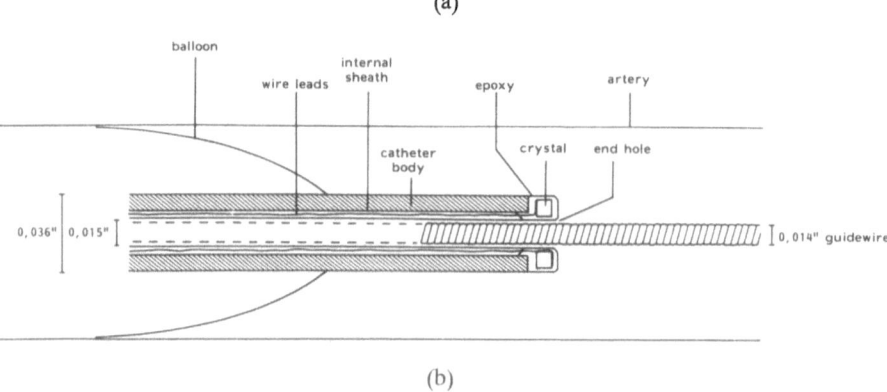

(b)

Figure 2. (a) Tip of a Doppler-balloon catheter showing the end-mounted ultrasonic crystal, and a radiopaque marker within the ballon. (b) Schematic cross-sectional drawing of Doppler-balloon catheter.

catheter between the original 0.5 mm lumen and a thin-walled tube which serves as a new 0.4 mm lumen. The leads exit near the proximal luer hub and are wired to a two pin plug for connection to the pulsed Doppler instrument. The connector cable contains an integral torroidal isolation transformer which insulates the patient from the instrument and which also provides impedance matching for more efficient energy transfer. The new inner lumen extends from the luer hub through the crystal providing a smooth unobstructed path for a guide wire. Blood flow velocity is measured from the catheter tip transducer using a range-gated 20 MHz pulsed Doppler-ultrasonic piezocrystal designed specially for this purpose (Baylor College of Medicine). The master oscillator frequency of 20 MHz is pulsed at a frequency of 62.5 kHz. Each pulse is approximately one millisecond in width and therefore contains 20 cycles of the master oscillator frequency.

The parameters chosen (master oscillator frequency = 20 MHz and pulse repetition frequency = 62.5 kHz) allow velocities up to 100 cm/s to be recorded at a distance of up to 1 cm from the catheter tip. The sampling window was individually adjusted to obtain the most optimal signal which (usually) resulted in a sampling window of 1.8 mm (range 1.5–2.0). The output of the pulsed Doppler is a frequency shift (f, kHz) which can be related to blood velocity by the Doppler equation:

$$f = 2F(V/c) \cos \alpha,$$

where F is the ultrasonic frequency (20 MHz), V is the velocity within the sample volume, c is the speed of sound in blood (1500 m/s), and α is the angle between the velocity vector and the sound beam. Using an end-mounted crystal with the catheter parallel ($\pm 20°$) to the vessel axis, $\cos \alpha = 1 \pm 6\%$, and the relation between the Doppler shift and velocity is approximately 3.75 cm/s per kHz [16]. Previous calibration experiments in canine femoral and coronary arteries have shown that the measured Doppler shift frequency is proportional to volume flow measured by timed collection [10–12, 16].

Coronary flow reserve measurements with digital subtraction cineangiography (CFR-DSC)

The coronary flow reserve measurement from 35 mm cinefilm has been implemented on the CAAS [14]. The heart was atrially paced at a rate just above the spontaneous heart rate. An ECG-triggered injection into the coronary artery was made with Iopamidol at 37°C through a Medrad Mark IV® infusion pump. The nonionic contrast agent has a viscosity of 9.4 cP at 37°, an osmolality of 0.796 osm/kg and an iodine content of 370 mg/ml. For the left coronary artery 7 ml of contrast was injected at a flow rate of 4 ml/s, and the coronary angiogram obtained in the left anterior oblique projection. For the right coronary artery 5 ml was injected at a flow rate of 3 ml/s, and the angiogram taken in the left or right anterior oblique projection. The injection rate of the contrast medium was judged to be adequate if backflow of contrast medium into the aorta occurred. The angiogram was repeated 30 s after PH, produced by a bolus injection of 12.5 mg papaverine into the coronary artery by way of the guiding catheter [8, 9]. Five or six consecutive end-diastolic cineframes were selected for analysis. Logarithmic nonmagnified mask-mode background subtraction was applied to the image subset to eliminate noncontrast medium densities. The last end-diastolic frame prior to the administration of contrast was chosen as the mask. From the sequence of background subtracted images, a contrast arrival time image was determined using an empirically derived fixed density threshold [14]. Each pixel was labeled with the sequence number of the cardiac cycle, numbered from the cycle of the ECG-triggered contrast injection, in which the pixel intensity level first exceeded the threshold. In addition to the contrast arrival time image, a density image was computed, with each pixel intensity value being representative of the maximal local contrast medium accumulation. The CFR-DSC was defined as the ratio of the regional flow computed from a hyperemic image divided by the regional flow of the corresponding baseline image.

Regional flow values were quantitatively determined using the following videodensitometric principle: regional blood flow (Q) = regional vascular volume/transit time. Regional vascular volume was assessed from logarithmic mask-mode subtraction images, using the Lambert-Beer relationship. CFR can then be calculated as:

$$\text{CFR} = \frac{Q_h}{Q_b} = \frac{CD_h}{AT_h} : \frac{CD_b}{AT_b}$$

where CD is the mean contrast density and AT the mean appearance time at baseline (b) and hyperemia (h). Mean contrast medium appearance time and density were computed within a user-defined region-of-interest, which was chosen so that the epicardial coronary arteries visible on the angiogram, the coronary sinus, and the great cardiac vein were all excluded from the analysis [14].

Quantitative analysis of the coronary artery

The determination of coronary arterial dimensions from 35 mm cinefilm was performed with a computer-based Cardiovascular Angiography Analysis System (CAAS), previously described in detail [14, 26, 27]. In essence, boundaries of a selected coronary artery segment are detected automatically from optically magnified and video digitized regions-of-interest of a cine-frame. The absolute diameter of the stenosis in mm is determined using the guiding catheter as a scaling device. This involves the automatic edge-detection of the boundaries of the catheter *in situ* and the comparison of this value with the actual diameter measurement of the catheter using a micrometer. Calibration of the diameter in absolute values (mm) is achieved by comparing the mean diameter of the guiding catheter in pixels with the measured size in millimeters. Each catheter is measured individually [28]. To correct the detected contour of the arterial and catheter segments for pincushion distortion, a correction vector is computed for each pixel based on a computer-processed cineframe with a centimeter grid placed against the input screen of the image intensifier [27]. Since the functional significance of a stenosis is related to the expected normal cross-sectional area of the vessel at the point of obstruction, we use a computer-estimation of the original arterial dimension at the site of the obstruction to define the inter-polated reference region [26, 27]. The interpolated percentage area stenosis (AS) and the minimal luminal cross-sectional area (mm^2) are then calculated from at least two, preferably orthogonal, projections. The length of the lesion is then determined from the diameter function on the basis of a curvature analysis. A mean of 2.3 angiographic projections/patient were used in this study.

Exercise thallium scintigraphy

In the second study group, exercise studies were performed 5 ± 0.4 months after angioplasty. The patients performed a symptom-limited exercise test on the bicycle ergometer with stepwise increments of 20 Watt/min. All patients exercised to more than 80% of their expected normal exercise capacity (normalized for age, sex and length). One minute before peak exercise 1.5 mCi thallium-201 was injected intravenously. Imaging was started 3 min later in 3 views: anterior, left anterior oblique 45° and 65°. Static planar images were obtained after exercise and 4 hours later and processed on a DEC Gamma-11 system with a quantification procedure developed at our institution [29]. The late image was corrected for acquisition time differences with respect to the early image. The exercise and redistribution images were registered on the basis of the detected positions of two point sources; for these purposes, the technician briefly holds a Cobalt-57 marker pen at the appropriate positions on the patient's chest immediately prior to the Tl-201 acquisition. After automated left ventricular contour detection and interpolative background correction, circumferential profiles were computed at 6° intervals. The profiles of the early and late images were normalized for the maximal value in the early image excluding the outflow tract of the left ventricle. The analog Polaroid® images from the gamma camera, the processed images and the circumferential profiles were analyzed prospectively on a routine basis by 3 experienced observers without knowledge of the angiographic data. Redistribution and persistent defects were considered abnormal [29, 30].

Statistical analysis

All comparisons between groups were made after variance analysis with the Student's *t*-test for paired or unpaired observations. Linear regression analyses were used to define the relationships between the various measurements and the angiographic parameters.

Results

Quantitative analysis of the coronary angiogram

In the first study group (Table 1), the minimal luminal cross-sectional area (mean ± s.d.) increased from 1.2 ± 0.8 to 3.6 ± 1.1 mm^2 as an immediate result of the angioplasty procedure. Percentage diameter stenosis (mean ± s.d.) decreased from 61 ± 11% to 29 ± 10%. Percentage area stenosis (mean ± s.d.) decreased from 83 ± 10% to 49 ± 14%. The interpolated reference area (mean ± s.d.) at the site of obstruction was 7.1 ± 1.6 mm^2.

In the second study group, the quantitative cineangiographic measurements were made before, immediately after and 5 months following angioplasty (Table 2). The changes in minimal cross-sectional obstruction area are shown in Fig. 3 and the changes in percentage diameter stenosis in Fig. 4. Percentage area stenosis (mean ± s.d.) decreased from 85 ± 7% to 49 ± 12% immediately following angioplasty. Five months later percentage area stenosis had further decreased to 38 ± 16% ($p < 0.05$).

Assessment of coronary flow reserve using pharmacologically induced hyperemia with digital subtraction cineangiography (PH-DSC, Table 1)

In the first study group, PH-DSC was measured before and after angioplasty in the myocardium supplied by the dilated coronary artery. PH-DSC (mean ± s.d.) increased from 1.1 ± 0.4 to 2.2 ± 0.4 ($p < 0.001$). PH-DSC was also measured in a coronary artery with no angiographically significant coronary artery disease. PH-DSC (mean ± s.d.) in these vessels was 3.3 ± 0.7

191

Table 1. Results: quantitative angiographic data and coronary flow reserve in the first study group.

Pat	vessel	no of dil	QACA before PTCA			after PTCA			CFR before PTCA		after PTCA		
			OA	DS	AS	OA	DS	AS	PH-DOP	PH-DSC	RH	PH-DOP	PH-DSC
1	LAD	3	1.1	64	87	5.4	19	35	–	1.4	2.2	2.1	2.0
	CX*									5.0			
2	LAD	3	2.3	54	79	4.8	30	51	1.0	–	2.9	2.9	3.3
3	RCA	6	0.6	71	91	2.9	40	64	–	–	2.8	3.0	2.8
4	RCA	3	0.3	76	94	2.2	41	66	–	–	1.4	1.1	1.2
5	LAD	4	1.9	53	78	3.3	39	63	0.9	0.6	2.8	2.9	2.4
6	LAD	4	0.9	63	86	3.5	22	40	0.9	1.0	2.0	1.8	2.0
	CX*									3.0			
7	LAD	4	1.6	47	72	3.5	30	51	1.8	2.0	2.6	2.7	2.4
	CX*									2.9			
8	LAD	4	0.7	65	88	3.7	13	24	1.1	0.8	2.2	2.3	2.2
	CX*									2.8			
9	LAD	4	1.2	59	83	4.5	21	37	1.3	1.1	3.0	2.3	3.0
	CX									3.3			
10	CX	6	0.5	74	93	2.5	28	49	–	1.0	2.0	1.9	1.7
	LAD*									3.9			
11	CX	4	0.6	69	90	2.7	45	69	–	0.9	1.7	2.0	2.2
	LAD*									3.1			
12	LAD	5	2.9	36	59	5.3	23	41	1.0	1.1	2.1	2.2	1.7
	CX*									2.6			
13	LAD	3	0.7	58	82	2.9	26	44	1.2	1.4	2.6	2.4	2.7
	CX*									3.5			

Pat = patient; no of dil = number of dilatations; QACA = quantitative analysis of the coronary angiogram; PTCA = percutaneous transluminal coronary angioplasty; DS = percentage diameter stenosis; OA = minimal obstruction area (mm²); AS = percentage area stenosis; CFR = coronary flow reserve; PH-DOP = ratio of maximal coronary blood flow velocity after intracoronary papaverine as compared to baseline; PH-DSC = digital subtraction cineangiographic measurement of CFR; RH = reactive hyperemia after the final dilatation; * = nondiseased coronary artery.

Table 2. Results: Coronary flow reserve and quantitative angiographic data in the second study group.

Pat	age	sex	vessel	PTCA before			after			5 months follow-up		
				OA	DS	CFR	OA	DS	CFR	OA	DS	CFR
1	54	M	LAD	1.2	53	1.0	5.4	14	3.0	5.2	6	2.9
			CX			3.9			3.7			4.3
2	31	M	LAD	0.5	70	1.0	3.7	15	2.3	3.1	19	2.5
			CX			3.3			2.5			3.1
3	53	F	LAD	0.5	72	0.6	3.3	27	2.8	5.9	7	3.7
			CX			2.6			2.5			2.2
4	36	M	LAD	0.4	70	1.2	3.7	14	3.3	2.8	20	2.9
			CX			3.2			3.4			3.3
5	62	M	LAD	0.8	66	1.0	2.5	44	2.1	3.8	32	3.8
			CX			2.6			2.8			2.9
6	42	M	CX	0.7	66	0.7	3.8	24	1.5	2.6	38	3.4
			LAD			3.8			3.6			4.1
7	53	M	RCA	1.3	65	0.9	3.6	31	2.2	2.9	35	3.9
8	66	M	LAD	0.7	58	1.4	2.9	26	2.7	3.1	12	2.9
			CX			3.5			3.8			3.4
9	36	M	LAD	1.1	59		3.4	34		6.0	14	4.8
			CX									4.9
10	39	M	LAD	1.2	65		3.0	45		5.2	25	4.1
			CX									3.9
11	56	M	LAD	0.8	72		3.6	39		4.9	27	4.0
			CX									4.4
12	45	M	LAD	0.7	72		3.3	35		3.1	38	3.9
			CX									3.2
13	47	M	LAD	1.2	46		3.4	27		4.7	14	3.9
			CX									5.6
14	58	M	LAD	1.8	58		4.9	27		5.7	20	3.4
			CX									4.1
15	36	M	LAD	1.5	60		5.1	27		4.0	33	2.5
			CX									2.5
16	61	M	RCA	1.7	53		3.1	26		5.0	15	6.3
17	54	F	LAD	1.9	51		3.6	32		6.8	8	6.4
			CX									5.7
18	60	F	LAD	0.4	70		2.4	28		2.4	27	3.4
			CX									3.7

PTCA = percutaneous transluminal coronary angioplasty; pat = patient; OA = minimal cross-sectional obstruction area (mm^2); DS = percentage diameter stenosis; CFR = coronary flow reserve; M = male; F = female; LAD = left anterior descending artery; CX = circumflex artery; RCA = right coronary artery.

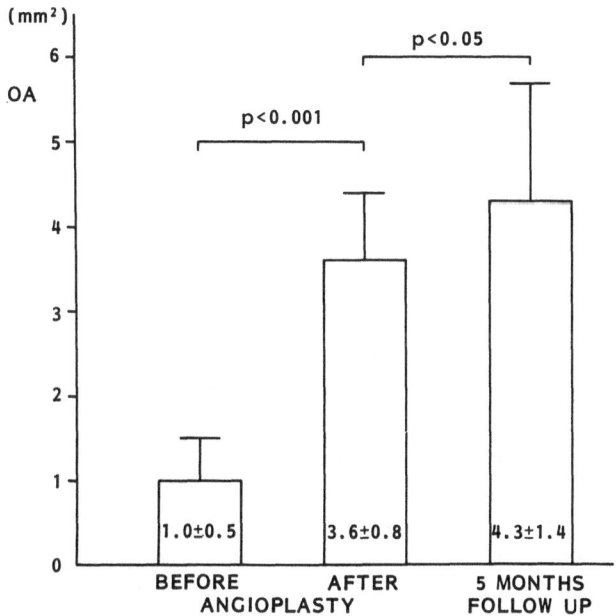

Figure 3. Results of quantitative analyses of coronary angiograms, before, immediately after and 5 months following angioplasty $N = 18$). OA = minimal cross-sectional obstruction area (mm²).

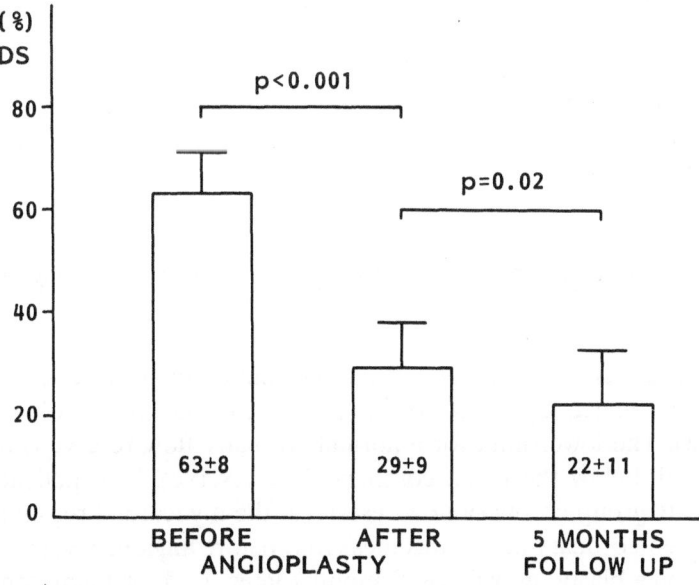

Figure 4. Results of quantitative analyses of coronary angiograms, before, immediately after, and 5 months following angioplasty ($N = 18$). DS = percentage diameter stenosis.

which differed significantly ($p < 0.01$) from the PH-DSC of the dilated coronary artery in the same patients (2.2 ± 0.4).

Assessment of coronary flow reserve, using pharmacologically induced hyperemia, with the Doppler probe (PH-DOP, Table 1)

In 8 patients of the first study group, PH-DOP was measured before and after angioplasty in the dilated coronary artery. The minimal luminal cross-sectional area was 1.5 mm^2 before angioplasty and 3.9 mm^2 after angio-plasty. PH-DOP (mean ± s.d.) increased from 1.2 ± 0.3 to 2.4 ± 0.4 ($p < 0.001$). In the remaining 5 patients no Doppler recording could be made before the angioplasty. They had a mean minimal luminal cross-sectional area before angioplasty of 0.6 mm^2, and 3.1 mm^2 after angioplasty. Since the guide wire (0.014 inch) with a cross-sectional area of 0.12 mm^2 had already been passed through the stenosis when these measurements were made, the absence of a recordable Doppler signal indicated an extreme reduction in blood flow velocity in the vessel proximal to the stenotic lesion. The mean PH-DOP after the angioplasty procedure was 2.0 in these 5 patients, which is comparable to the CFR-DOP of the other 8 patients.

Relation between the pharmacologically induced hyperemia (PH) measured by digital subtraction cineangiography (DSC) and by the Doppler probe (DOP)

In 7 patients of the first study group, PH-DSC and PH-DOP were measured before angioplasty and in all 13 patients both measurements were made after the procedure. PH-DSC and PH-DOP were linearly related, (Fig. 5): PH-DOP = 0.9 × PH-DSC + 0.3, $r = 0.91$, SEE = 0.3.

Coronary flow reserve before angioplasty, immediately following angioplasty and five months later

In the 24 patients with angiographically normal coronary arteries, coronary flow reserve ranged from 3.4 to 6.5 (Table 3). The mean value was 5.0 (s.d. = 0.8). The lower limit for a normal coronary flow reserve is therefore 3.4 (2 × s.d. below the mean coronary flow reserve). In 8 patients of the second study group coronary flow reserve in the myocardial region supplied by the dilated coronary artery was measured before angioplasty, immediately following angioplasty, as well as 5 months later. In 7 of them consecutive measurements were also obtained of an adjacent myocardial region supplied by a nondilated coronary artery (Table 2 and Fig. 6). The coronary flow

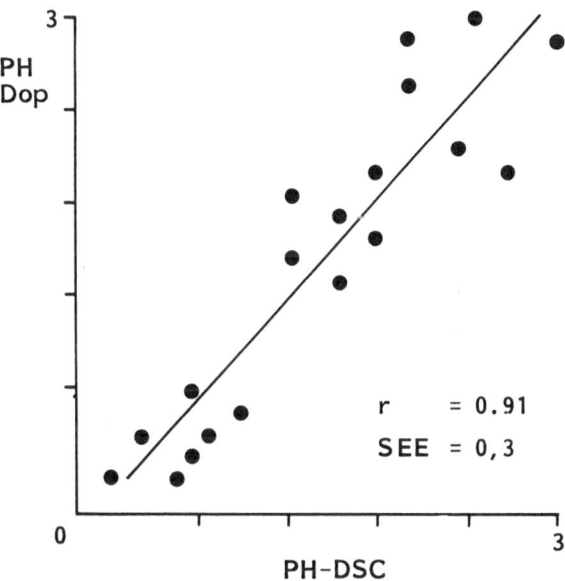

Figure 5. Relationship between pharmacologically induced hyperemia assessed by Doppler (PH-DOP) and pharmacologically induced hyperemia assessed by digital subtraction cine-angiography (PH-DSC). The dotted line is the line of identity. The solid line corresponds to the linear regression equation: PH-DOP = 0.9 × PH-DSC + 0.3 with a regression coefficient of 0.91 and a standard-error-of-the-estimate (SEE) of 0.3.

reserve of these adjacent myocardial regions remained unchanged immediately following angioplasty as well as after 5 months follow-up. Coronary flow reserve (mean ± s.d.) in the myocardial region supplied by the dilated coronary artery increased from 1.0 ± 0.3 to 2.5 ± 0.6 immediately following angioplasty ($p < 0.001$). In none of these patients coronary flow reserve was restored to a normal level immediately following angioplasty. A substantial late improvement ($p < 0.01$) in coronary flow reserve had occurred 5 months later. Coronary flow reserve in the myocardial region supplied by the dilated coronary artery 5 months after angioplasty was of the same magnitude at the coronary flow reserve in the myocardial region supplied by a nondilated and angiographically nondiseased coronary artery.

In all 18 patients of the second study group, coronary flow reserve (mean ± s.d.) was measured 5 months after angioplasty in the myocardial region supplied by the dilated coronary artery, and was 3.8 ± 1.1. In 16 patients of the second study group, coronary flow reserve was also measured in the myocardial region supplied by a nondilated and angiographically nondiseased coronary artery and was 3.8 ± 1.0. In 13 of the 18 patients (72%) coronary flow reserve of the dilated coronary artery was restored to a normal level of at least 3.4, whereas in 5 of 18 patients (28%) coronary flow reserve was still abnormal (Figs. 7 and 8).

Table 3. Results: Coronary flow reserve (CFR) of patients with angiographically normal coronary arteries.

Pat	age	sex	vessel	CFR
1	38	M	LAD	6.5
2	41	M	CX	6.2
3	62	F	LAD	5.3
4	31	M	RCA	5.2
5	60	M	CX	5.0
6	63	M	CX	5.0
7	54	M	CX	5.0
8	48	M	CX	4.0
9	66	F	CX	4.5
10	52	M	LAD	4.0
11	59	M	LAD	5.0
12	59	M	CX	4.8
13	47	M	CX	4.9
14	58	M	LAD	3.7
15	59	M	LAD	4.3
16	54	F	CX	6.4
17	61	M	LAD	4.9
18	62	M	RCA	4.8
19	58	M	LAD	4.7
20	57	M	RCA	4.6
21	64	M	LAD	4.5
22	61	M	LAD	3.4
23	50	M	LAD	6.3
24	58	M	LAD	4.0

CFR = coronary flow reserve; M = male; F = female; LAD = left anterior descending coronary artery; CX = circumflex artery; RCA = right coronary artery.

Linear regression analysis between coronary flow reserve and percentage diameter stenosis showed no significant correlation (Fig. 7), whereas the correlation between coronary flow reserve and the minimal cross-sectional obstruction area was significant (Fig. 8, $r = 0.57$, $p = 0.014$). Coronary flow reserve 5 months after angioplasty was significantly related ($r = 0.74$, $p < 0.001$) to the change in minimal cross-sectional obstruction area occurring between immediately after angioplasty and at follow-up (Fig. 9). In 10 patients the minimal cross-sectional obstruction area 5 months after angioplasty was larger than immediately following the procedure (late improvement). Only one of them had a coronary flow reserve of less than 3.4. In 7 patients of the second study group, the minimal cross-sectional obstruction area 5 months after angioplasty was smaller than the area immediately following the procedure (late deterioration). The percentage of patients showing normalization of coronary flow reserve 5 months after angioplasty

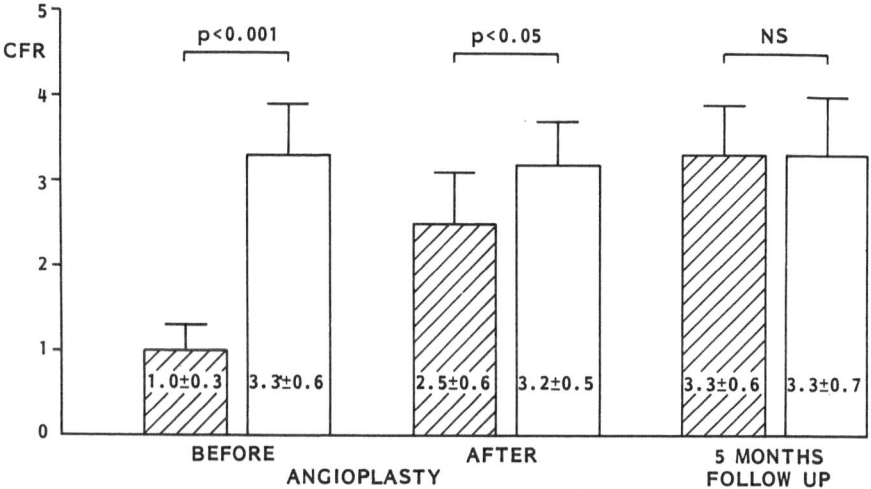

Figure 6. Coronary flow reserve (CFR) measured with digital subtraction cineangiography, before, immediately after and 5 months after angioplasty. The shaded bars represent the CFR of the myocardial region supplied by the dilated coronary artery ($N = 8$). The white bars represent the CFR of an adjacent myocardial region supplied by a nondilated and angiographically normal coronary artery ($N = 7$).

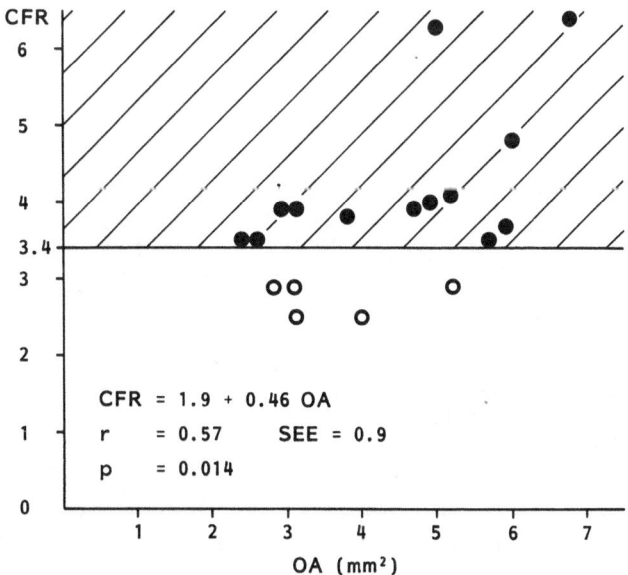

Figure 7. Coronary flow reserve (CFR) plotted against minimal cross-sectional obstruction area (OA) of all 18 patients five months after angioplasty. The lower limit of the normal value for CFR as measured with the digital subtraction cineangiographic technique is 3.4.

198

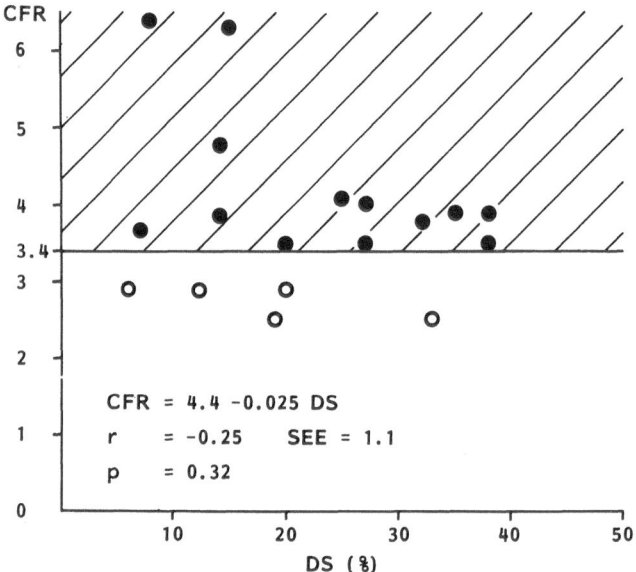

Figure 8. Coronary flow reserve (CFR) plotted against percentage diameter stenosis (DS) of all 18 patients five months after angioplasty. The lower limit of the normal value for CFR as measured with the digital subtraction cineangiographic technique is 3.4.

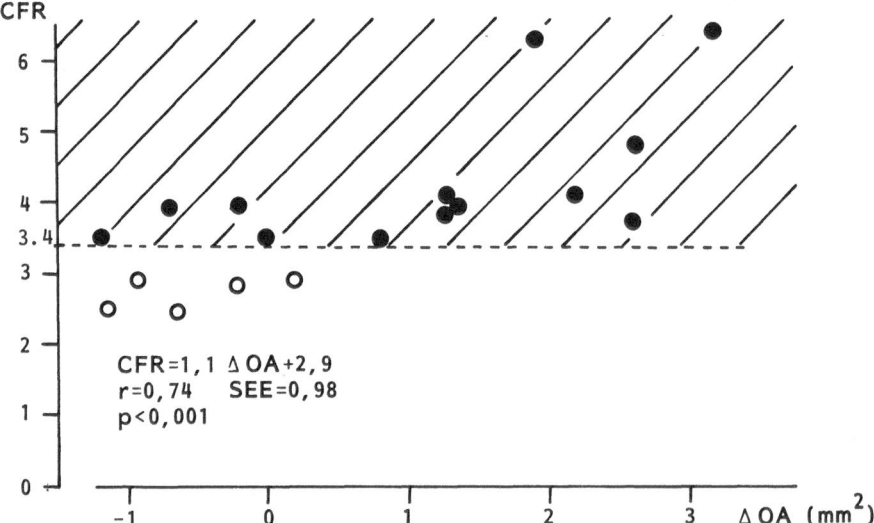

Figure 9. Relationship between coronary flow reserve (CFR) five months after angioplasty and the change that occurred in minimal cross-sectional obstruction area (ΔOA) between immediately after angioplasty and 5 months later. The lower limit of the normal value for CFR as measured with the digital subtraction cineangiographic technique is 3.4.

is substantially higher (p < 0.05, Chi Square test) in the group with late angiographic improvement (90%) compared to the group with late deterioration (43%).

Discussion

The purpose of the present study was twofold. First, to compare before and after an angioplasty procedure in the same individuals two different techniques of assessing regional coronary blood flow; secondly, to establish whether coronary flow reserve in a myocardial region supplied by a stenotic coronary artery could be restored to normal by percutaneous transluminal coronary angioplasty.

Comparison between the intracoronary Doppler blood flow velocity measurements and the radiographic determination of coronary blood flow during hyperemia

Over the last ten years the relationship between volume and Doppler shift measured from the tip of an intravascular catheter has been extensively validated in peripheral and coronary arteries of anesthetized animals [10–12, 16]. The relationship between the Doppler shift (ranging from 0.5 to 8 kHz) and the volume flow (ranging from 15 ml to 400 ml/min) is linear with correlation coefficients generally equal to or greater than 0.95 [10–12, 16]. These results have been obtained irrespective of whether the Doppler crystal was end- or side-mounted on the tip of the catheter. Although excellent correlations between flow velocity and volume flow have been reported in these studies, no attempts have been made to quantify volume flow from the velocity data. Only changes in flow velocity were measured as catheter tip position, crystal angle and vessel diameter cannot be determined with sufficient accuracy to allow volume flow calculations. Similarly, only relative coronary flow rates can be assessed in myocardial regions-of-interest by the quantitative digital radiographic determination of time-density curves. Despite the difficulties associated with the use of contrast media and the densitometric rather than geometric assessment of relative vascular volume, a good correlation (r = 0.92) between electromagnetic flow measurements in the proximal coronary artery and the digital radiographic determinations have been found [31]. As emphasized by Vogel, the individual ratios must be interpreted bearing in mind the 95% confidence limits which result in a standard deviation of 0.35 [15]. The two approaches have methodologically nothing in common and their respective regions-of-interest (myocardial for the radiographic technique and intravascular for the Doppler technique) are basically different. Since the coronary artery lesions selected in this study were discrete, focal and not associated with distal narrowing, it is assumed that the flow ratio measured in the myocardial region-of-interest by the radiographic technique distal to the stenotic lesion, reflects the flow velocity ratio measured proximal or distal to the stenotic lesion in the coronary artery. A similar assumption was made by Hodgson *et al.* in their validation study of the radiographic technique [31]. Despite these limitations we felt justified in comparing both techniques in the same individuals. A reasonable correlation ($r = 0.91$, SEE $= 0.3$) between the two methodological approaches was found, suggesting that both techniques are valuable in measuring changes in regional coronary blood flow reserve as a result of an acute intervention.

Why is the coronary flow reserve not normalized immediately after the angioplasty?

Although coronary flow reserve in the myocardial region supplied by the dilated vessel increased substantially after the angioplasty procedure, it was not restored to normal. This is in accordance with previous reports in the literature [21, 22, 32—36].

In our patients we measured the coronary flow reserve of the adjacent myocardial region supplied by a nonstenotic coronary artery and found a marked difference in response to a vasodilator. This indicates that the abnormal vasodilatory response is restricted to the myocardium supplied by the dilated coronary artery. There are several potential explanations for this phenomenon.

1. Since coronary flow reserve is a ratio between maximal coronary blood flow and resting flow, any increase in resting flow results in a decrease of this ratio. Neither of the techniques we used provided us with absolute measurements of volume flow and we therefore cannot draw any conclusion regarding the resting coronary volume flow after the angioplasty procedure. However, several authors using the thermodilution technique in the coronary sinus or the great cardiac vein have reported comparable resting volume flows before and after angioplasty [37—41].

2. Metabolic, humoral or myogenic factors could potentially play a role in limiting coronary flow reserve after angioplasty [42]. The metabolic derangements (lactate, hypoxanthine, potassium) due to the angioplasty seem quickly reversible [37, 41, 43], and are therefore not likely to be of major significance in this regard. Although humoral factors such as thromboxane release [44] may influence vasoactive regulation in a specific subgroup of patients with complicated angioplasty, so far no scientific evidence has been presented for the persistence of humoral derangements after angioplasty.

However, the long-standing reduction in perfusion pressure distal to the stenotic lesion may induce alterations in the complex mechanism of auto-nomic coronary blood flow autoregulation [13]. A prolonged period of time might be needed before these abnormalities subside. Finally, Bates *et al.* postulated that the difference in coronary flow reserve in men with normal arteries and those who underwent revascularization is related to the athero-sclerotic disease process, affecting the microvascular reactivity [13].

3. The impaired coronary flow reserve could be directly related to the severity of the residual stenosis. Cross-sectional area as measured immedi-ately after angioplasty generally is about threefold increased as a result of the procedure, but it remains grossly abnormal [45]. In a previous study in our laboratory the relationship between cross-sectional obstruction area and coronary flow reserve in patients with stable angina and single vessel coro-nary artery disease has been established [9]. In Fig. 10 this relation is shown with the results of the sequential coronary flow reserve and obstruction area measurements of the present study superimposed. The large majority of data of the present study are within the 95% confidence limits of the relation between flow reserve and obstruction area. Therefore, the persisting reduced

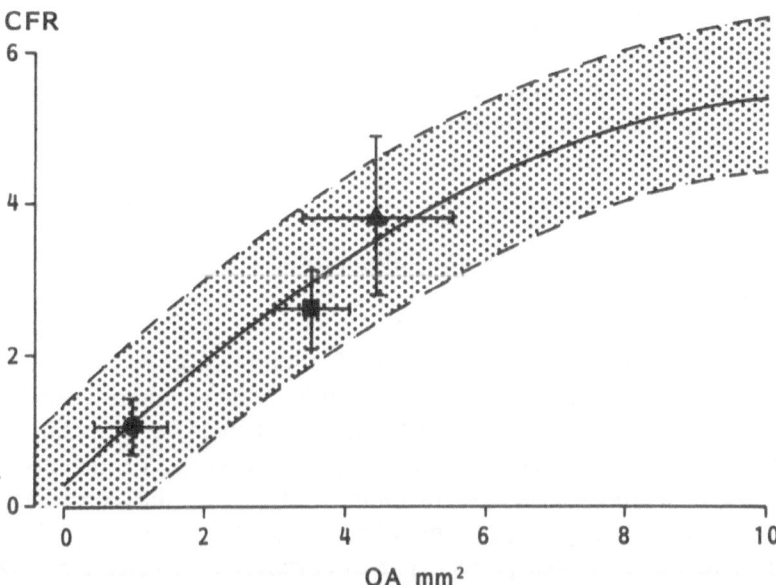

Figure 10. Relationship between coronary flow reserve (CFR) and cross-sectional obstruction area (OA) as previously reported [14]. The solid line is the best-fit curve and the shaded area corresponds to the 95% confidence limits. The mean values and standard deviations of coronary flow reserve and obstruction area as obtained in the present study, before (circle, $N = 8$), immediately after (square, $N = 8$) and five months later (triangle, $N = 18$) are plotted on this diagram.

obstruction area is by itself a sufficient explanation for the limited restoration of coronary flow reserve, although it does not rule out other contributing pathophysiological mechanisms.

Limitations

There are two important limitations of coronary angiography in the setting of angioplasty. Firstly, the changes in luminal size of an artery following the mechanical disruption of its internal wall may be difficult to assess by angiographic means [2, 3]. The irregular shape with intimal tears that fill with contrast medium to a variable extent will result in some overestimation of the true functional luminal size immediately following angioplasty.

Secondly, the extent of coronary atherosclerosis may be difficult to delineate angiographically. McPherson *et al.* [46] documented that substantial intimal atherosclerosis resulting in diffuse obstructive disease that involves the entire length of an epicardial artery, is often present, even when angiograms reveal only discrete lesions. As a consequence, relative measurements of stenosis severity are an inadequate approach to assessing the severity of coronary obstructions. This may explain why 5 of our angioplasty patients with only very mild residual percentage diameter stenoses 5 months after angioplasty still had an abnormal vasodilatory reserve. Also, the fact that cross-sectional obstruction area correlated better with coronary flow reserve than percentage area stenosis suggests the presence of diffuse coronary artery disease in our angioplasty patients [47].

What mechanism is responsible for the normalization of coronary flow reserve 5 months after angioplasty?

Johnson *et al.* [45] as well as Serruys *et al.* [5] found that important morphological changes may take place in the 6 months after angioplasty. In about one-third of Johnson's patients a substantial late increase in minimal cross-sectional obstruction area occurred. In our selected group of patients with no angina and a normal exercise thallium scintigraphy, the percentage of patients with late angiographic improvement was even higher (56%). We have found that in 13 of our patients (72%) coronary flow reserve 5 months after angioplasty was restored to a normal level and this late restoration of vascular reserve is correlated with late angiographic improvement. Of the patients with late angiographic improvement, 90% had a normalization of coronary flow reserve, whereas only 43% of patients with late angiographic deterioration had a normal coronary flow reserve 5 months after angioplasty.

Conclusion

The data inferred from digital subtraction cineangiography have been corroborated by the subselective intracoronary flow velocity measurements and established this technique as a practical means of assessing regional coronary blood flow reserve in the setting of interventional cardiology. Coronary flow reserve is not restored to normal following angioplasty, but its substantial improvement is consistent with the changes in coronary geometry brought about by angioplasty.

In 72% of our patients without angina and with normal exercise thallium scintigraphy 5 months after angioplasty for single vessel coronary artery disease, coronary flow reserve is restored to normal despite the fact that flow reserve immediately after angioplasty is not normalized. Late changes in stenosis geometry (increase in minimal obstruction area) are likely to be the major determinants of the improvement in coronary flow reserve.

Acknowledgement

We are indebted to R. v.d. Perk, J. Ligthart, N. Bruining and R. de Ruiter for their expert technical assistance.

References

1. Grüntzig AR, Senning A, Siegenthaler WE: Nonoperative dilatation of coronary-artery stenosis: percutaneous transluminal angioplasty. N Engl J Med 301: 61—68, 1979.
2. Block PC, Myler RK, Stertzer S, Fallon JT: Morphology after transluminal angioplasty in human beings. N Engl J Med 305: 382—385, 1981.
3. Serruys PW, Reiber JHC, Wijns W, Brand M van den, Kooijman CJ, Katen HJ ten, Hugenholtz PG: Assessment of percutaneous transluminal coronary angioplasty by quantitative coronary angiography: Diameter versus densitometric area measurements. Am J Cardiol 54: 482—488, 1984.
4. Leimgruber PP, Roubin GS, Hollman J, Cotsonis GA, Meier B, Douglas JS, King III SB, Grüntzig AR: Restenosis after successful coronary angioplasty in patients with single-vessel disease. Circulation 73: 710—717, 1986.
5. Serruys PW, Wijns W, Reiber JHC, Feyter P de, Brand M van den, Piscione F, Hugenholtz PG: Values and limitations of transstenotic pressure gradients measured during percutaneous coronary angioplasty. Herz 10: 337—342, 1985.
6. Klocke FJ: Measurements of coronary blood flow and degree of stenosis: current clinical implication and continuing uncertainties. J Am Coll Cardial 1: 31—41, 1983.
7. Hoffman JIE: Maximal coronary flow and the concept of coronary vascular reserve. Circulation 70: 153—159, 1984.
8. Wilson RF, White CW: Intracoronary papaverine: an ideal coronary vasodilator for studies of the coronary circulation in conscious humans. Circulation 73: 444—451, 1986.

9. Zijlstra F, Serruys PW, Hugenholtz PG: Papaverine: the ideal coronary vasodilator for investigating coronary flow reserve? A study of timing, magnitude, reproducibility, and safety of the coronary hyperemic response after intracoronary papaverine. Cathet Cardiovasc Diagn 12: 298—303, 1986.

10. Cole JS, Hartley CJ: The pulsed Doppler coronary artery catheter. Preliminary report of a new technique for measuring rapid changes in coronary artery flow velocity in man. Circulation 56: 18—25, 1977.

11. Wilson RF, Laughlin DE, Ackell PH, Chilian WM, Holida MD, Hartley CJ, Armstrong ML, Marcus ML, White CW: Transluminal, subselective measurement of coronary artery blood flow velocity and vasodilator reserve in man. Circulation 72: 82—92, 1985.

12. Hartley CJ, Cole JS: An ultrasonic pulsed Doppler system for measuring blood flow in small vessels. J Appl Physiol 37: 626—629, 1974.

13. Bates ER, Aueron FM, LeGrand V, LeFree MT, Mancini GBJ, Hodgson JM, Vogel RA: Comparative long-term effects of coronary artery bypass graft surgery and percutaneous transluminal coronary angioplasty on regional coronary flow reserve. Circulation 72: 833—839, 1985.

14. Zijlstra F, Ommeren J van, Reiber JHC, Serruys PW: Does the quantitative assessment of coronary artery dimensions predict the physiologic significance of a coronary stenosis? Circulation 75: 1154—1161, 1987.

15. Vogel RA: The radiographic assessment of coronary blood flow parameters. Circulation 72: 460—465, 1985.

16. Sibley DH, Millar HD, Hartley CJ, Whitlow PL: Subselective measurement of coronary blood flow velocity using a steerable Doppler catheter. J Am Coll Cardiol 8: 1332—1340, 1986.

17. Kent KM, Bentivoglio LG, Block PC, Cowley MJ, Dorros G, Gosselin AJ, Grüntzig A, Myler RK, Simpson J, Stertzer SH, Williams DO, Fisher L, Gillespie MJ, Detre K, Kelsey S, Mullin SM, Mock MD: Percutaneous transluminal coronary angioplasty: Report from the Registry of the National Heart, Lung and Blood Institute. Am J Cardiol 49: 2011—2020, 1982.

18. Scholl J-M, Chaitman BR, David PR, Dupras G, Brévers G, Val PG, Crépeau J, Lespérance J, Bourassa MG: Exercise electrocardiography and myocardial scintigraphy in the serial evaluation of the results of percutaneous transluminal coronary angioplasty. Circulation 66: 380—390, 1982.

19. Kent KM, Bonow RO, Rosing DR, Ewels CJ, Lipson LC, McIntosh CL, Bacharach S, Green M, Epstein SE: Improved myocardial function during exercise after successful percutaneous transluminal coronary angioplasty. N Engl J Med 306: 441—450, 1982.

20. Zijlstra F, Reiber JHC, Juillière Y, Serruys PW: Normalization of coronary flow reserve by percutaneous transluminal coronary angioplasty? Am J Cardiol 61: 55—60, 1988.

21. O'Neill WW, Walton JA, Bates ER, Colfer HT, Aueron FM, Lefree MT, Pitt B, Vogel RA: Criteria for successful coronary angioplasty as assessed by alterations in coronary vasodilatory reserve. J Am Coll Cardiol 3: 1382—1390, 1984.

22. Wilson RF, Aylward PE, Talman CL, White CW: Does percutaneous transluminal coronary angioplasty restore normal coronary vasodilator reserve? Circulation 72 (Supp III): III-397, 1985 (Abstract).

23. Marcus ML: Effects of cardiac hypertrophy on the coronary circulation. In: The coronary circulation in health and disease, McGraw-Hill Book Co, New York, 1983, pp 285—306.

24. Marcus ML: Effects of anemia and polycythemia on the coronary circulation. In: The coronary circulation in health and disease. McGraw-Hill Book Co., New York, 1983, pp 307—319.

25. Marcus ML, Doty DB, Hiratzka LF, Wright CB, Eastham CL: Decreased coronary reserve: a mechanism for angina pectoris in patients with aortic stenosis and normal coronary arteries. N Engl J Med 307: 1362—1367, 1982.

26. Reiber JHC, Serruys PW, Kooijman CJ, Wijns W, Slager CJ, Gerbrands JJ, Schuurbiers JCH, Boer A den, Hugenholtz PG: Assessment of short-, medium-, and long-term variations in arterial dimensions from computer-assisted quantitation of coronary cineangiograms. Circulation 71: 280—288, 1985.

27. Reiber JHC, Kooijman CJ, Slager CJ, Gerbrands JJ, Schuurbiers JCH, Boer A den, Wijns W, Serruys PW, Hugenholtz PG: Coronary artery dimensions from cineangiograms-methodology and validation of a computer-assisted analysis procedure. IEEE Trans Med Imaging, MI-3: 131—141, 1984.

28. Reiber JHC, Kooijman CJ, Boer A den, Serruys PW: Assessment of dimensions and image quality of coronary contrast catheters from cineangiograms. Cathet Cardiovasc Diagn 11: 521—531, 1985.

29 Reiber JHC, Lie SP, Simoons ML, Wijns W, Gerbrands JJ: Computer quantitation location, extent and type of thallium-201 myocardial perfusion abnormalities. In: Proc Int Symposium on Medical Imaging and Image Interpretation ISMIII. IEEE, Cat No·82 CH1804-4: 123—128, 1982.

30. Lie SP, Reiber JHC, Simoons ML, Gerbrands JJ, Kooy PPM, Bakker WH: Computer processing of thallium-201 myocardial scintigrams. In: Proc 2nd Int Conf Visual Phychophysics and Medical Imaging. IEEE, Cat No 81CH 1676—6: 19—25, 1981.

31. Hodgson JMcB, LeGrand V, Bates ER, Mancini GBJ, Aueron FM, O'Neill WW, Simon SB, Beauman GJ, LeFree MT, Vogel RA: Validation in dogs of a rapid digital angiographic technique to measure relative coronary blood flow during routine cardiac catheterization. Am J Cardiol 55: 188—193, 1985.

32. Wilson RF, Aylward PE, Leimbach WH, Talman CL, White CW: Coronary flow reserve late after PTCA — Do the early alterations persist? J Am Coll Cardiol 7: 212A, 1986 (Abstract).

33. Hodgson JMcB, Williams DO: Characterization of coronary flow reserve pre and post successful angioplasty. Circulation 72 (Supp III): III-456, 1985 (Abstract).

34. Sibley D, Bulle T, Baxley W, Dean L, Chandler J, Whitlow P: Acute changes in blood flow velocity with successful coronary angioplasty. Circulation 74 (Supp. II), II-193, 1986 (Abstract).

35. Johnson MR, Wilson RF, Skorton DJ, Collins SM, White CW: Coronary lumen area immediately after angioplasty does not correlate with coronary vasodilator reserve; a videodensitometric study. Circulation 74 (Supp II): II-193, 1986 (Abstract).

36. Bates ER, McGillem MJ, Beats TF, DeBoe SF, Mickelson JK, Mancini GBJ, Vogel RA: Angioplasty induced medial injury, but not endothelial denudation, impairs coronary reactive hyperemia. Circulation 74 (Supp II): II-498, 1986 (Abstract).

37. Serruys PW, Wijns W, Brand M van den, Meij S, Slager C, Schuurbiers JCH, Hugenholtz PG, Brower RW: Left ventricular performance, regional blood flow, wall motion, and lactate metabolism during transluminal angioplasty. Circulation 70: 25—36, 1984.

38. Feldman RL, Conti CR, Pepine CJ: Regional coronary venous flow responses to transient coronary artery occlusion in human beings. J Am Coll Cardiol 2: 1—10, 1983.

39. Rothman MT, Baim DS, Simpson JB, Harrison DC: Coronary hemodynamics during percutaneous transluminal coronary angioplasty. Am J Cardiol 49: 1615—1622, 1982.

40. Friedman HZ, McGillem MJ, Mancini GBJ, Vogel RA: A new method to measure absolute coronary blood flow using standard angioplasty technique. Circulation 74 (Supp II): II-497, 1986 (Abstract).

41. Serruys PW, Piscione F, Wijns W, Harmsen E, Brand M van den, Feyter P de, Hugenholtz PG, Jong JW de: Myocardial release of hypoxanthine and lactate during percutaneous transluminal coronary angioplasty: a quickly reversible phenomenon, but for how long?". In: Transluminal coronary angioplasty: an investigational tool and a nonoperative treatment of acute myocardial ischemia, Serruys PW (Doctoral Thesis, Erasmus University), 1986 pp 75—92.

42. Marcus ML: The coronary circulation in health and disease. McGraw-Hill Book Co. New York: 1983, pp 65 and 147.
43. Webb SC, Canepa-Anson R, Rickards AF, Poole-Wilson PA: Myocardial potassium loss after acute coronary occlusion in humans. J Am Coll Cardiol 9: 1230—1234, 1987.
44. Peterson MB, Machaj V, Block PC, Palacios I, Philbin D, Watkins WD: Thromboxane release during percutaneous transluminal coronary angioplasty. Am Heart J III: 1—6, 1986.
45. Johnson MR, Brayden GP, Ericksen EE, Collins SM, Skorton DJ, Harrison DG, Marcus ML, White CW: Changes in cross-sectional area of the coronary lumen in the six months after angioplasty: a quantitative analysis of the variable response to percutaneous transluminal angioplasty. Circulation 73: 467—475, 1986.
46. McPherson DD, Hiratzka LF, Lamberth WC, Brandt B, Hunt M, Kieso RA, Marcus ML, Kerber RE: Delineation of the extent of coronary atherosclerosis by high-frequency epicardial echocardiography. N Engl J Med 316: 304—309, 1987.
47. Harrison DG, White CW, Hiratzka LF, Doty DB, Barnes DH, Eastham CL, Marcus ML: The value of lesion cross-sectional area determined by quantitative coronary angiography in assessing the physiologic significance of proximal left anterior descending coronary arterial stenoses. Circulation 69: 1111—1119, 1984.

13. Theoretical and practical aspects of digital angiography for quantitative coronary flow studies

JOACHIM H. BÜRSCH

SUMMARY. Digital angiography offers the potential benefits of densitometric parameter extraction for functional studies of the coronary circulation. Special emphasis is placed on coronary flow and flow reserve measurements for assessment of the severity of critical coronary stenoses. Basically, two approaches are discussed: (1) the use of a large region-of-interest (ROI) for summated density measurements of the total amount of contrast medium that traverses the vascular bed of a myocardial perfusion segment; and (2) the analysis of temporal variations in contrast mass at each picture element allowing the display of functional information in a parametric image.

ROI-densitometry is used to derive numerical data on contrast flow, vascular volume and myocardial transit-time, while functional imaging provides information on myocardial appearence time of the contrast bolus as well as regional thickness of the perfused vasculature. There is theoretical and practical evidence, that the reliability of angiographically determined flow is essentially dependent on specific angiographic requirements, among which selective coronary injections with high flow rates and concomitant backflow of contrast medium into the aorta are of particular importance. Nevertheless, experimental studies with nonstenosed vessels demonstrate great variability in flow data indicating that the extent of coronary flow reserve is not solely determined by the degree of maximal vasodilatation but also by the spontaneous and highly variable resistance in the control state. In view of these findings it is perhaps now appropriate to reconsider the need for methodologic improvements in quantitative flow studies and to focus on the physiologic and angiographic factors affecting the flow.

Introduction

Recent advances in digital angiography and roentgen densitometry have focused attention on the potential benefits of parameter extraction for functional studies of the coronary circulation [2, 3, 6, 7, 9, 10, 14, 15]. Special emphasis have been placed on the new approaches for the assessment of coronary flow reserve in the presence of a critical coronary stenosis [5]. A variety of digital imaging techniques are under investigation for optimizing these specific tasks and to quantitate coronary and myocardial perfusion.

Basically two methods are feasible: the first one utilizes manual outlining

J. C. Reiber & P. W. Serruys (eds.), New Developments in Quantitative Coronary Arteriography,
207—224.

of regions-of-interest (ROI's) for the measurements of summated densities in anatomically defined segments (Fig. 1). This technique was originally developed for 'videodensitometric' studies. Usually, a numerical value is obtained. Either a single digital subtraction image or a sequence of images may be analyzed to establish a density-time curve (densogram). The second technique is based upon the analysis of numerous densograms from the entire field of picture elements in a digital matrix. An equivalent number of parameter values is derived. A unique feature of this technique is the reconversion of parametric data into video signals for final display on the TV-monitor, thus providing angiographic interpretation of hemodynamic parameters (Fig. 2).

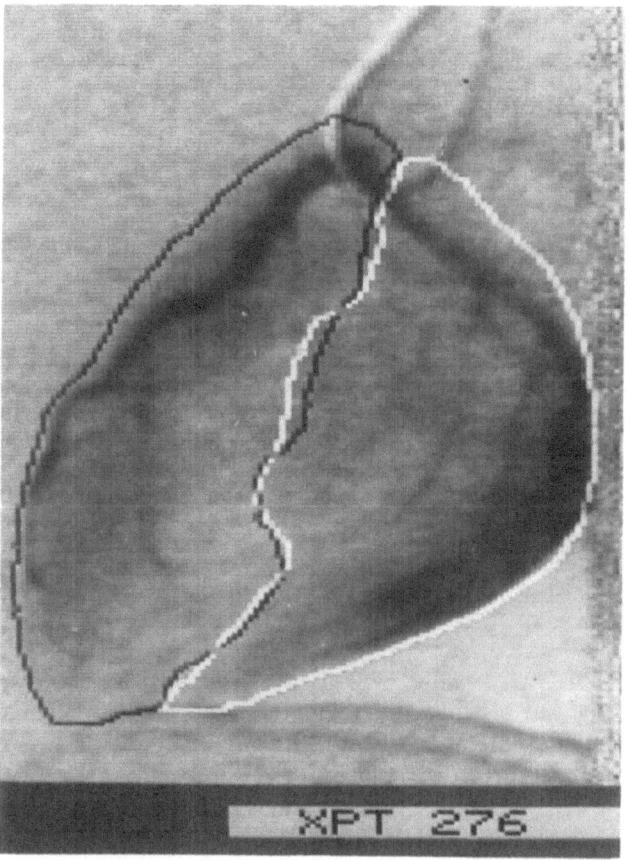

Figure 1. Mask-mode subtraction image of a digital coronary angiogram showing myocardial opacification shortly after selective contrast injection into the left coronary artery. The contours were manually outlined to define regions-of-interest for densitometric analysis of the anterior wall (black contour) and of the posterior wall (white contour). Experimental study in a 20 kg pig.

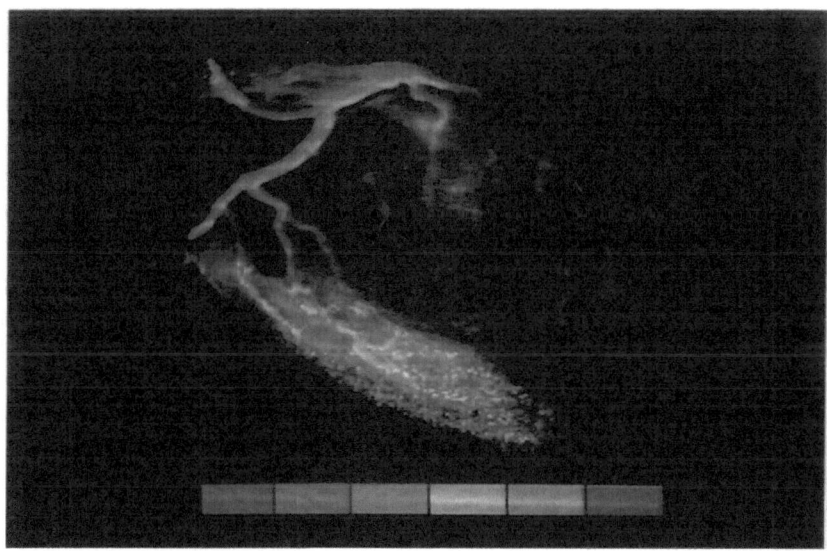

Figure 2. Parameter image of a coronary angiogram indicating the temporal course of contrast opacification in different colors. This information was derived from the sequence of ECG-gated enddiastolic images in an animal study.

To apply these techniques and to utilize the advantages of quantitative coronary flow analysis requires consideration of a number of specific conditions of this particular vasculature. It is the purpose of this paper to outline the theoretical and practical aspects for coronary flow studies, as well as to indicate interactions of the angiographic procedures on flow measurements.

General considerations

A fundamental consideration in densitometric contrast studies relates to the theory of indicator dilution.

Basically, the time course of the *concentration* of an indicator provides a quantitative index of flow. However, compared to conventional techniques of indicator sampling, the mass rather than the concentration of contrast medium is estimated by densitometry. Accordingly, this paper will primarily deal with the diagnostic potentials of *mass measurements* and its temporal and regional course for the quantitative assessment of coronary hemodynamics. Furthermore, contrast injections for coronary angiography have certain limitations in reference to the theory of classical indicator dilution:

1. Large volumes (relative to absolute flows) are injected resulting in significant disturbance of the intravascular flow patterns.
2. The mechanical properties of contrast medium are quite different from

blood. Consequently, the motion of contrast medium is not necessarily representative of blood flow.

Nevertheless, diagnostic conclusions can be drawn, particularly if parameters calculated in different sections of the circulation or under variable hemodynamic conditions, are compared among themselves.

Thereby, many of the inherent deficiences will cancel out and reproducible data of relative flow in the coronary circulation can be obtained.

The different approaches to be described here will follow a dimensional order for angiographic analysis relative to the size of the ROI, thus beginning with the application of large areas for indicator sampling in order to finally come to the use of minute picture elements.

Concepts

ROI-densitometry

The largest possible ROI that can be applied encloses the entire projection area of the perfused myocardium. Figure 3 schematically depicts the network of the coronary circulation with a vascular entrance (I) and exit (E). Suppose, that a certain mass of contrast medium enters the vascular bed at (I) and subsequently traverses the system until it finally leaves the network at

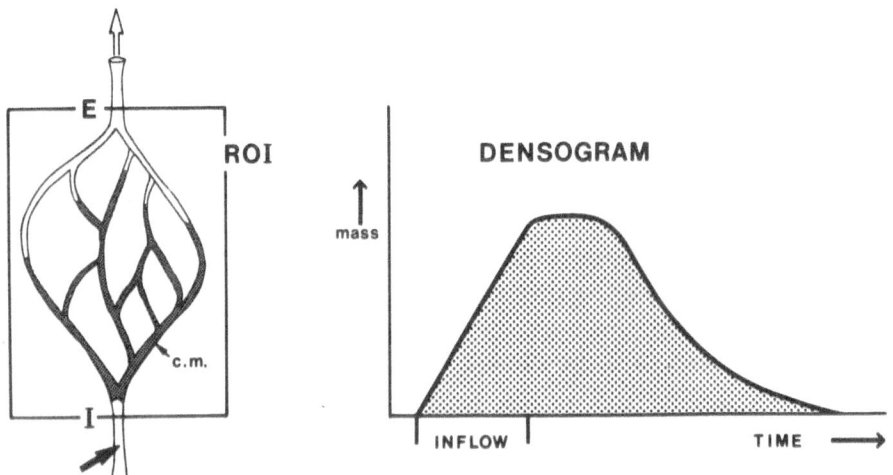

Figure 3. Schematic drawing for illustration of contrast bolus flow through the coronary vascular bed encompassed by a large region-of-interest (ROI). It is assumed that the contrast bolus (c.m.) has completely entered the ROI projection area before runoff occurs. I: entrance; E: exit. The densogram depicts an idealized mass-time curve of contrast bolus flow through the vasculature.

(E). Assume, that the mass has totally entered the container before runoff at the exit (E) occurs. These conditions provide for the detection of the total mass of contrast medium. Practically, mask subtraction images are used for the display of pure contrast density information on a homogeneous (zero) image background, hence nonspecific density variations are completely eliminated. Considering the mass-time curve that has been constructed from sequential subtraction images, the maximum amplitude represents the total mass of the indicator.

Total mass (M) is related to flow (Q) according to the degree of indicator dilution. Thus relative flow can be assessed by considering the indicator concentration (C) and its temporal course (t).

$$Q = \frac{M}{\int C \, dt} \tag{1}$$

This approach allows the measurement of relative flow if the concentration-time product is not variable in studies to be compared with each other. Coronary angiography can meet these requirements, since relatively large contrast volumes in relation to the native coronary blood flow are injected selectively, thus a bolus of almost pure contrast medium will enter the system. This condition is indicated by visualization of continuous (systolic and diastolic) reflux of contrast medium into the aorta during the time-course of injection. Quantitation of the total amount of contrast medium entering the coronary vasculature may serve as an indicator of flow and its respective changes, e.g. induced by physical or pharmacologic interventions. In this particular application the mass of contrast medium is used as a 'flow-parameter'.

A potential advantage of this method is the estimation of angiographic contrast flow data in absolute units of volume per time [4]. The mass of contrast medium entering the coronary bed is a fraction of the total amount injected. This fraction is equivalent to the ratio of coronary flow to the injection flow rate. Since the latter is known, absolute data of coronary volume flow during the time course of injection can be calculated. It is necessary in this application to calibrate the summated density signal in units of contrast volume by a separate measurement.

A second parameter, the transit-time of the contrast bolus flowing through the vascular bed can be estimated. This information is derived from the difference between contrast accumulation and venous runoff. Dividing the curve area by the maximum amplitude yields the time interval of bolus travel. Limitations in this analysis may result from practical difficulties in defining precisely the curve area. Usually the descending limb of the denso-gram will not reach the pre-injection baseline level. Therefore, either an arbitrary definition of the correct time to cease density collection, or a modality to extrapolate the indicator washout is required. Finally, the estimation of the curve area itself may serve as another important parameter, namely the volume of the vascular bed containing contrast material.

The description in the preceding section can be applied to the understanding of angiographic parameter extraction from any small ROI.

A stepwise reduction of a large ROI to infinitely small picture element areas would consistently alter the hight and the temporal course of densograms: no longer does the maximum amplitude reflect total mass, nor does the temporal course correspond to vascular transit-times. The latter rather relates to the length and speed of the bolus passing the site of sampling. Consequently, the information of contrast mass or the temporal course alone cannot contribute to flow measurements. However, as a specific parameter the mass-time product, i.e. the area under the densogram, is directly related to the vascular volume delineated by the ROI irrespective of its size (Fig. 4). Theoretical and experimental evidence indicates that even the density-time product of individual picture elements is proportional to the size of the respective vascular volume element. The validity of this 'volume-parameter' implies the fundamental assumption that the concentration-time product is not variable in measurements that are compared to each other, i.e. as long as $\int C \, dt$ is constant, the volume (V) can be estimated from the mass-time product $\int M \, dt$.

$$V = \frac{\int M \, dt}{\int C \, dt} \, . \tag{2}$$

This consideration holds for indicator sampling at any site in one individual angiogram. However, if two or more angiograms are analyzed for comparison to each other, the contrast injection mode must account for the same degree of indicator dilution. As has been explicitly outlined earlier, coronary angiography can meet these requirements if pure contrast medium enters the coronary bed under the described 'overflow' conditions. At present, the diagnostic value of volume parameters cannot be judged definitely, whether these data are derived from manually outlined ROI's or displayed as parameter images (picture element processing).

Parameter calculation of myocardial vascular volume has been combined with time parameter imaging in order to improve the diagnostic information on studies of hyperemic vascular response. Another possible application is to combine the volume parameter, e.g. from a coronary artery segment, with geometric measurements of the respective vessel dimensions. According to formula (2) a measure of the concentration-time product is obtained. Further experimental and clinical evaluation is necessary to confirm the practicality of this measurement.

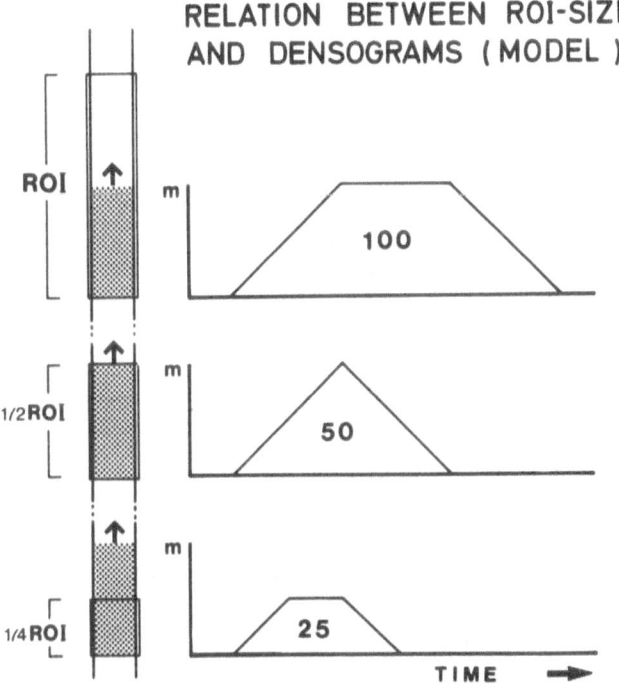

Figure 4. Schematic drawing for illustration of the relationship between the extent of a region-of-interest (ROI), the length of a contrast bolus and the derived densograms. For simplicity it is assumed that the bolus contains a homogeneous distribution of indicator and traverses a straight tube with a constant flow rate. Three typical situations are illustrated. *Top*: The length of the ROI is twice the length of the bolus. The hypothetical densogram on the right has an area of 100 units. *Center*: The ROI used in this example has a length equal to that of the contrast bolus. The resulting densogram reveals an area of 50 units. *Bottom*: The ROI is reduced to half the length of the bolus. The densogram accordingly reveals 25 area units. These examples indicate the significant variation in the shape of the densograms, as well as the linear relationship between vascular volumes encompassed by the ROI and the curve areas.

Parametric imaging

It is obvious from the preceding discussion that useful information of regional flow cannot be obtained from a *single* densogram of any small ROI. However, multidimensional analysis from the entire field of picture elements (matrix) can be used to extract temporal information of the regional progression of contrast flow. Time values of the contrast appearance may be calculated from each site in the vasculature (Fig. 5).

The display of these calculated temporal data allows for the estimation of time intervals along the arterial vessels [3, 8]. Excellent flow information was

214

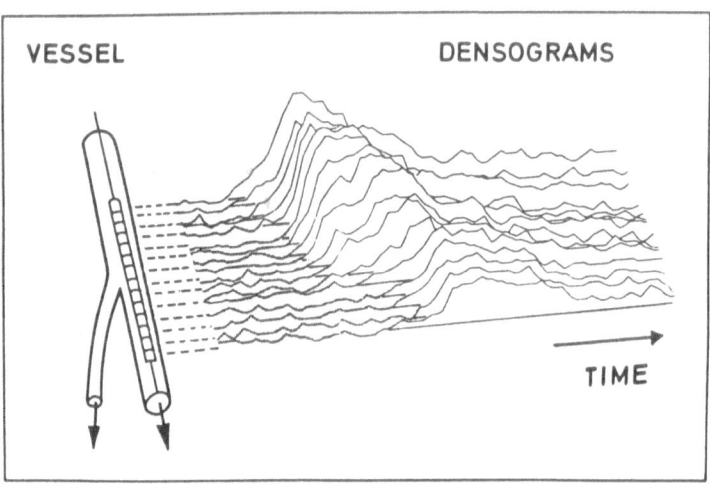

Figure 5. Semi-schematic drawing of sequential densograms of picture elements along a straight vessel. The progressive delay of contrast appearence (shaded area) from subsequent picture elements may be used to analyze the temporal and regional aspects of vascular perfusion.

obtained particularly from larger vessels such as the aorta, the renal and iliac arteries. The dimensional size, the straight course and immobility of these vessels are favorable for densitometric analysis.

Obviously, the coronary arteries do not lend themselves to comparable assessment due to their complex spatial orientation, their small size, and significant motion. A major concern relates to the latter effects of phasic motion of this vasculature. Most frequently, analysis of time-sequenced angiographic images has been based on the ECG-gated image acquisition mode, occasionally combined with electrical pacing to minimize misregistration and motion artefacts. The resulting discontinuity of density information (one per cardiac cycle) definitely limits the accuracy with which time data are finally calculated. Nevertheless, an estimation of temporal events can be achieved, thus forming the basis for studies of flow velocities in a variety of clinical applications [12, 16, 17]. A rather simple version of gated image processing is depicted in Fig. 6. This schematic drawing illustrates that different colors are assigned to the sequence of serial images. If one considers this set to be contrast images after mask subtraction, subsequent density values of each picture element reflect the density of the contrast medium bolus at the respective site. A simple mathematical operator may be used to detect the particular image containing the *maximal value* of regional densities, thereby selecting the appropriate color for each picture element in the parameter image. In addition, the degree of maximal absorption may be converted into color intensity for the final display. This method requires only

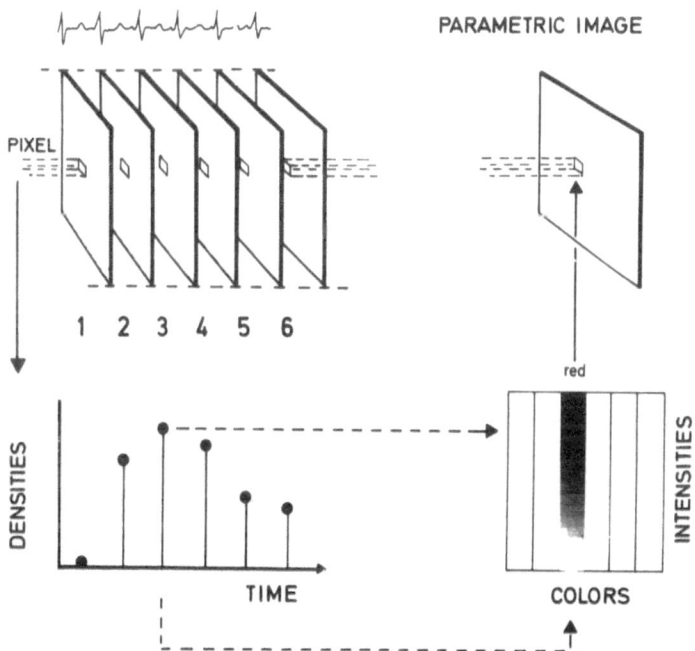

Figure 6. Schematic illustration of time parameter extraction. Temporal variations in density of a picture element (pixel) are depicted in the lower left panel. A computer program automatically detects the maximum density values, thus selecting a particular image and the corresponding time of maximal opacification. Different colors are assigned to subsequent images, thus providing the conversion of temporal information into a color coded parameter image. In addition, the degree of maximal contrast absorption may be used to vary the color intensities.

short processing times and reveals parameter images indicating bolus progression in time intervals of one cardiac cycle length.

Similarly, criteria other than the maximal density have been used. Vogel and coworkers [11, 17] applied the parameter of maximum change in contrast densities as the representative time value. We have preferred using the mean rise time of densograms with the advantage that time interval processing can be performed independently of the cardiac cycle length [1, 3].

Another problem that needs further consideration is the high flow velocity of the initial contrast front, possibly traversing the epicardial coronary arteries within less than one cardiac cycle length. In order to assess mean velocities over an adequate distance from the site of injection, the onset of myocardial opacification (myocardial appearence time) has been used to overcome these particular circulatory conditions. But one cannot define the velocity of flow in the epicardial vessels from the myocardial appearence time. This restricts the general use to comparative studies in the same individual.

In summary, time parameter imaging has been applied to estimate myocardial appearance times for estimation of changes in coronary flow, potentially induced by reactive hyperemia. Very recently 'volume parameters' were also used by estimating changes of the mass-time product from small myocardial ROI's [16]. This combined temporal and densitometric analysis apparently has improved the reliability of flow reserve measurements.

Practical aspects

Linear density recording

Linearity of densitometric recording systems is an essential requirement for quantitation of contrast mass. Therefore, filtering of the incident radiation is necessary in order to narrow the spectral distribution of X-rays. The use of a 0.1 mm sheet of copper has been found to be adequate in coronary angiography. Digital imaging processing must provide for adequate logarithmic conversion of density data to account for the exponential attenuation of X-rays. In order to assure linear density recording one must test the equipment by use of a simple test object. We prefer to inflate a balloon with a constant flow rate of 4 ml/s up to a volume of 40 ml using a 10% contrast solution. The balloon is kept in a water bath of 10 cm height. Ideally one can expect an increase of ROI density values linearly related to contrast volume.

Myocardial overlapping

Flow parameters can be assessed for each of the three main arterial vessels. From a practical viewpoint, it is necessary to avoid overlapping of myocardial regions that are supplied by the left LAD and LCX coronary arteries. In order to discriminate between these perfusion areas, right anterior obliquity is the preferred roentgen projection mode. However, complete and free projection of the separately perfused wall segments is difficult to achieve in routine diagnostic studies. In order to partly overcome such practical limitations, superselective injections into either the LAD or LCX coronary arteries have been applied. Consequently, the noncatheterized artery will obtain relatively small amounts of contrast medium (by overflow) resulting in low opacification, that in turn reduces the effects of superimposing structures.

Overflow conditions

An additional advantage of superselective injections is to satisfy the demands for retrograde contrast flow with tolerable injection flow rates. This may otherwise become a critical problem in left main coronary artery injections, which occasionally require flow rates of more than 10 ml/s, particularly in hyperemic flow studies.

The feasibility and safety of superselective injections for the described purpose has so far not yet been fully explored clinically. The latter is of considerable importance for successful angiographic comparisons of flow and volume parameters using contrast mass measurements. Otherwise, time parameter extraction alone does not necessarily require the aforementioned conditions. Nevertheless, adequate contrast volumes are likewise necessary to achieve the appropriate signal-to-noise relationship for the analysis of small density variations from picture elements. In fact, a critical situation may arise in hypoperfused vessel segments when the contrast density signal is naturally reduced. Thus time parameter imaging may occasionally fail to indicate subnormal flow conditions.

Motion artefacts

A final aspect concerns the possible misregistration of vessel contours even if ECG-gated image acquisition is applied. An analysis of time-sequenced images is extremely sensitive to cardiac arrhythmia which may cause erroneous parametric data and false temporal information. The high resolution image matrix (e.g. 1024^2 matrix) is not particularly useful; the 256^2 matrix format usually resolves temporal data with adequate distinction. The preferred image acquisition rate is 25 images/s from which corresponding images are selected according to the pre-systolic phase in order to optimally match opacified vessels. Temporal data from myocardial ROI's are naturally only little affected by nonoptimal matching and last, but not least, it has become the prevailing technique for time parameter analysis. It is noteworthy that the approach of total myocardial contrast mass measurements (large ROI) is least affected by possible misregistration. Basically, this method requires only one pair of images for mask mode subtraction and subsequent densitometric analysis.

The practicality of these and other alternative techniques will be of considerable importance to the success of quantitative flow measurements in future clinical studies.

Experimental data

We have had the opportunity to test the described techniques in animal experiments comparing coronary flow studies in hyperemic and control states. Initial studies were performed with simultaneous recordings of coronary artery flow by electromagnetic flowmetry (EMF). These data were obtained immediately prior and subsequent to selective left coronary artery injections with volumes and flow rates comparable to conventional diagnostic coronary angiography (volume ⩽ 6 ml Solutrast).

Analysis of the flowmeter recording *during* contrast injections was not feasible due to the disturbance of the electromagnetic signal. But a significant increase of coronary artery flow was observed shortly *after* injection (on the order of 2—2.5 fold of the pre-injection flow values). Figure 7 depicts these flow ratios 5 and 8 seconds after the onset of injection. During this time period the highest flow values were observed as an expression of flow response to the injection, followed by a much longer period of slowly decreasing coronary flow ($t \geqslant 60$ s) to baseline values. Even though simultaneous comparison of EMF data with angiographically determined flow rates was not possible, the described data provided for the scheme in which angiographic data would fit.

Since the approach of myocardial densitometry using a large ROI encompassing the total myocardium allowed for the calculation of flow rates in absolute units (ml/min), we applied this technique for the validation of angiographic flow measurements. Thus, relating the DSA densitometric data

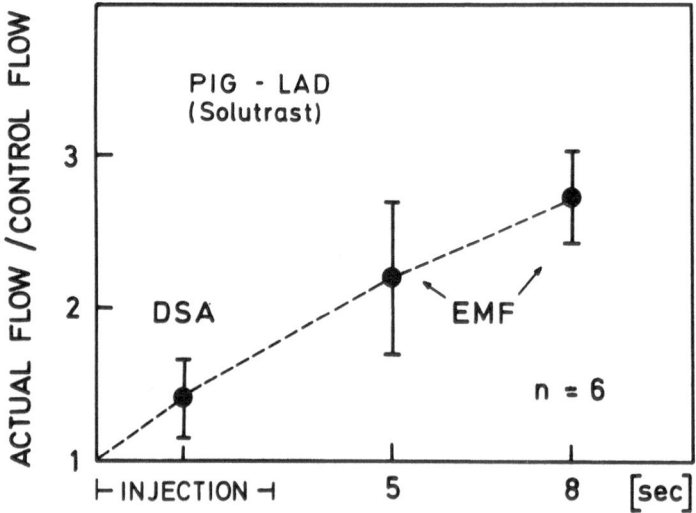

Figure 7. Diagrammatic presentation of the increase in coronary blood flow (left anterior descending artery = LAD) during and following selective contrast injection in animal studies. Flow data at 5 and 8 seconds after onset of injection were obtained from the electromagnetic flowmeter (EMF). Flow data during the injection were derived from densitometric analysis of mask subtraction images (DSA).

with the electromagnetic pre-injection flow, we estimated an increase by about 1.3. The early DSA measurements fit with the later EMF values confirming the early and steady increase in flow following the contrast injection.

Angiography is in itself an intervention with a pronounced coronary circulatory response [13]. These well-known effects have previously been used as an interventional stimulus; duplicate contrast injections were performed using the first injection (control angiography) as the stimulus for the hyperemic response [17]. We have followed this scheme in our experimental studies. The second contrast injection was performed about 15 seconds after the initial one.

Figure 8 indicates absolute values of flow rates of the left anterior descending (LAD) coronary artery in the control state and as an equivalent for coronary flow reserve.

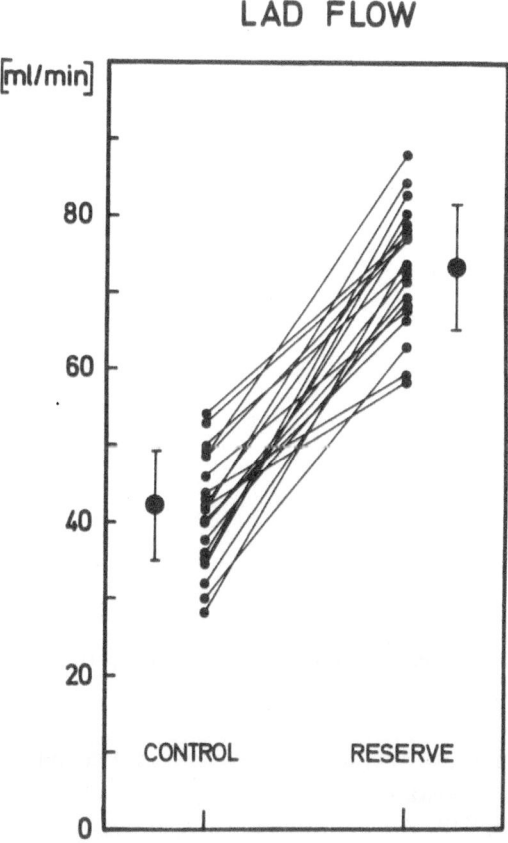

Figure 8. Diagram depicting LAD coronary flow reserve data in experimental pigs (20 kg body weight). Hyperemic response was induced by the initial angiographic contrast injection (Solutrast).

Comparative measurements in each pair of angiograms revealed an increase in flow rates by a factor of 1.8 ± 0.36 (mean ± s.d.). The variability in the data in both the control and the reserve state was comparable (about 20%). Similarly, the individual increase in flow showed significant variations. In order to elucidate this variability, mean aortic pressures were also measured during coronary angiography. Figure 9 illustrates the similar degree of variations.

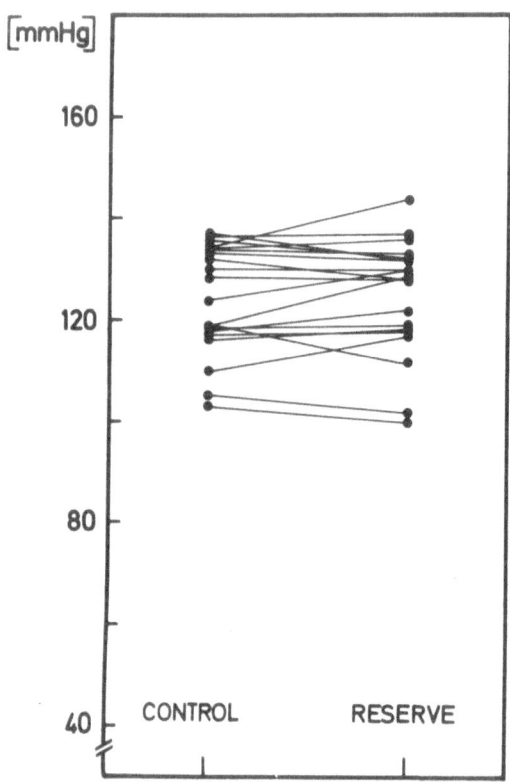

Figure 9. Variations in mean aortic pressure according to the flow data of Fig. 8.

Mean aortic pressure was also related to LAD coronary flow in order to estimate vascular resistance and the respective changes in the coronary vascular bed (Fig. 10). As a result, the resistance data varied over a wide range during the control state. But during the hyperemic state LAD resistance systematically dropped to values that showed a significantly smaller variation of 6%. The consistency of the latter *resistance* data signifies a much

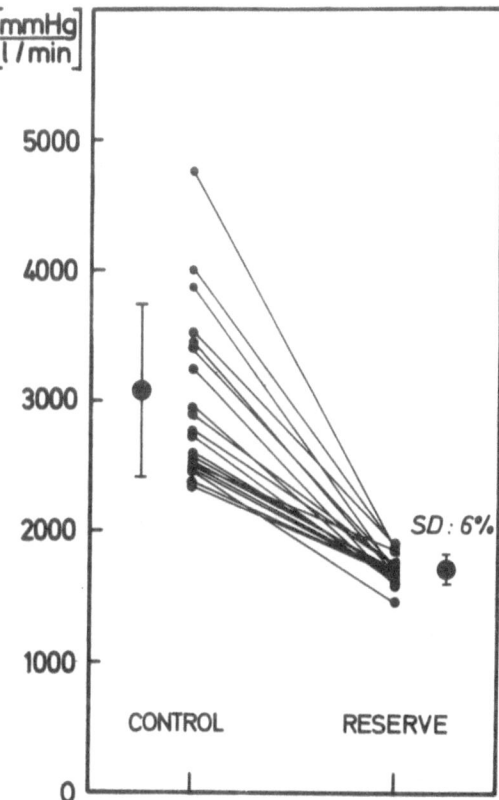

Figure 10. Data on mean resistance according to Figs. 8 and 9 showing rather little variation in the hyperemic state with a standard deviation (SD) of 6%.

better reproducibility than hyperemic *flow* data. Apparently, coronary flow reserve is affected by the aortic pressure. It is important that in future studies pressure data and vascular resistance both be considered, since the latter appears to be more appropriate for studies of vascular response to phar-macologic interventions.

Finally, we calculated the change in vascular resistance as a function of the resistance during the control state. Figure 11 depicts an extraordinary linear relationship between these two parameters.

Extrapolation to a level of zero change in vascular resistance may indicate the basal tone of that vasculature. It appears from this graph that many of these angiographic studies produce vasodilatation not too far off from the basal tone. On the other hand, it seems likely, that vascular reserve is partially exhausted by the angiographic examinations that usually included repeated injections over a several hour period.

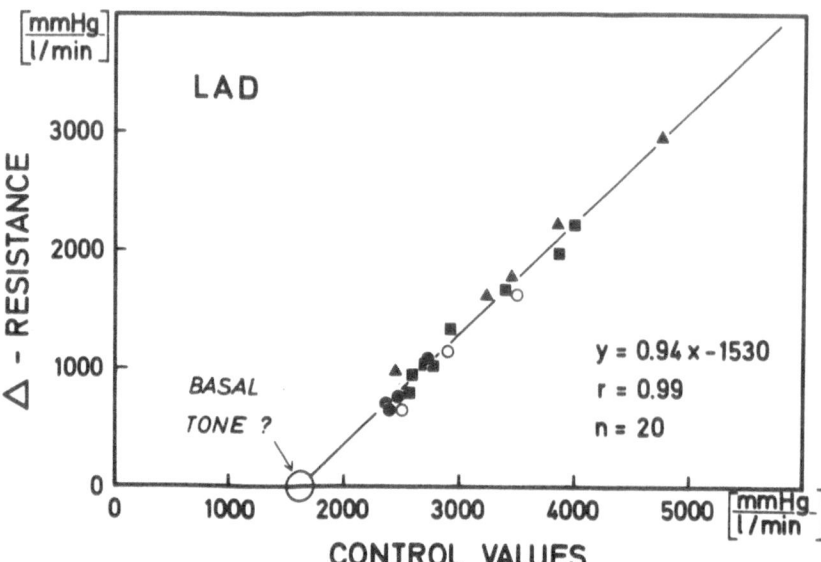

Figure 11. Demonstration of a linear relationship between the change in mean resistance (reserve data minus control data) and LAD mean resistance in the control state. The intersection of this linear function with the x-axis may possibly indicate the basal tone of that vasculature.

In summary, the vascular resistance in the resting state may vary due to a number of factors including aortic pressure, ventricular diastolic pressure, hematocrit, vasoactive substances, and last, but not least the contrast medium itself usually injected several times during the course of the angiographic procedures.

It appears that the extent of coronary flow reserve is not solely determined by the degree of 'maximal vasodilatation', but also by the spontaneous and variable resistance in the 'control state'. In view of these findings, it is doubtful that flow reserve data can quantitatively reflect the degree of proximal vascular stenosis. However, the demonstration of an almost abolished flow reserve might indicate a severe obstruction.

Though there is unquestionably.a hypothetical relationship between vascular reserve and proximal arterial stenosis, the measurement of control coronary flow is complicated by so many factors that the variability in the control flow may significantly affect the estimation of hyperemic response. This makes it difficult to draw clinically significant conclusions from a single patient study. Perhaps it is appropriate now to reconsider the need for methodologic improvements of quantitative flow studies and focus rather on the physiologic and anatomic factors affecting the flow.

Acknowledgement

I wish to express my gratitude to Prof. P. Heintzen, M.D. whose ideas contributed to the development of these techniques and to my many collagues, particularly G. Fischer, D. Balzer, U. Bürsch, G. Gonschior, J. Müller and K. Moldenhauer, M.D. for their assistance in the experimental studies and validation of digital coronary angiography.

References

1. Brennecke R, Bürsch JH: Functional analysis of angiograms by digital image processing techniques. In: Nalcioglu O, Chow ZH, (eds). Selected topics in image science: Applications to medical diagnosis and physical sciences. Springer, Berlin/Heidelberg/New York, 1984, pp 182—220.
2. Bürsch JH, Hahne HJ, Beyer C, Seemann S, Meissner L, Brennecke R, Heintzen PH: Myocardial perfusion studies by digital angiography. Comput Cardiol, 343—346, 1983.
3. Bürsch JH, Heintzen PH: Parametric imaging. Radiol Clin North Am 23: 321—333, 1985.
4. Bürsch JH: Densitometric studies in digital subtraction angiography: Assessment of pulmonary and myocardial perfusion. Herz 10: 208—214, 1985.
5. Gould KL, Lipscomb K, Hamilton GW: Physiologic basis for assessing critical coronary stenosis. Instantaneous flow response and regional distribution during coronary hyperemia as measures of coronary flow reserve. Am J Cardiol 33: 87—94, 1974.
6. Heintzen PH and Bürsch JH: Roentgen-video-techniques for dynamic studies of structure and function of the heart and circulation. Georg Thieme Publishers, Stuttgart, 1978.
7. Heintzen PH, Brennecke R: Digital imaging in cardiovascular radiology. Georg Thieme Vcrlag, Stuttgart/New York, 1983.
8. Heintzen PH, Bürsch JH, Hahne H-J, Brennecke R, Budach W, Lange P: Assessment of cardiovascular function by digital angiocardiography. J Am Coll Cardiol 5: 150s—157s, 1985.
9. Heintzen PH and Bürsch JH: Progress in Digital Angiocardiography. Martinus Nijhoff Publishers, Dordrecht/Boston/Lancaster, 1987.
10. Lantz BMT: Video Dilution Technique; A Radiological Approach to Hemodynamics. In: Everett J (ed.). Digital Image Processing in Radiology. Williams ands Wilkens Publ, 1984, pp 138—158.
11. LeFree MT, Vogel RA, O'Neill WW, Bates ER, Smith DN, Pitt B: A digital radiographic technique for visualization and quantitation of regional myocardial perfusion. Comput Cardiol 153—156, 1982.
12. Ratib O, Chappuis F, Rutishauser W: Digital angiographic technique for the quantitative assessment of myocardial perfusion. Ann Radiol, 28: 193—197, 1985.
13. Rutishauser W, Bussmann W-D, Noseda G, Meier W, Wellauer J: Blood flow measurement through single coronary arteries by roentgen densitometry. Part I. A comparison of flow measured by a radiologic technique applicable in the intact organism and by electromagnetic flowmeter. Am J Roentgenol 109: 12—20, 1970.
14. Reiber JHC, Serruys PW: State of the art in quantitative coronary arteriography. Martinus Nijhoff Publishers, Dordrecht/Boston/Lancaster, 1986.
15. Spiller P, Jehle J, Pölitz B, Schmiel FK: A digital X-ray image processing system for measurement of phasic blood flow in coronary arteries. Comput Cardiol 223—226, 1982.

224

16. Vogel RA: The radiographic assessment of coronary blood flow parameters. Circulation 72: 460–465, 1985.
17. Vogel R, LeFree M, Bates E, O'Neill W, Foster R, Kirlin P, Smith D, Pitt B: Application of digital techniques to selective coronary arteriography: Use of myocardial contrast appearence time to measure coronary flow reserve. Am Heart J 107: 153–164, 1984.

14. Three-dimensional reconstruction and flow measurements of coronary arteries using multi-view digital angiography

DENNIS L. PARKER, J. WU, D. L. POPE, R. VAN BREE, G. R. CAPUTO, and H. W. MARSHALL

SUMMARY. In this paper we discuss three-dimensional reconstruction and flow measurements of the coronary artery vascular bed from multiple view coronary angiography. The reconstruction generates densitometric centerline and cross-sectional area measurements of the major branches of the arterial bed from two view ECG correlated digital angiograms for all images obtained throughout the cardiac cycle. The completeness of the reconstruction is well suited to allow computation of absolute flow through the major branches.

The arterial bed is represented as a branching tree structure. A projected structure including vessel branching and other recognizable node points is specified on all images of both views. Dynamic programming with subsequent operator verification is used to determine the true vessel centerline and projected cross section in each image of each view. Each pair of computer determined structures is used to generate a three-dimensional representation of the arterial bed centerlines. The conversion factor between digital density value and vessel thickness is obtained from an average of all vessel profile measurements after correction for orientation and magnification. Segments which are too steeply inclined for orientation correction or which overlap other segments are not included in the averaging process. Absolute lumen area is then obtained from the densitometric profiles. Absolute flow measurements are obtained by tracking the leading edge of the iodine bolus down the known volume of the arterial tree.

Introduction

Coronary arteriography is currently the standard technique for evaluating the state of the coronary arteries to determine the need for and/or success of bypass surgery and coronary angioplasty. Because the cost and risk of revascularization procedures are substantial, it is important that an accurate assessment of coronary artery anatomy be included in the decision for such interventions. The ability to perform accurate dimensional measurements is also critically needed to assess the relatively newer coronary angioplasty and thrombolysis procedures which change the morphology and flow characteristics of vessels with lesions. The ability to perform such measurements is necessary to accurately assess changes in lesion size and thus the long term efficacy of the procedures.

J. C. Reiber & P. W. Serruys (eds.), New Developments in Quantitative Coronary Arteriography,
225—247.

Developments in quantitative coronary artery analysis include the pioneering work of Brown [1] and Sandor *et al.* [2, 3] for geometric analysis of coronary arteries from magnified cinefilm. The use of biplane views allows some correction for projection angle for the proper measurement of asymmetric lesions. Absolute changes in vessel morphology due to disease progression, drug therapy and vascular spasm have been measured geometrically [4]. Other techniques have been developed which refine edge information with densitometric information obtained from a predetermined relationship between the film density and X-ray exposure [5—9]. Most of these systems analyze a short segment of a single arterial branch. A recent review of coronary analysis techniques has been published by Reiber [10].

The technique discussed in this paper relates specifically to three-dimensional reconstruction of the major branches of the coronary arterial bed. The technique has been described in detail in other publications [11—16]. The three-dimensional position of the vessel centerline and a measure of the vessel lumen is determined at each point in the reconstructed structure. The reconstruction is obtained for each image in at least one cardiac cycle giving a complete determination of the arterial bed at all points in time throughout the cardiac cycle. Flow is then determined by tracking the leading edge of the iodine bolus in a set of images obtained when iodine is entering the arterial bed. The technique as developed has similarities to and builds in some sense on work of many other researchers [17—23].

This paper gives a brief review of the general concepts of three-dimensional reconstruction of the vascular tree as implemented in our system. The problem of densitomety is addressed and the effects of X-ray scatter are specifically added. The potential for blood flow measurements is discussed. Finally, the reconstruction process is illustrated with a recent clinical example.

Theory

The three-dimensional reconstruction consists of the determination of the three-dimensional vessel centerline and then the vessel lumen area at all points along the major branches of the arterial bed. The centerline determination is a geometric problem that requires the determination of corresponding anatomic points of reference (node points) in the vascular structure in at least two views. The current implementation of the algorithm is limited to two views with additional views available for determination of measurement accuracy. The centerline determination also requires that the geometry of view acquisition be determined as accurately as possible. As this part of the reconstruction algorithm has been described previously, we will discuss certain novel features of the specific implementation with the clinical example.

Vessel densitometry

The densitometric determination of lumen area has also been discussed previously [12, 14, 15]. However, in order to include the effects of scatter we review the derivation. Conventional X-ray densitometry is based on the assumption that X-ray scatter has been corrected or can be neglected. The digital values d_{ij} are then proportional to the iodine contrast density and the length of the X-ray path through the artery, x_{ij}:

$$d_{ij} = -k' \ln[I_0 \exp(-\mu_I \rho_{Iij} x_{ij}) + I_s] + k' \ln[I_0 + I_s] \approx k' \mu_I \rho_{Iij} x_{ij} \quad (1)$$

where μ_I and ρ_{Iij} are the mass attenuation coefficient and mass density of iodine, respectively, k' is a constant of the image system, I_0 is the X-ray intensity detected in the absence of iodine, I_s is the detected scattered X-ray intensity and the indices i and j represent the position in the image. It has been our experience that contrast injections which last 2 to 3 seconds result in relatively uniform opacification over a large portion of the arterial tree. For the extent over the image where the iodine concentration is uniform we define a conversion factor, k, from digital density value to thickness (in mm) as:

$$k = x_{ij}/d_{ij}. \quad (2)$$

If we define the indices i and j such that i is along the length of the vessel and j is orthogonal to the vessel (in practice this requires sub-pixel sampling with some form of interpolation such as bilinear) we can obtain the cross-sectional area from the integral of the digital density values across the vessel width:

$$A_i = k \sum_j d_{ij} \Delta x_i = k a_i. \quad (3)$$

The factor Δx converts from unit distances in the pixel matrix to distance (in mm) at the position i of the artery segment. Because of the three-dimensional structure of the artery bed, there is variability in the position and thus magnification of the vessel at point i. The factor Δx is thus a function of position along the vessel and can be computed from the three-dimensional reconstruction of the vessel centerline. Using a vessel segment of circular cross section that is parallel to the imaging plane, it is possible to obtain densitometric measures of the vessel diameter D, as well as the conversion factor k. Using the fact that the area A is equal to $\pi D^2/4$ and the fact that the maximum density value d_{max} is proportional to the diameter:

$$D_i = k d_{max\,i}. \quad (4)$$

Eqs. (3) and (4) can be combined to give:

$$D_i = \frac{4 \sum\limits_{j} d_{ij} \Delta x_i}{\pi d_{\max i}} . \tag{5}$$

The same relations can also be used to solve for the conversion factor k:

$$k = \frac{4 \sum\limits_{j} d_{ij} \Delta x_i}{\pi d^2_{\max i}} . \tag{6}$$

The above relationships only hold if the vessel is parallel to the imaging plane. In the case of small angulations relative to the imaging plane, it is possible to correct for the orientation of the vessel, assuming that the lumen cross section does not change too rapidly. In fact, the rate of change of the vessel lumen determines the maximum angle that can be corrected for a given segment. If x is assumed to be the vessel thickness perpendicular to vessel long axis, Eq. (1) can be written:

$$d_{ij} = k' \mu_1 \rho_{1ij} x_{ij} / \cos \theta_i , \tag{7}$$

where θ_i is the angle of the vessel relative to the imaging plane.

The area is corrected as:

$$A_i = k_i \sum\limits_{j} d_{ij} \Delta x_i \cos \theta_i . \tag{8}$$

The densitometric diameter D (Eq. 5) remains unchanged, but the conversion factor k is obtained as:

$$k_i = \frac{4 \sum\limits_{j} d_{ij} \Delta x_i}{\pi d^2_{\max i} \cos \theta_i} . \tag{9}$$

Equation (9) can be used to determine the conversion factor k from any round vessel segment that is at some small angle from the imaging plane. Due to imaging noise (photon statistics, etc.) determinations of k from a single vessel cross section may be significantly in error. It is, therefore, advantageous to determine k with some form of averaging over many vessel cross sections. It is also not possible to determine, *a priori*, if the vessel segments are of circular cross section. We make the assumption that most vessel segments are nearly round and that, over the course of the three-dimensional vascular tree, the direction of elongation is randomly distributed with respect to the imaging plane. With these assumptions, it can be shown [12–15] that an average value of k can be obtained by computing Eq. (9) for positions along the vessel segments that satisfy the validity of Eq. (9) (e.g. for which the vessel is not too greatly inclined and not obscured by other vessels) and then taking the average of all these estimates of k.

In conventional angiography systems, scatter is a significant fraction of the primary X-ray intensity and may not be negligible. In the following we solve for the error that occurs when it is neglected. Rearranging Eq. (1) we have:

$$d'_{ij} = k'\mu_1\rho_{1ij}x_{ij} + k' \ln[(1 + f)/(1 + f \exp(\mu_1\rho_{1ij}x_{ij}))] \tag{10}$$

where f is defined as the ratio of the scattered X-ray intensity I_s to the detected primary X-ray intensity I_0. The error in densitometry is seen to increase with f as well as with iodine density and vessel thickness. As x is the thickness traversed by the X-rays, the error also increases with the angle of inclination of the vessel relative to the imaging plane. For $f = 0.5$, $\mu = 0.1$ mm^{-1} and $x = 5$ mm, the error in d in nearly 20%.

The error in diameter and area measurements may be somewhat less because the conversion factor k is computed from the same image that it is used on. This can be shown numerically by substituting d' from Eq. (10) for d in Eq. (9). We then assume that k is computed as the average of determinations of k_i from a large, randomly oriented arterial bed. If the vessels were truly randomly oriented, the number at any angle, θ, would be proportional to $\cos \theta$. Averaging over all possible allowed orientations and vessel diameters, k would then have a value nearly equal to:

$$\bar{k} = \frac{\displaystyle\int_{t_{min}}^{t_{max}} dt \int_0^{\theta_{max}} d\theta\, w(t, \theta)k(t, \theta)}{\displaystyle\int_{t_{min}}^{t_{max}} dt \int_0^{\theta_{max}} d\theta\, w(t, \theta)} \tag{11}$$

If all thicknesses are equally likely, the weights $w(t, \theta)$ are just $\cos \theta$. The average value of k will be a function of the scatter fraction f only.

Equation (11) was used to obtain an estimate of k for values of f equal to 0, 0.2, and 0.5. The image was assumed to be composed of randomly oriented vessels of thicknesses between 0.5 and 5.0 mm with an iodine attenuation coefficient of 0.1 mm^{-1}. The maximum angle used was 60°. The vessel diameter was obtained from the computed area of Eq. (8) as well as from the maximum vessel density of Eq. (4). The error in vessel diameter is plotted as a function of diameter in Fig. 1. For the diameter obtained from the area, the maximum error is still only 0.2 mm for the 5 mm vessel or 4%. For the diameter obtained directly from the maximum vessel density, the error increases to 0.6 mm for the 5 mm vessel, or 12%.

One might conclude from the above discussion that, although scatter is a significant problem, it may be of less significance than errors due to subtraction artifacts (or other overlying structures if subtraction is not used). The problem is compounded because the ratio f may not be uniform across the image and vessel orientations may not be sufficiently random.

Because the three-dimensional reconstruction is accomplished from at

230

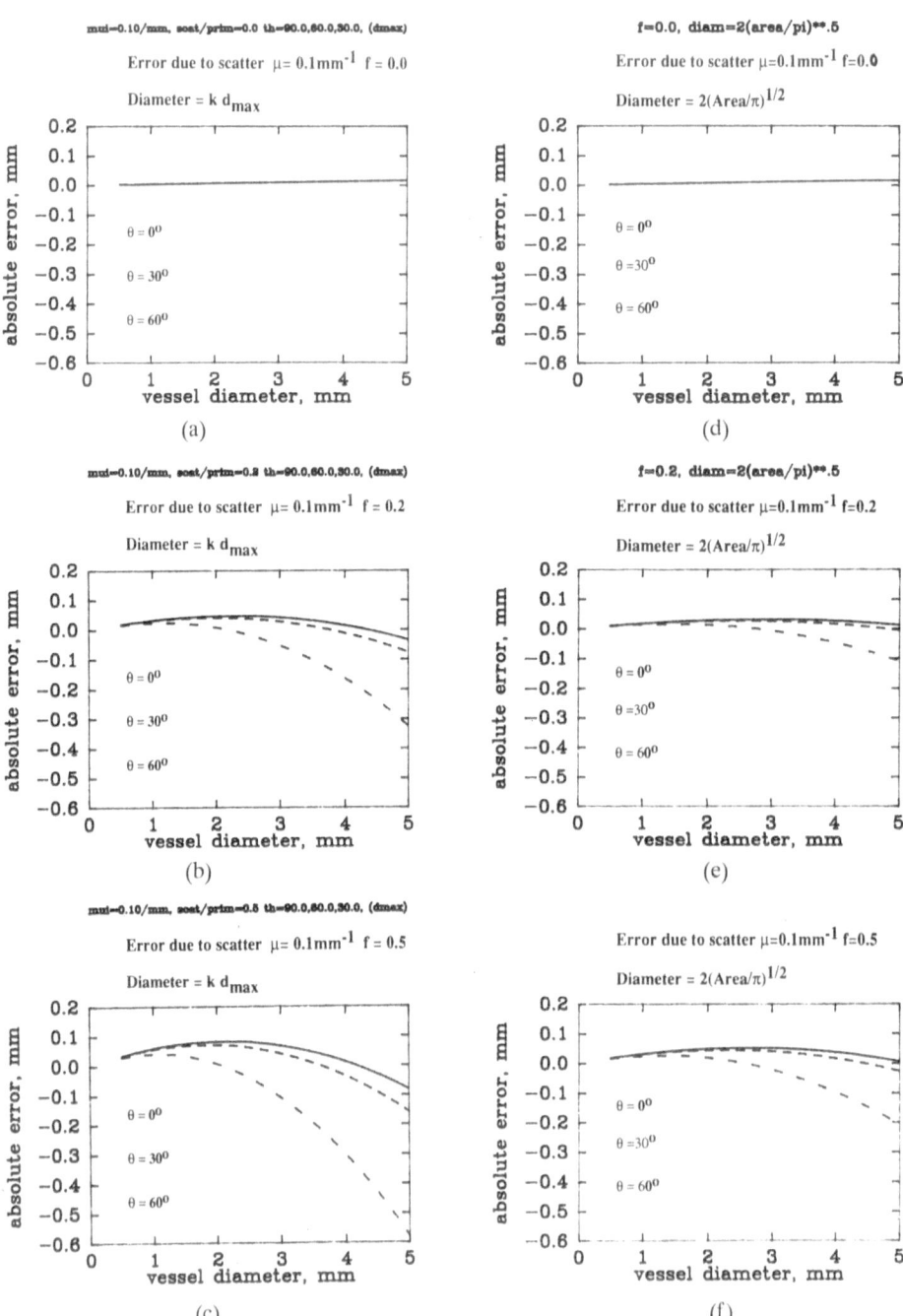

Figure 1. Absolute error in diameter measurements for vessel inclination angles of 0°, 30°, and 60°. The errors are determined for diameters obtained from the maximum central density (parts a—c) and the integrated densitometric area (parts d—f). The ratio f of scattered X-ray intensity I_s, to detected primary X-ray intensity I_0 is 0.0 (parts a and d), 0.2 (parts b and e) and 0.5 (parts c and f).

least two views, it is possible, using Eq. (8), to obtain an estimate from each view of the vessel cross-sectional area at each point in each vessel. In our current implementation of the algorithm, these two values are averaged to obtain a 'better' estimate of the true vessel lumen area. It is, however, possible to use the densitometric measures from both views to obtain a refinement to the lumen shape. Reiber has proposed an elaborate method that obtains an estimate of absolute vessel cross-sectional shape [22]. In this paper we propose a simple method of obtaining an estimate of vessel elonga-tion. The method assumes an elliptical cross section and determines the magnitude and direction of ellipse elongation. For this procedure the con-version factor k will be determined for each image as outlined above for absolute area determinations. In deriving the following expressions, we simplify by assuming the vessel is parallel to the imaging planes. The general-ization to arbitrary orientations proceeds as was done above. For an ellipse the cross-sectional area is obtained as:

$$A_i = k \sum_j d_{ij} \Delta x_i = \pi ab \tag{12}$$

where a and b are the semi-minor and semi-major axes, respectively. If the long axis of the ellipse is oriented along the X-ray path, the central density value will be:

$$2a = kd_{max}. \tag{13}$$

The densitometric diameter obtained from Eq. (5) would be $2b$, or the diameter parallel to the imaging plane. The ratio of the minor to the major axis could be obtained as the ratio ε of the area to the square of the central maximum diameter:

$$\frac{4k \sum_j d_j \Delta x}{\pi k^2 d_{max}^2} = \frac{4\pi ab}{\pi 4a^2} = \frac{b}{a} = \varepsilon. \tag{14}$$

If the minor axis of the ellipse is at an angle β with respect to the imaging plane, the area measured is still πab while the maximum central dimension is:

$$kd_{max} = \frac{ab}{\sqrt{b^2 \cos^2 \beta + a^2 \sin^2 \beta}}. \tag{15}$$

The ratio ε obtained in analogy to Eq. (14) is:

$$e(\beta) = \frac{b}{a} \cos^2 \beta + \frac{a}{b} \sin^2 \beta. \tag{16}$$

The vessel orientation relative to each view is determined by the centerline reconstruction algorithm. Although the angle β is not known, the relative change in β can be computed from the view orientations. By measuring the ratio ε for two or more angles, it is possible to solve for the ratio b/a as well as β. From the ratio and the absolute area, the absolute major and minor axes can also be determined.

Blood flow

Once the three-dimensional reconstruction of the vascular bed is obtained, blood flow is measured by tracking the leading edge of the iodine contrast bolus through the arterial tree structure in a sequence of images. Flow Q through a branch is then defined as the volume traversed divided by the time between images:

$$Q = \Delta V / \Delta t. \tag{17}$$

Although the iodine bolus may pass rapidly through a short vessel segment, it is still possible to compute the flow through the segment by adding the volume traversed by the bolus through all sub-branches of the segment of interest [14]. Such measurements require that the sub-branches be included in the reconstruction and can only be made while the bolus is contained within reconstructed sub-branches.

The determination of bolus position is a difficult problem because of the arbitrary orientation of the vessels relative to the imaging plane and because of potential turbulence and dispersion effects. We have developed a technique which corrects for vessel orientation but neglects potential effects due to mixing and dispersion [16]. In the absence of mixing, the vessel profile will move uniformly as a function of volume traversed. We thus assume that the bolus density $\rho_I(s, t)$ has some shape as a function of volume along the vessel:

$$\rho_I(s, t) = \rho_I(V(s) - V_f(s, t)). \tag{18}$$

This equation indicates that the bolus density at a position s, is a function of the volume of bolus that has passed the point s at time t. This volume of passage is given here by $V(s) - V_f(s, t)$ where both volumes are measured from the same reference position. $V(s)$ is a measure of volume from some initial position to the point s on the vessel:

$$V(s) = \sum_{i=0}^{n(s)} A(s_i) \Delta s_i \tag{19}$$

and V_f is the volume of flow through the point s from time 0 to time t:

$$V_f(s, t) = \int_0^t Q(s, t') \, dt'. \tag{20}$$

In any of the digital projection X-ray images, the digital density value of the profile is proportional to iodine density as well as to the thickness of the vessel through which X-rays pass:

$$d_j(s_i) = k' \mu_I \rho_I(s_i) x_j(s_i)/\cos \theta_i. \tag{21}$$

The density at the position s at the center of the profile can be found as:

$$\rho_I(s_i) = \frac{d_{max}(s_i)}{k' \mu_I D(s_i)} \cos \theta_i. \tag{22}$$

Using Eq. (22) it is possible to determine the density profile along the artery segment, with correction for change in cross section. Measurement of the iodine bolus profile as a function of volume along the length of the artery segment can then be used to determine the location of the profile. Currently in our system we use Eq. (22) to determine a single point of specified density on the leading edge of the bolus. Trying to match an extended profile shape would require corrections for branching where flow rates differ between branches. Such corrections may prove unnecessary if simple single point detection methods prove adequate.

Methods

Images for reconstruction were obtained from a Siemens Angioskop D interfaced to a Digitron II digital image acquisition system. This system is currently able to acquire images simultaneously with conventional cinefilm acquisition and thus requires no change in cath lab procedure. The images are then transfered to a VAX 11/750 for image processing. Reconstruction requires two views of known orientation. Although the views do not need to be orthogonal, best results appear to occur when the angle between views is between 40° and 90°.

Centerline reconstruction

The centerline reconstruction algorithm which has been described in some detail previously [11—13] consists of a collection of operators which operate on and interconvert between related data structures. The principle data structures are the original image, the planar vessel representation (plane_tree) and the three-dimensional vessel representation (tree). Each element in the tree structure contains the three-dimensional position, orientation and size (radius) of the vessel at that point. The plane_tree contains the same information for two dimensions in the coordinate system of the image. The tree structures also contain the branching hierarchy for all elements. The reconstruction process consists of the operations: 1. Specification (or recognition) of the primary vessel branching structure (i.e. the number and inter-relationships of the branches); 2. determination of the plane_tree for each projection image; and 3. construction of the 3D tree from the plane_trees. Pseudo inverse operations which can be of significant utility, include projection of the 3D tree to form a plane tree and conversion of a plane_tree to a projection image.

The internal consistency of the algorithms is tested by projecting a mathematical representation of a three-dimensional tree onto two images at different orientations. These images are then input into the reconstruction process and the resulting tree is compared with the original.

Results

The features of the 3D reconstruction algorithm are illustrated in the following case study. An example of algorithm validation by simulation is also included.

Clinical example

In Fig. 2 we show 2 views of a left coronary artery. The approximate view orientations are obtained from image intensifier position and angle readout displays on the Angioskop controls. Table position is not controlled, but an approximate magnification is obtained from measurements of the patient relative to the image intensifier face.

The images are then viewed in motion both on the digital display device and cinefilm in order to determine which points and vessel branches correspond between views. Sets of these points are then entered (Fig. 3) and the view geometry is evaluated as shown in Fig. 4. The square dots are points entered on the view shown and the line segments represent the X-ray path of the corresponding point from the other view projected onto the view shown. The short line segment between the small square and the X-ray path gives a measure of the deviation due to geometry misalignment. Geometry adjustment is currently accomplished by minimizing the sum of the squares of the deviations. This is done using an algorithm that assesses small adjustments to angles, position offset and view magnification. Improvements in geometry alignment due to this procedure are illustrated in parts b and c of Fig. 4.

After geometric alignment has been accomplished, vessel centerlines and edges are determined using operator directed automated algorithms [14, 24, 25]. Node points (vessel branch points and other recognizable points) must currently be accurately specified in each image of each view. Target lines along segments between node points are entered on the first image of each

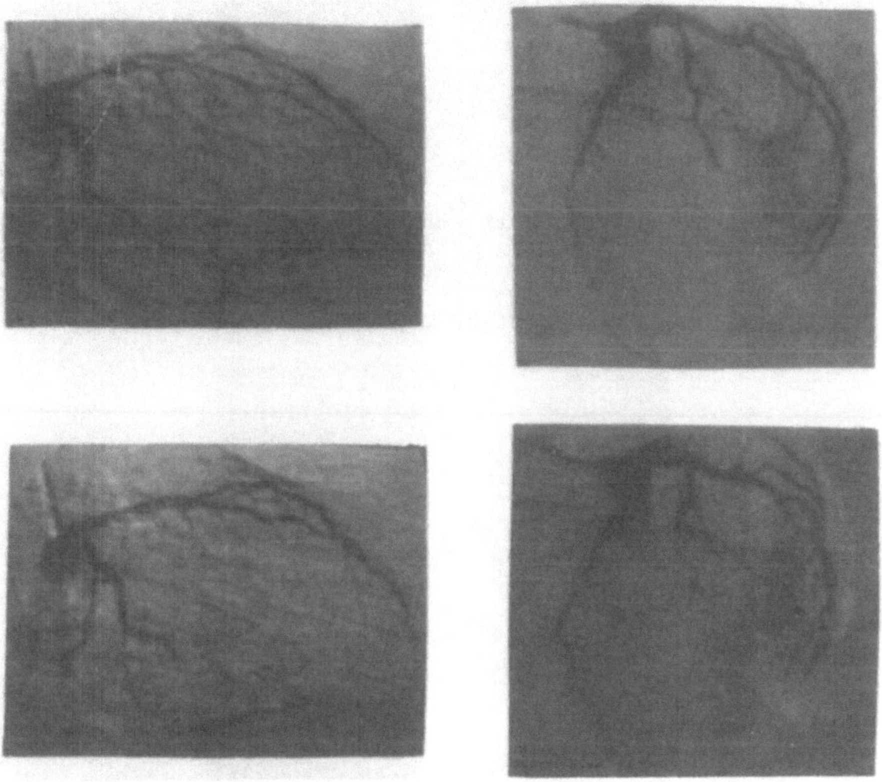

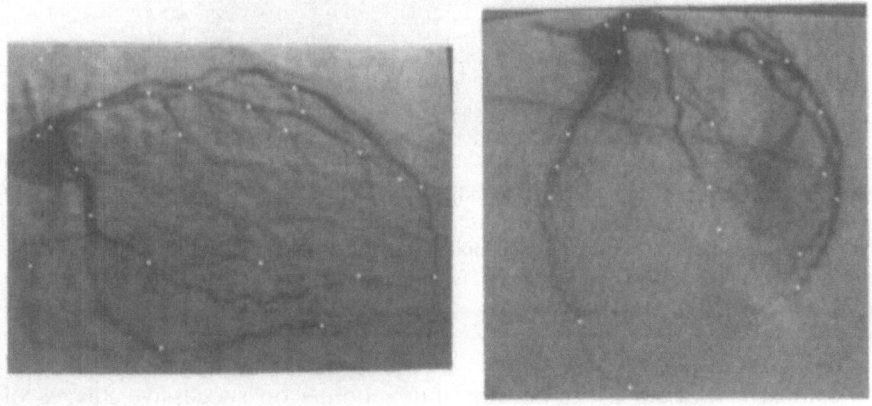

Figure 2. Original RAO (left) and LAO (right) views of left coronary artery system. Images are at diastole (top) and systole (bottom).

Figure 3. Corrresponding points indicated by bright dots on the RAO (left) and LAO (right) views.

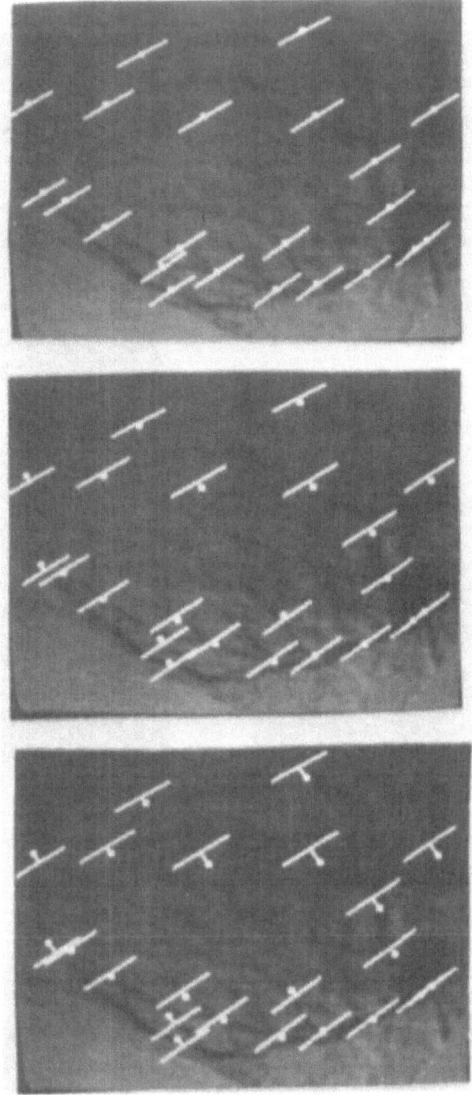

Figure 4. Using corresponding points to adjust imaging system geometry. Small squares represent points entered on the RAO view. The line segments represent segments of the projected X-ray path for the corresponding points in the LAO view. The distance between the points and the line segments is minimized from top to bottom by adjusting the assumed imaging geometry.

view and are 'warped' to fit between node points on successive images of each view (see Fig. 5). Boundary detection based on dynamic programming is used to search for centerlines and edges near each target line on each image (Fig. 6). The boundary detection is currently an iterative process

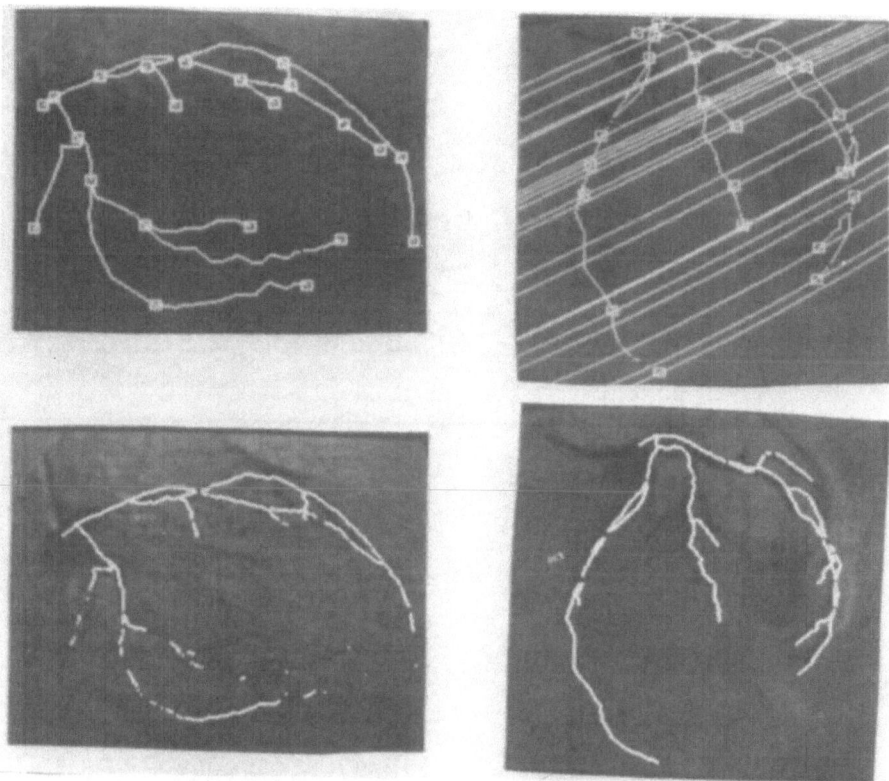

Figure 5. Vascular structure and target entry on RAO (left) and LAO (right) images. The original target is entered on the diastolic RAO image (upper left). The target is then warped by specifying branch point position on subsequent RAO images (lower left). The target is entered on the first image of the LAO view by moving node positions (vessel branch points) along X-ray path lines from the RAO view (upper right). The LAO target is warped by specifying branch positions for subsequent images (lower right).

where a rough centerline is first located, then both edges. Currently a new centerline is defined as the midpoint of the two edges. It is anticipated that a densitometric technique, such as center of mass, may improve centerline location results. After all edges in all images have been determined operator interaction is used to correct any mistakes in the computer determined centerlines and edges.

Once the vessel centerlines are known, 3D reconstruction is accomplished by matching all vessel points between views, projecting these points back to the X-ray source positions and determining the 3D positions closest to each pair of 'intersecting' lines. From the 3D reconstruction, the orientation of each vessel position relative to the imaging orientation in each view can be determined. Specifically, the angle θ of the vessel relative to the imaging plane is computed for each point along the projected vessel structure. Using

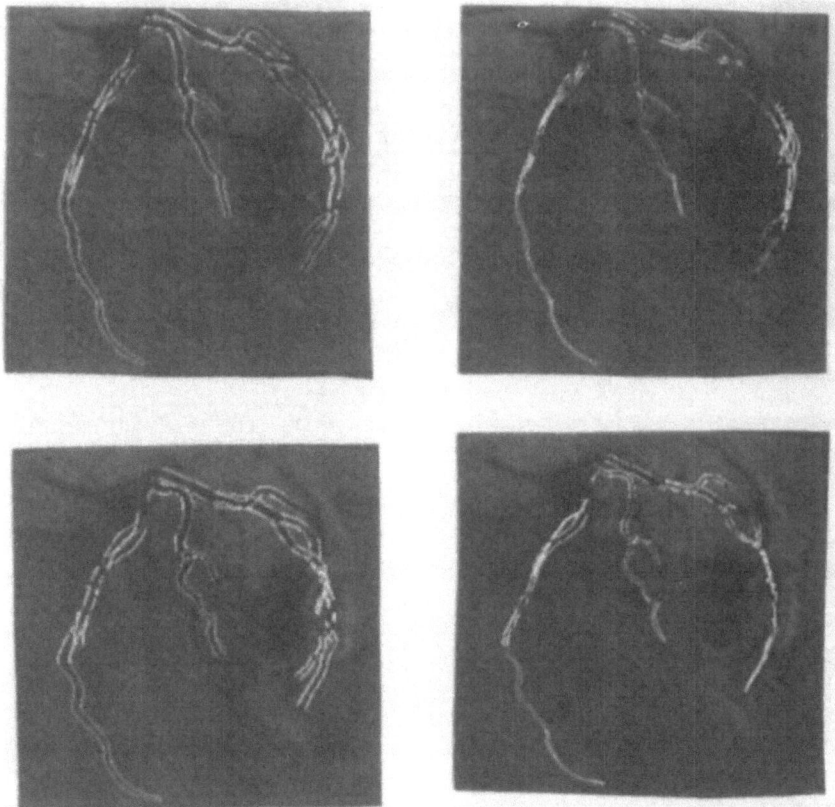

Figure 6. LAO vessel edges are first determined automatically using a matched filter perpendicular to the target and a dynamic programming search parallel to the target (left images). These edges are then recomputed (right images) using the cross-sectional area obtained from the densitometric profile as described in the text.

this angle and the densitometric profile orthogonal to the vessel, Eq. (9) is used to compute the conversion factor k for each image. Equation (8) is then used to compute the cross-sectional area and a measure of the radius is obtained from this area. Edges based on this corrected radius are displayed in Fig. 7. The measurements from the two views are then combined to generate the measure of the 3D tree. Finally, the measurements are averaged, on a point-by-point basis, over all instants in time throughout the cycle to reduce measurement noise.

Motion of a three-dimensional structure is difficult to portray on a single two-dimensional image. An attempt at showing the motion is given in Fig. 8 for various orientations of the arterial bed. The first two images are from two different points in the cardiac cycle. Each of the other images show the

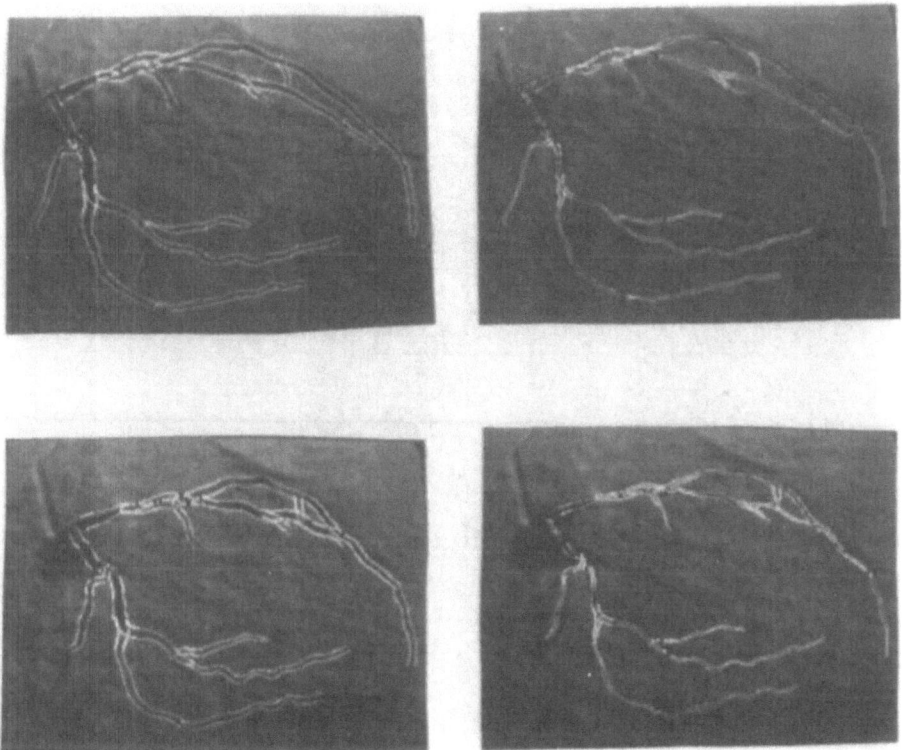

Figure 7. Same edge determinations (as described in Fig. 6) for the RAO view.

vessel in the same orientation at 3 points in time from end-diastole to end-systole. The vessel increases in brightness from diastole to systole to give the impression of motion.

The accuracy in reconstructed vessel centerline position cannot be directly assessed in clinical studies. The internal consistency of the reconstruction can be assessed by projecting the centerline onto the images of a third view (Fig. 9). The projected centerlines match reasonably well on nearly all vessels. In this case there is some discrepancy in the proximal LAD and distal circumflex branches. The left main, which was not clearly seen in either of the original views is not well reconstructed.

Flow measurements require that the reconstructed tree structure project uniformly to the vessel images for flow computation. For this study, the best images for flow computation were those of the third view. However, because of the misalignments between the actual and expected vessel locations the automated algorithm is not able to follow the bolus down the artery segments. In Fig. 10 some attempts at flow computation are given.

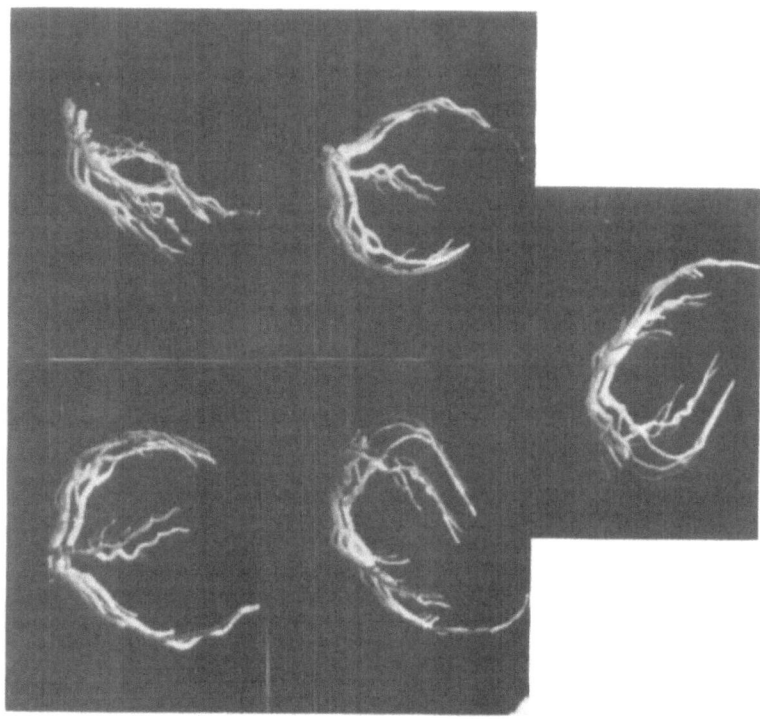

B:

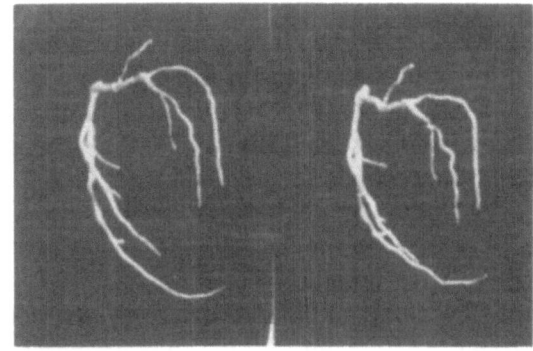

A:

Figure 8. Shaded surface displays of the 3D reconstructions of the vascular bed. The first two images (Fig. 8A) represent the vascular bed at two points in the cardiac cycle. The remaining images (Fig. 8B) attempt to portray motion of the arterial bed from five different view orientations. In each image, the artery is shown at three instants in time: end diastole (darkest), mid systole, and end systole (brightest).

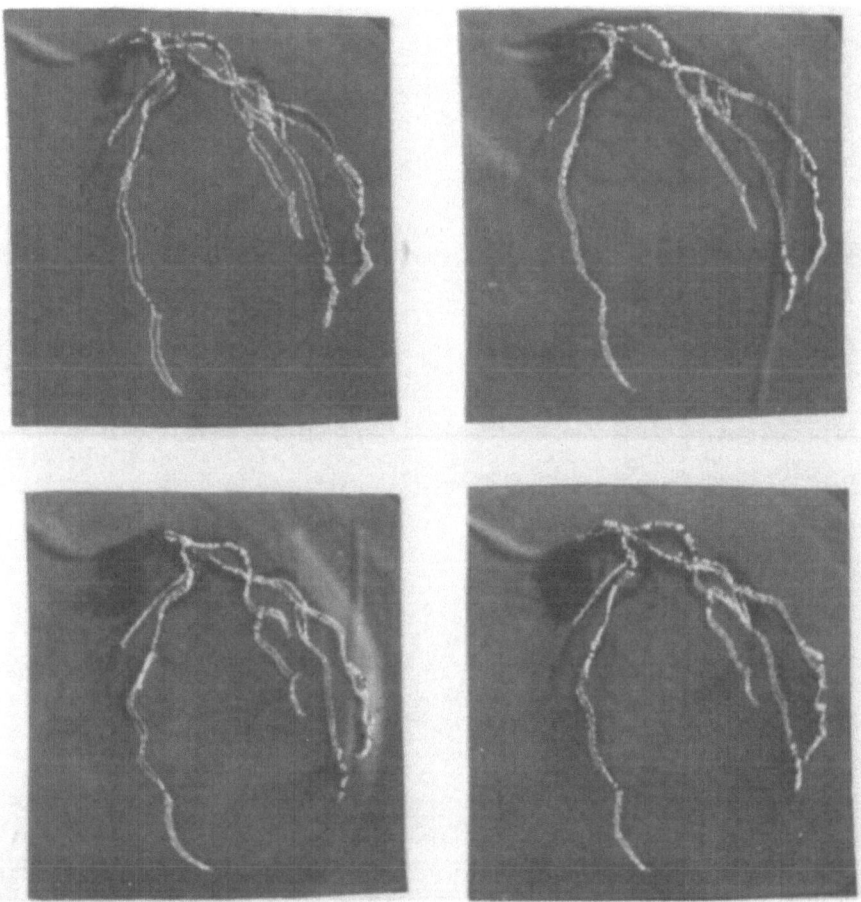

Figure 9. The consistency of the 3D reconstruction is illustrated by projecting edges from the 3D reconstruction at four different instants in the cardiac cycle onto 4 images (from corresponding times in the cardiac cycle) of a third view.

Simulation study

The internal consistency of the reconstruction algorithm is being tested by generating projection images of a three-dimensional vessel structure and by comparing reconstructions obtained from the projected images with the known dimensions of the original images. We give briefly some preliminary results of a simulation study to assess algorithm accuracy. Two projection views of a simple mathematically defined artery are given in Fig. 11. A small amount of scatter ($f = 0.2$) has been added to each image. The pixel dimensions are about 1 mm, referred back to the plane of the vessel.

242

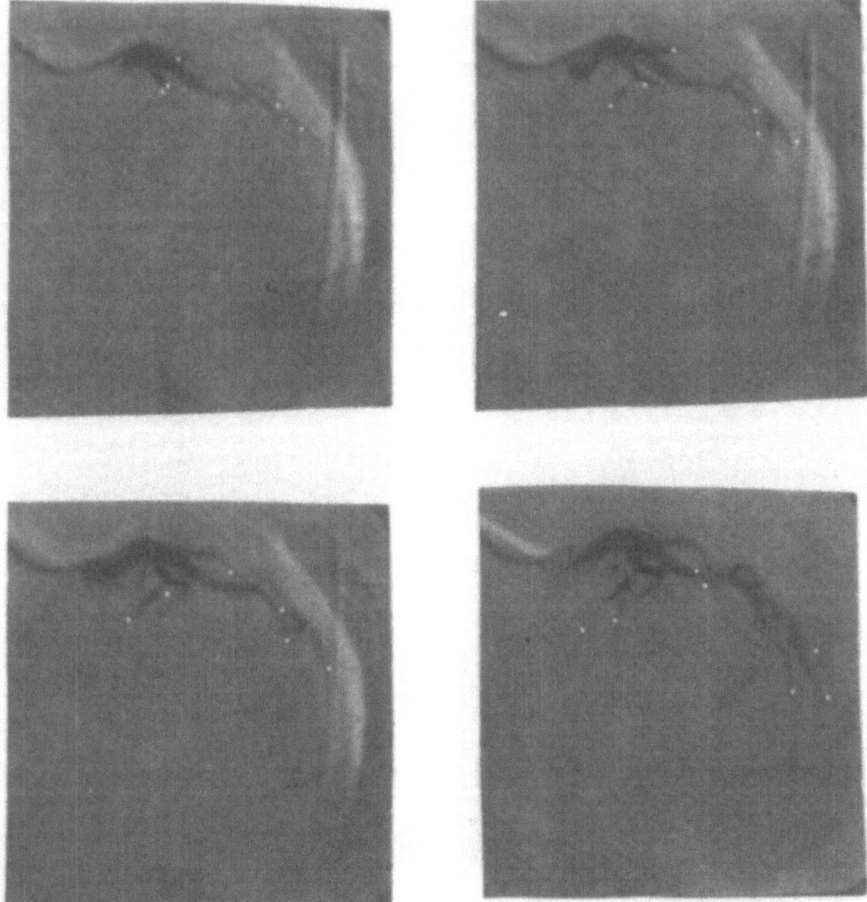

Figure 10. Four images from the early phase of iodine contrast injection from the sequence of images of the third view. Flow is determined by tracking the bolus leading edge down the reprojected vascular tree. The position of the bolus leading edge is indicated by the white dots. (Time sequence: top row followed by bottom row).

These images were then processed to generate a three-dimensional reconstruction. The radius determined from the matched filter dynamic program algorithm is shown as the top dotted line in the graphs of Fig. 12. The radii determined from the orientation corrected densitometric measurements are plotted as the lower dotted line. The calibration factor k is determined as described in this paper by averaging over the entire vessel structure and correcting for vessel orientation. The true radius is the solid line in each plot.

These preliminary experiments indicate that the densitometric measurements of vessel radius are much more accurate and precise than the dimensions of a single pixel. The effect of scatter has been found to be negligible

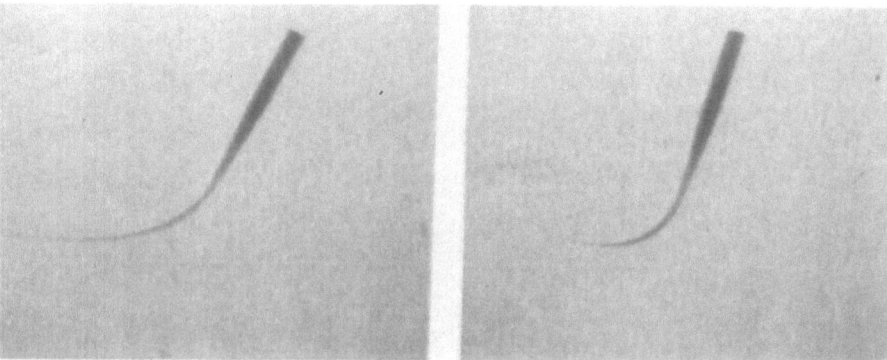

Figure 11. a and b. Two densitometric projection views of a computer generated artery segment. Views are generated with an angular separation of 30°. The top half of the vessel is a straight segment and is nearly parallel to the imaging plane of part a. A scatter fraction of $f = 0.2$ has been used.

compared to the effect of change in view orientations. Changes in view orientation appear to cause a minor shift in densitometrically determined vessel dimensions. This shift is still much smaller than the dimensions of a pixel and the causes of this shift are being investigated. It is likely that the shift results from minor inadequacies in the forward projection algorithm.

Discussion

The results presented in this paper are very preliminary. The problem of three-dimensional reconstruction of the arterial bed is very difficult because of the branching and overlapping of vessels. Although two clear views of a single vessel are sufficient for densitometric measurements, our initial experience indicates that two views cannot show all vessel segments clearly. It is expected that the inclusion of information from a third view, if properly oriented, will provide a significant increase in the number of vessels that are clearly resolved in at least two of the three views.

The time required for the complete reconstruction and display process is also quite long on our VAX 11/750. The time required is directly related to the number of images included in the cardiac cycle. The time also increases greatly when vessels are not clearly visualized in both views or when artifacts cause the automated vessel detection algorithm to stray. Operator interaction time has been greatly decreased by performing batch mode processing. The first reconstruction of the vessels shown in this paper took about 8 hours of operator time and another 20 to 30 hours of computer time. Projection onto the third view at that time caught a mistake in vessel recognition and matching between the other two views.

244

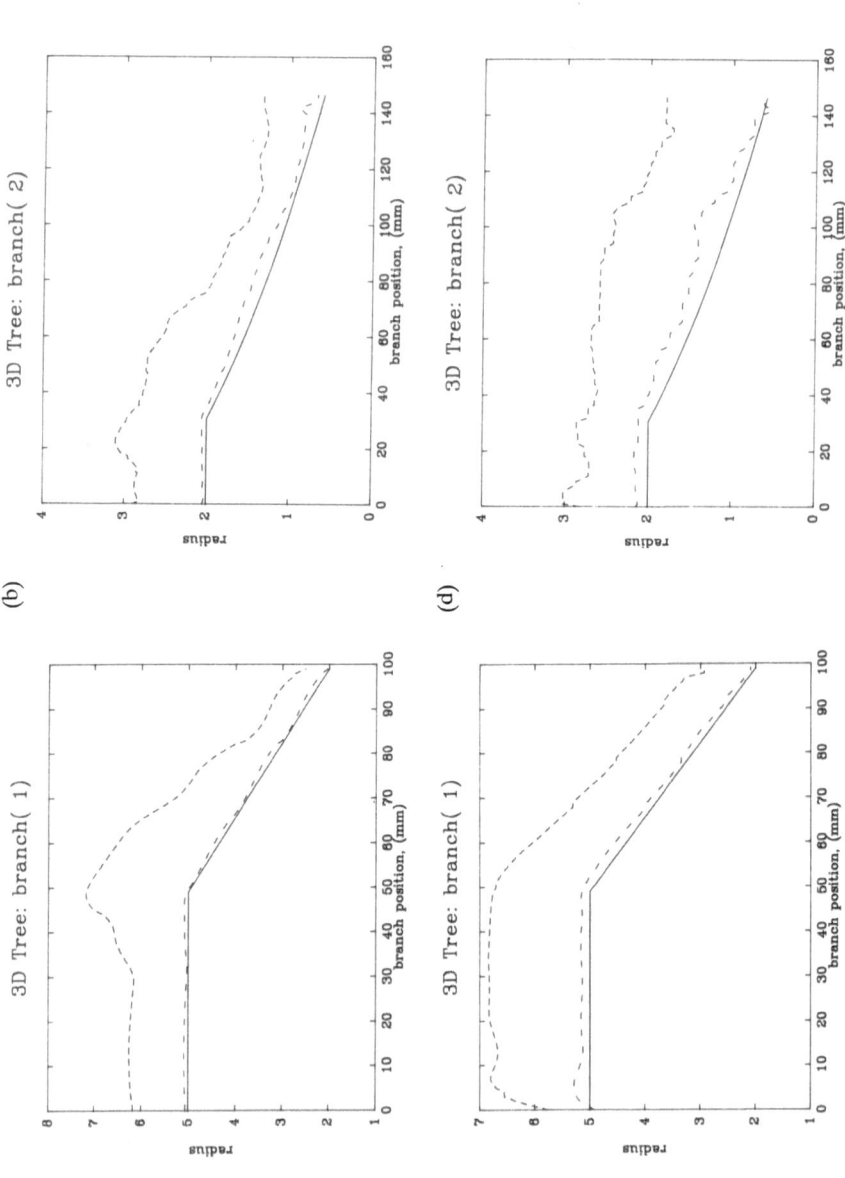

Figure 12. a and b: Radius measurements obtained from the 3D reconstruction of the projection images of Figure 11. The solid line is the true vessel radius. The top dotted line is the radius determined from the matched filtered edges and dynamic programming. The lower dotted line is the radius determined from the densitometric cross-sectional area. c and d: Radius measurements obtained from the 3D reconstruction of the computer generated artery segment using different view orientations (not shown). The straight vessel segment (the top half of the vessel in Fig. 11) is vertical and parallel to the imaging plane in both views and the two views are separated by 60°.

In spite of the problems still to be solved, we feel that these preliminary results are very encouraging. There are many algorithm modifications to be studied that may increase accuracy and reduce time required for operator involvement. Hardware improvements such as array processors and faster, dedicated image processing computers can also be expected to greatly increase speed. Finally, the goals to be addressed (e.g. following changes in general vascular morphology over time and measuring absolute coronary blood flow) are very important and justify continued research in this area.

Conclusions

We have presented an overview of a system designed to reconstruct coronary artery centerline position and lumen area at multiple points in time throughout the cardiac cycle. The preliminary results are encouraging and justify further research.

Acknowledgements

The authors acknowledge significant help from the cardiologists and technologists in the cardiac catheterization laboratory of LDS hospital. The work has been supported by Siemens Medical Systems and by grants from the Utah and Montana Heart Associations.

References

1. Brown BG, Bolson E, Frimer M, Dodge HT: Quantitative coronary arteriography. Estimation of dimensions, hemodynamic resistance, and atheroma mass of coronary artery lesions using the arteriogram and digital computation. Circulation 55(2): 329—337, 1977.
2. Sandor T, Spears JR, Paulin S: Densitometric determination of changes in the dimensions of coronary arteries. SPIE 314: 263—272, 1981.
3. Spears JR, Sandor T, Als AV, Malagold M, Markis JE, Grossman W, Serur JR, Paulin S: Computerized image analysis for quantitative measurement of vessel diameter from cineangiograms. Circulation 68(2): 453—461, 1983.
4. Brown BG, Petersen RB, Pierce CD, Bolson EL, Dodge HT: Arteriographic assessment of coronary disease: advantages, limitations, and clinical uses of a computer-assisted method. In: Cardiology Update, Reviews for Physicians, Elsevier Biomedical, New York, 1983, pp 67—98.
5. Doriot P-A, Rasoamanambelo L, Honegger H-P, Mérier G, Bopp P, Rutishauser W: Measurement of the degree of coronary stenosis by digital densitometry. Comput Cardiol, 329—332, 1981.
6. Nichols AB, Gabrieli CFO, Fenoglio JJ, Esser Jr PD: Quantification of relative coronary arterial stenosis by cinevideodensitometric analysis of coronary arteriograms. Circulation 69(3): 512—522, 1984.

246

7. Kruger RA: Estimation of the diameter of and iodine concentration within blood vessels using digital radiography devices. Med Phys 8(5): 652—658, 1981.

8. Reiber JHC, Gerbrands JJ, Booman F, Troost GJ, Boer A den, Slager CJ, Schuurbiers JCH: Objective characterization of coronary obstructions from monoplane cineangiograms and three-dimensional reconstruction of an arterial segment from two orthogonal views. In: Schwartz MD (ed): Applications of Computers in Medicine, 1982, pp 93—100.

9. Reiber JHC, Slager CJ, Schuurbiers JCH, Boer A den, Gerbrands JJ, Troost GJ, Scholts B, Kooijman CJ, Serruys PW: Transfer functions of the X-ray-cine-video chain applied to digital processing of coronary cineangiograms. In: Heintzen PH, Brennecke R, (eds): Digital Imaging in Cardiovascular Radiology. Georg Thieme Verlag, Stuttgart, 1983, pp. 89—104.

10. Reiber JHC, Kooijman CJ, Slager CJ, Gerbrands JJ, Schuurbiers JCH, Boer A den, Wijns W, Serruys PW: Computer assisted analysis of the severity of obstructions from coronary cineangiograms: a methodological review. Automedica 5: 219—238, 1984.

11. Parker DL, Pope DL, White KS, Tarbox LR, Marshall HW: Three dimensional reconstruction of vascular beds. In: Bacharach SL (ed): Proc Information Processing in Medical Imaging, Martinus Nijhoff Publishers, Dordrecht/Boston/Lancaster, 1985, pp. 414—430.

12. Parker DL, Pope DL, Van Bree R, Desai R: Three dimensional reconstruction of vascular beds from digital angiographic projections. Intrnl Workshop on Physics and Eng in Comp Multi-dimensional imaging and processing, Newport Beach, CA, 1986 (in press).

13. Parker DL, Pople DL, van Bree RE, Marshall HW: Flow measurements from 3D reconstruction of moving arterial beds from digital subtraction angiography. Comput Cardiol, 1986 (in press).

14. Parker DL, Pope DL, van Bree R, Marshall HW: Three dimensional reconstruction of moving arterial beds from digital subtraction angiography. Comput Biomed Res, 1987 (in press).

15. Parker DL, Pope DL, van Bree RE, Marshall HW: Three dimensional reconstruction and cross section measurements of coronary arteries using ECG correlated digital coronary arteriography. In: Heintzen PH (ed): Progress in Digital Angiocardiography. Martinus Nijhoff Publishers, Dordrecht, 1987 (in press).

16. Parker DL, Pope DL, van Bree RE, Marshall HW: Blood flow measurements in digital cardiac angiography using 3D coronary artery reconstructions. In: Heintzen PH (ed): Progress in Digital Angiocardiography. Martinus Nijhoff Publishers, Dordrecht, 1987 (in press).

17. MacKay SA, Potel MJ, Rubin JM: Graphics methods for tracking three-dimensional heart wall motion. Comp Biomed Res 15: 455—473, 1982.

18. Garrison JB, Ebert WL, Jenkins RE, Yionoulis SM, Malcom H, Heyler GA: Measurement of three-dimensional positions and motions of larger numbers of spherical radiopaque markers from biplane cineradiograms. Comput Biomed Res 15: 76—96, 1982.

19. Potel MJ, MacKay SA, Rubin JM, Aisen AM, Sayre RE: Three-dimensional left ventricular wall motion in man. Coordinate systems for representing wall movement direction. Invest Radiol 19(6): 499—509, 1984.

20. Kim HC, Min BG, Lee TS, Lee SJ, Lee CW, Park JH, Han MC: Three-dimensional digital subtraction angiography. IEEE Trans Med. Imaging MI-1(2): 152—158, 1982.

21. Colchester ACF, Hawkes DJ, Brunt JNH, Du Boulay GH, Wallis A: Pulsatile blood flow measurements with the aid of 3-D reconstructions from dynamic angiographic recordings. In: Bacharach SL (ed): Proc Information Processing in Medical Imaging, Martinus Nijhoff Publishers, Dordrecht/Boston/Lancaster, 1986: pp 247—265.

22. Reiber JHC, Gerbrands JJ, Troost GJ, Kooijman CJ, Slump CH: 3-D reconstruction of coronary arterial segments from two projections. In: Heintzen PH, Brennecke R (eds): Digital Imaging and Cardiovascular Radiology, Georg Thieme Verlag, Stuttgart, 1983, pp 151—163.

23. Mol CR, Colchester ACF, Hawkes DJ, O'Laoire SA, Hart G: 3-D reconstruction from biplane X-ray recordings: application to arterio-venous malformations. In: Jordan MM, Perkins WJ (ed): Computer-Aided Biomedical Imaging and Graphics. London: Biol Engin Soc, 1984 (abstract).
24. Pope DL, Parker DL, Gustafson DE, Clayton PD: Dynamic search algorithms in left ventricular border recognition and analysis of coronary arteries. Comput Cardiol, 71—75, 1984.
25. Pope DL, Parker DL, Clayton PD, Gustafson DE: Left ventricular border recognition using a dynamic search algorithm. Radiology 155: 513—518, 1985.

15. Coronary angioscopy during cardiac catheterization and surgery

THOMAS WENDT, L. ECKEL, M. KALTENBACH, E. KRAUSE, T. MÜLLER, N. RADÜNZ, K. SARAI, P. SATTER, R. SCHRÄDER, H. SIEVERT, C. VALLBRACHT, and G. KOBER

SUMMARY. Using angioscopes of 1.0 and 1.5 mm outer diameter (o.d.) coronary angioscopy was performed in 42 patients with coronary heart disease during cardiac catheterization and cardiac surgery without severe complications.

Our success rate of angioscopy was 47% during cardiac catheterization and 86% intraoperatively.

Angioscopy provides novel information concerning the morphology of atherosclerotic plaques, represents the best method for immediate, direct control of surgical interventions, and guarantees the performance of intraoperative balloon dilatation. Current indications for angioscopy lie in the area of intraoperative application. In the cardiac catheterization laboratory this method must still be regarded as experimental, because of unsolved technical problems.

Angioscopy may provide a means for delivering visually directed intravascular laser irradiation.

Introduction

Angiography presents pathologic changes of vessels, cardiac chambers and cardiac valves as photographic negatives. Now, for the first time, angioscopy has enabled the physician to look at these structures directly.

Since 1984, following experimental studies and *in-vitro* examinations with postmortem human hearts, angioscopy has been performed in our clinic in more than 100 patients with cardiovascular disease.

This report describes the procedures and results in coronary angioscopy in 42 patients, who underwent either cardiac catheterization (group 1) or cardiac surgery (group 2).

Our aims were:

(1) to optimize the angioscopic equipment utilization and the examination technique,
(2) to identify areas that require additional technical and methodical improvements and,
(3) to define the clinical indications for angioscopy.

J. C. Reiber & P. W. Serruys (eds.), New Developments in Quantitative Coronary Arteriography, 248—260.

Patients and methods

Patient population in group 1

Angioscopy was performed during cardiac catheterization in 16 coronary arteries and three vein grafts of 17 patients, aged 34 to 73 years (mean age 54, 14 males, 3 females).

In 13 patients with stable angina pectoris angioscopy was used for diagnostic purposes, in two patients it was applied pre and post PTCA and in two additional patients pre and post selective thrombolytic therapy.

Angioscopic equipment in group 1

Two fiberoptic angioscopes with outer diameters measuring 1.0 mm and 1.5 mm were utilized (Edwards Labs). Both have a working length of 150 cm and contain 12 illuminating bundles arranged in a circle. The 1.0 mm angioscope has approximately 2000 optical fibers with diameters between 5—7 μm, whereas the 1.5 mm angioscope contains 8000 fibers, 8—10 μm in diameter. Their field of view is 55 degrees in air and 42 degrees in saline solution. Depth of field is 1—15 mm with an optimal visual distance of 4 mm.

Behind the tip of the angioscope we fixed two metal markers for enhanced X-ray visibility; for some special cases an additional metal loop was attached, which accepted a 0.12 inch wire. In the beginning, the visualizations were documented with an Olympus 35 mm single lens reflex camera, thereafter with a NTSC color video camera with monitor and light source (Edwards), and finally exclusively with the PAL Endovision System 533 (Storz). Illumination was provided by the light sources (Storz) 600 BA (150 Watt), 488 B (205 Watt) or 484 BI (300 Watt). Permanent recordings were made with a 3/4 inch videotape recorder (Sony) and a VHS 5 head VT 8 E (Hitachi); for publications still photographs were obtained from this video material.

Cold sterilization was accomplished by immersing the flexible part of the angioscope in a plexiglas tube, which was filled with a 10% Gigasept® solution. The non-sterile angioscope eyepiece and the video camera were placed in a long sterile, transparent plastic covering.

Catheterization technique in group 1

During fluoroscopy the angioscope was inserted into an 8.0 or 8.5 F guiding catheter (Cook, Sterzer), which was inserted via a brachial or femoral artery approach into the coronary ostium. The tip of the angioscope was carefully pushed forward into the coronary artery in one of three ways A, B or C (Fig. 1):

Method A: Without additional materials, flushing was done through the guiding catheter.

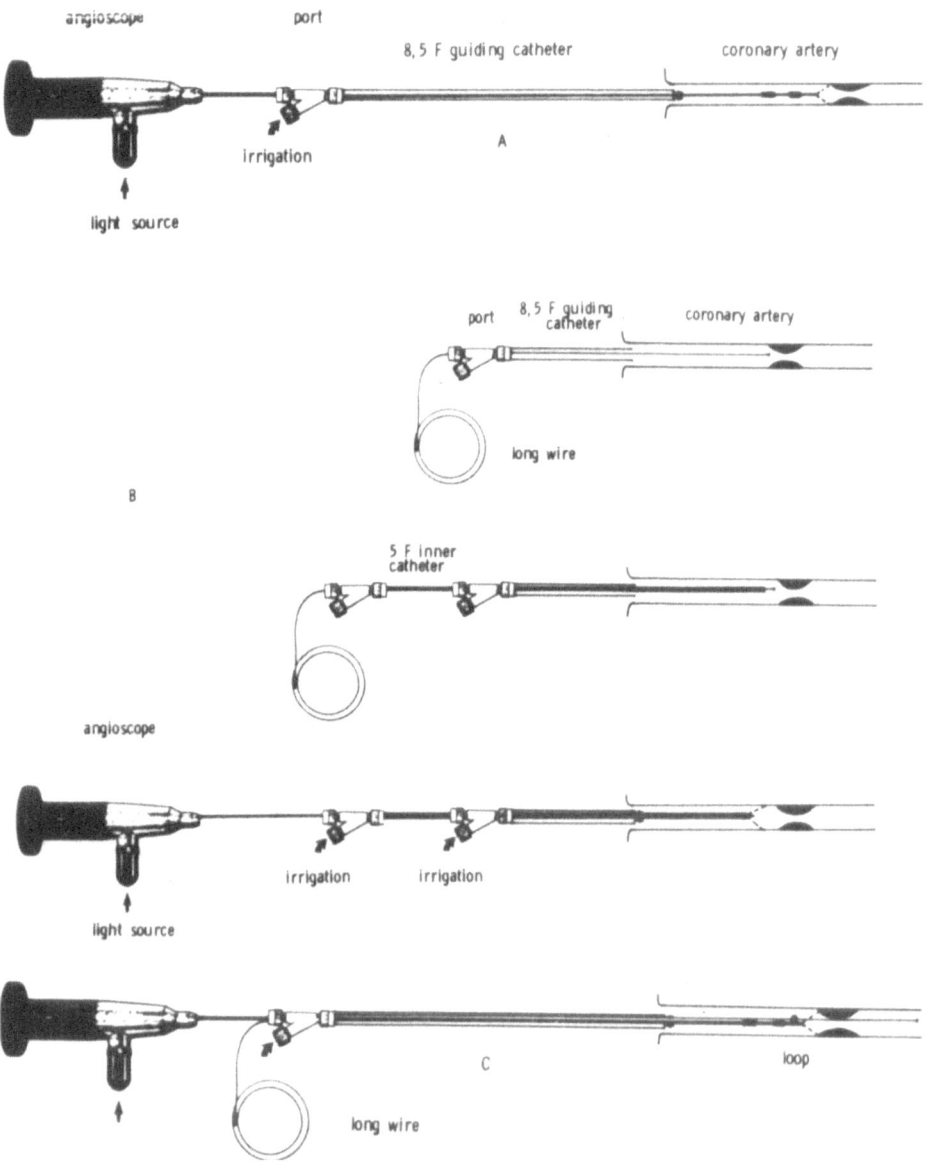

Figure 1. Angioscopic techniques during cardiac catheterization. A: Simple flushing through the guiding catheter. B: Double flushing through the guiding catheter and the inner catheter, which is placed over a long guide wire. C: Long-wire guided, loop assisted angioscopy.

Method B: After placement of the 8.5 F guiding catheter a 0.12 inch long-guide-wire was positioned in front of the stenosis, followed by a 5 F high flow angiography catheter (Krauth, Angiomed). As a next step, the guide wire was removed and exchanged for the angioscope. Irrigation was performed through both catheters simultaneously.

Method C: The 0.12 inch long-guide-wire was passed through the stenosis and the angioscope with the metal loop at the tip was pushed along the guide wire using it as a rail. Flushing was carried out through the 8.5 F guiding catheter.

All irrigations were done manually within 15 seconds using a 50 ml syringe containing Ringers solution at a temperature of 22°C. A maximum of 250 ml within 15 minutes was used per patient. Ringers solution proved best as a flushing fluid. Following the injection of isotonic saline solution some patients complained of angina. Contrast media were too viscous and produced streaking artifacts.

Patient population in group 2

Angioscopy was performed during aortocoronary bypass grafting in 25 patients aged 38—73 years (mean age 58 years, 22 males, 3 females). From this patient population one patient underwent emergency surgery following a PTCA complication, one suffered from unstable angina, while all others had stable angina. In two of the stable angina patients PTCA prior to surgery was unsuccessful.

Angioscopic equipment and operative technique in group 2

For intraoperative coronary angioscopy the angioscope was inserted into a 5 F high flow irrigation catheter (Krauth, Angiomed). If surgery was performed with blood cardioplegia or during hypothermia induced ventricular fibrillation, the orthograde blood flow was blocked temporarily from the outside with a swab. If surgery was performed with crystalloid cardioplegic solution, irrigation was not necessary. The angioscope-holding catheter was inserted by the surgeon through the arteriotomy and moved either orthograde or retrograde with a gentle rotating motion. For angioscopy of the distal anastomosis a second, 1.5 mm o.d. angioscope (Edwards), placed in a 7 F irrigation catheter, was inserted into the proximal end of the vein. In the same manner, desobliterated right coronary arteries were inspected.

A 1.7 mm o.d. Trimedyne angioscope with a Sony videocamera was used in two occasions.

Results

Group 1

In 8 of the 17 patients the selected vessel could be visualized, although not always completely inspected. With increasing experience, refinement in technique and changes in patient selection the success rate rose.

Angioscopy demonstrated, that stenotic or occluded vein grafts could be examined most easily, as they originate tangentially from the ascending aorta and have a relatively low flow rate. Of the native coronaries, the LCA was easier to probe than the RCA due to its straight proximal course. Because of the high flow rates in these arteries, clear visualization after irrigation was only possible for a short period of time.

Of the three angioscopic techniques described above, method A was most suitable for the inspection of aortocoronary bypasses and the RCA. In these cases movement of the heart during systole and diastole helped to push the angioscope forward without resistance.

Method B proved to be unsatisfactory. The inner 5 F catheter reduced the lumen of the guiding catheter to such extent, that adequate flushing could not be accomplished.

Procedure C was appropriate for peripheral stenoses of the LCA. The guide wire was not as stiff as the tip of the angioscope, which sometimes caused the wire to move in another direction. In addition, the metal loop sometimes worked like a barb when trying to pull the angioscope back into the guiding catheter. Therefore we gave up this technique.

The video camera system was indispensable. All examiners could watch the angioscopic picture at the same time, especially the one, who had to introduce the angioscope. Furthermore, structures that were only visible for a very short time could be replayed instantly in slow motion (frame by frame).

Angioscopy prolonged the cardiac catheterization procedure on the average by 15 minutes. Of the tested equipment only the American NTSC video system was inferior, because of poor resolution and unnatural colors in comparison to the Storz system. The variable and automatic light intensity regulator in the Storz light source 484 BI was very useful. In cases with only a short focusing distance to the structure of interest, the light intensity had to be reduced almost to zero to produce good pictures. The various appearances of atherosclerosis which we had learned from our examinations in peripheral arteries could not yet be demonstrated in the coronary arteries, as the number of successful examinations is still small and as there are greater technical difficulties to cope with.

We did, however, succeed in demonstrating that angiographically normal mainstems of LCA and RCA are smooth and pink angioscopically. Furthermore, we could determine that a bypass occlusion was caused by a red thrombus and could observe the results of subsequent thrombolytic therapy, which left angioscopically identifiable small fibrin remnants, which had not been noted angiographically. The other examinations did not produce satisfactory recordings. Complications did not occur.

Group 2

In 25 patients we experienced a success rate of 86%. After an introductory phase, in which the surgeon familiarized himself with the technique, the time necessary for an examination decreased to 5 minutes. By externally manipulating the inserted angioscopic device with a swab, little angulation of the tip could be accomplished. Light shining through the catheterized vessel proved to be advantageous.

Our experiences demonstrated, that the LAD could be visualized more easily than the LCX, which required that the heart be rotated. Artery irrigation could be improved by shortening the 5 F irrigation catheter to a minimal length of 15—20 cm. Additional holes made in the walls of this catheter increased the irrigation flow rate without improving the view in front of the lens. The view was best during withdrawal of the angioscope due to the more coaxial position of the scope in the lumen.

In the patient requiring emergency surgery following a PTCA dissection, the retrograde inspection of the LAD segment showed a circumferential protrusion of intimal tissue. During vigorous retrograde flushing the occlusion was forced open.

Angioscopy in the preoperative unstable patient showed an ulcus with a wall-adherent thrombus in the offending LAD. The two patients, in whom PTCA was unsuccessful despite correctly positioned and inflated balloons, showed a severe, excentric stenosis without peculiarities such as ulcus or thrombus, which could have explained the failure.

Three occluded LADs, which had been illuminated only partially with contrast medium during angiography, showed no additional plaques. Eighteen stenoses diagnosed preoperatively underwent intraoperative balloon dilatation. The distance from the stenosis to the incision was measured angioscopically. Therefore, the intraoperative dilatation was performed and finally, a follow-up angioscopy was carried out. A case example in a 48 year old woman is described below.

In the preoperative RAO angiogram a groove at the end of a proximal LAD stenosis could be seen (Fig. 2, arrows). Angioscopically, a wing like structure was demonstrated, which spread into the lumen laterally from the right (Fig. 3). After dilatation with an Edwards 2.0 mm intraoperative balloon catheter at 8 atm (125 psi) over a period of two minutes, the wing

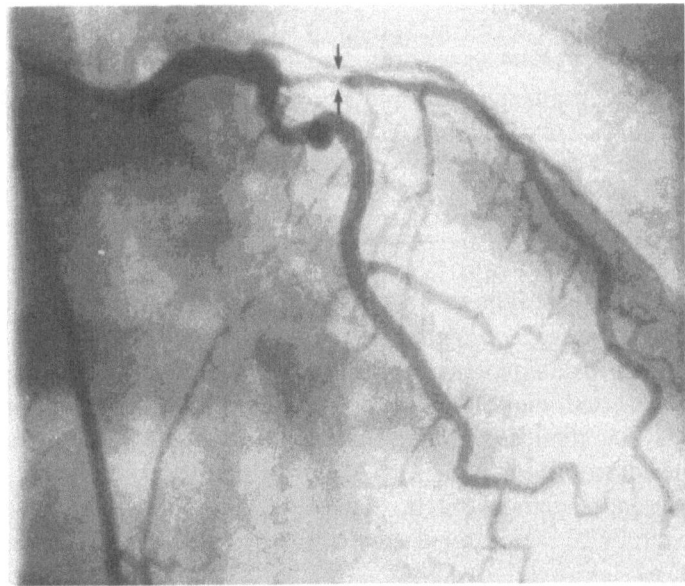

Figure 2. Preoperative right anterior oblique projection of a LCA in a 48 year old woman showing a proximal LAD stenosis with a groove at its end (arrows).

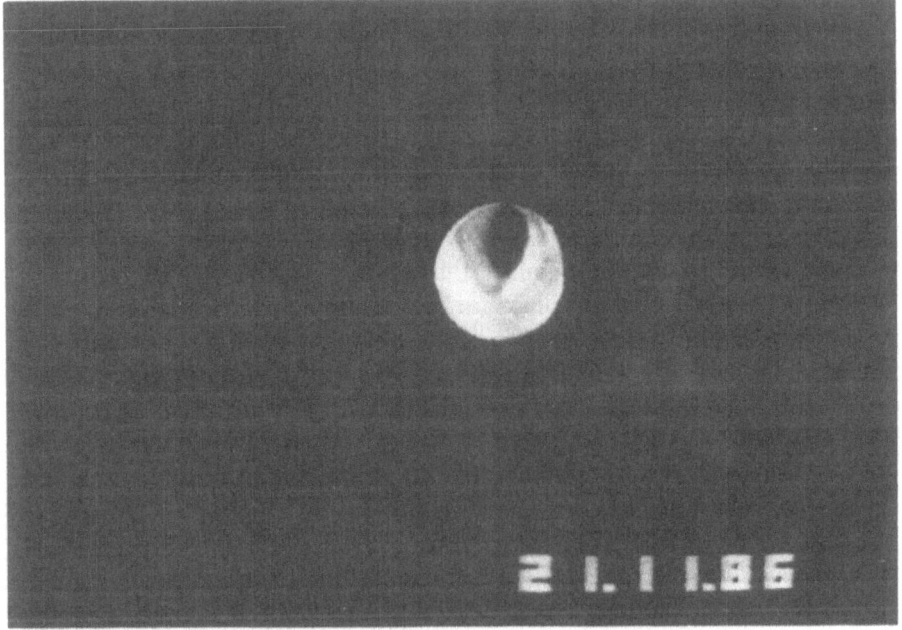

Figure 3. Intraoperative retrograde view of this groove, showing a wing like structure on the right half; the vessel segment behind this notch is oval stenotic.

was torn, so that it fluttered in the lumen during irrigation (Fig. 4). The follow-up angiogram obtained six days later showed the result (Fig. 5): the proximal stenosis was dilated and the wing had disappeared. However, the LAD was occluded distal to the incision as was the vein graft. Whether this was a complication caused by the angioscopic and dilatation manipulations at the incision, or due to the surgical technique, could not be ascertained.

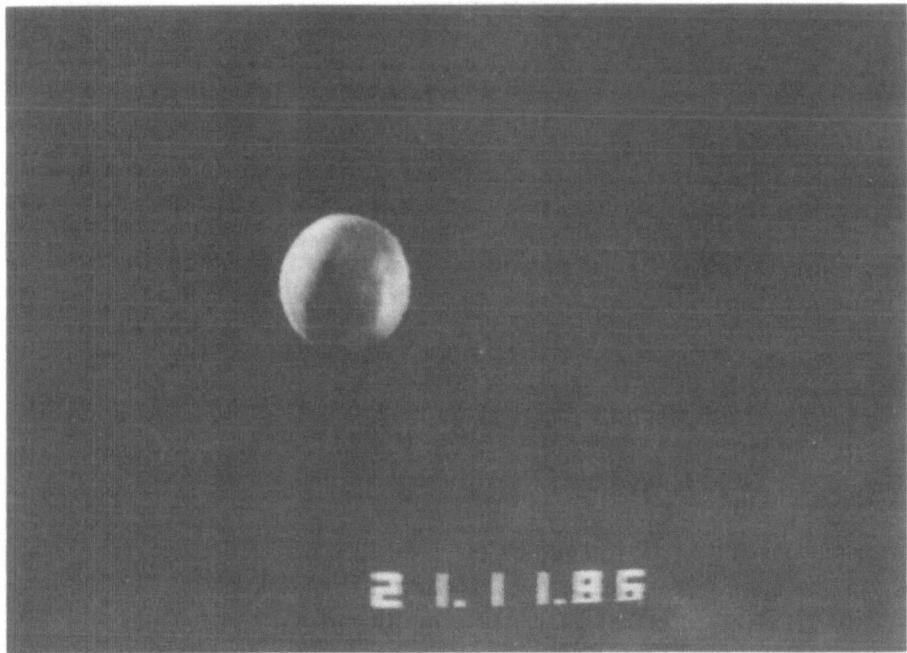

Figure 4. In the view identical to the one in Figure 3 but now following balloon dilatation the wing is still visible; it is torn at its upper and lower parts and flutters in the irrigation stream.

The remaining balloon dilatations demonstrated phenomenons we had seen in our *in-vitro* studies: smooth, raised, yellow-white plaques were pressed flat retaining their intact smooth surfaces, while ulcerated plaques remained rough following dilatation.

The angioscopic examination following six desobliterations of RCA's showed small remaining intimal shreds; in one case they could be removed with a Fogarty catheter.

All 23 angioscoped anastomoses were open; however, in one patient we found a large waving flap, which was excised. At the same time the vein grafts were examined for twisted sections, torsions and intima lesions, none of which were found.

Following the inspection of an internal mammarial artery that had not

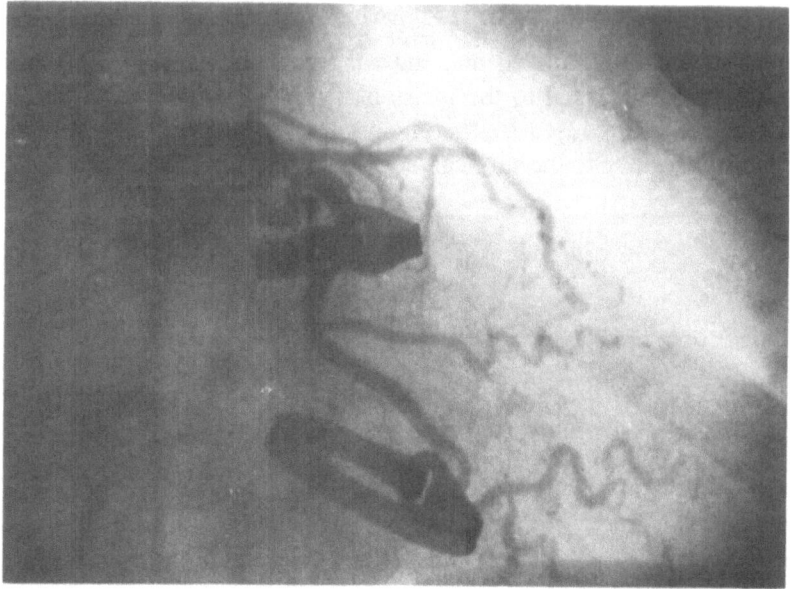

Figure 5. The angiographic follow-up six days later shows the dilated LAD stenosis; the groove is not visible anymore, but the distal LAD is occluded.

been angiogrammed preoperatively, a large ulcerous bed was found. This vessel was used as a bypass graft and was found completely occluded at the time of the follow-up angiogram. We cannot conclude whether this was due to the angioscopic manipulation, or to the preexisting ulcus. Complications directly related to the angioscopic procedure were not seen.

Discussion

Since 1982 various working groups have reported on coronary angioscopy during cardiac catheterization [1—3] and intraoperatively [1, 3—14]. They all agree, that this new procedure offers many advantages.

Intraoperatively

Vessels which have not been angiogrammed preoperatively such as an internal mammary artery, or those which only had an obscure angiographic visualization due to occlusion, can be inspected for further significant stenoses and plaques. Furthermore the transplanted vein can be examined for intimal lesions [14], injured valves or poorly ligated side branches. Finally, the result of any surgical intervention on the vessel can be controlled instantly, which allows immediate revision. Until to date, this desirable follow-up has only been possible with limited precision. The peripheral run-off and integrity of an implanted bypass graft can only be roughly ascertained by injection of a fluid into the proximal end of the vessel.

Electromagnetic flow measurement [15—17], which is performed after complete anastomosis of the graft, depends on many different parameters of which the most important is the hemodynamic condition of the patient [18, 19]. In addition, only severe stenoses influence flow rates quantitatively under intraoperative resting conditions [20]. However, long-term patency rates are greatly influenced by small intimal lesions and suture irregularities.

Intraoperative angiography, which is at present only utilized on a regular basis during peripheral vascular surgery is cumbersome and produces false negative results in 10—15% of the cases [20]. The recently proposed intraoperative visualization of coronary arteries with high-frequency ultrasound also gives only rough information [23].

The same is true for traditional lumen-control methods such as the ring-stripper or inflated balloon check-up, as well as for macroscopic judgements, to determine whether the extracted cylinder is complete and the level of dissection is maintained [24]. In our experience, angioscopy can detect the smallest intima stumps, floating intimal flaps, wall adherent thrombi, plaques, suture irregularities and bypass torsions.

In addition, it has been found useful for the localisation and identification of stenoses during intraoperative balloon dilatation [25], which we have confirmed.

Cardiac catheterization

During cardiac catheterization only special stenoses or occlusions can be inspected. In comparison to the results described by Hombach, our success rate has been lower, probably because of his use of a wider (9F) guiding catheter, which fully occluded the coronary ostium allowing easier irrigation [1]. This technique, however, allows little time for manoeuvering the angioscope to the segment of interest, because of arising ischemia.

The quantification of stenoses, which has been performed intraoperatively by Lee [7], cannot be achieved at present during cardiac catheterization, as the distance between object and lens is unknown; this has also been mentioned by Hombach [1].

Although several technical improvements were advanced by our group, routine coronary angioscopy during cardiac catheterization will not be possible before the following additional improvements are realized:

(1) The tip of the angioscope must be more flexible and must have an external angulation system.
(2) The guiding catheter should have a balloon on top to block the blood stream.
(3) The measurement of the distance between the lens and the object should be made possible for quantitating stenoses.

Similar to reports by other authors in other studies [1, 4, 6, 10, 13, 24], no severe complications occurred in our study. However, Chaux [4] reported two cases of intima dissections, which probably were caused by manipulations with the angioscope and which seem to be similar to the complications we had. Therefore, the possible occurrence of such complication should not be forgotten or disregarded.

Our experiences, although modest in comparison to the number of examinations already performed by the Cedars Sinai working group, supports the paradigm of Sherman [10], Litvack [8], Forrester [5, 27] and Grundfest (personal communication), which describes the relationship between clinical symptoms and the appearance of coronary endothelium. These authors report, that in stable angina the coronary arteries have smooth, yellow-white atheroma on the endothelial surface, in accelerated angina they develop endothelial ulcerations and in acute ischemia platelet aggregation and thrombus formation complicating the ulcus is seen. This stage leads either to a complete occlusion followed by infarction or to ulcus healing, which is followed by stenosis progression and stable angina at a lower level of exercise tolerance.

If this is true, it would have important therapeutical implications concerning the choice between PTCA, thrombolytic therapy, surgery, low speed rotational angioplasty [28], catheter affected atherectomy [29] or laser angioplasty [30—35].

Conclusion

Coronary angioscopy is a relatively simple and safe procedure and provides clinically relevant information. Intraoperatively it has found its place already in the immediate control of surgical interventions and it can be of assistance during balloon dilatation. Before it takes its place in routine cardiac catheterization, further technical improvements are necessary. In combination with laser angioplasty it may provide a valuable new alternative for the treatment of occlusive vascular disease.

Acknowledgements

This study was supported by the Riese and the Dr. Carl Wilder Foundations. Special thanks are due to Edwards, Storz, W. Bamberg and Monica Meyer.

References

1. Hombach V, Höher M, Hannekum A, Hügel W, Buran B, Höpp HW, Hirche Hj: Erste klinische Erfahrungen mit der Koronarendoskopie. Dtsch Med Wochenschr 111: 1135—1140, 1986.
2. Spears JR, Spokojny AM, Marais HJ: Coronary angioscopy during cardiac catheterization. J Am Coll Cardiol 6: 93—97, 1985.
3. Wendt T, Müller T, Eckel L, Krause E, Rauber K, Riemann H, Sarai C, Satter P, Sievert H, Stauder M, Vallbracht C, Kober G, Kaltenbach M: In vivo Angioskopie: Technik, Indikationen und Ergebnisse beim Menschen. Z Kardiol 76 (Suppl 1): 51, 1987 (Abstract).
4. Chaux A, Lee ME, Blanche C, Kass RM, Sherman TC, Hickey AE, Litvack F, Grundfest W, Forrester J, Matloff J: Intraoperative coronary angioscopy. J Thorac Cardiovasc Surg 92: 972—976, 1986.
5. Forrester J, Grundfest W, Litvack F, Lee M, Chaux A, Matloff J, Carroll R, Foran R, Berci G, Morgenstern L: Intraoperative vascular endoscopy using flexible fiberoptics. Circulation (Suppl II) 70: 297, 1984 (Abstract).
6. Grundfest WS, Litvack F, Sherman T, Carroll R, Lee M, Chaux A, Kass R, Matloff J, Berci G, Swan HJC, Morgenstern L, Forrester J: Delineation of peripheral and coronary detail by intraoperative angioscopy. Ann Surg 202: 394—400, 1985.
7. Lee G, Garcia JM, Corso PJ, Chan MC, Rink JL, Pichard A, Lee KK, Reis RL, Mason DT: Correlation of coronary angioscopic to angiographic findings in coronary artery disease. Am J Cardiol 58: 238—241, 1986.
8. Litvack F, Grundfest WS, Lee ME, Carroll RM, Foran R, Chaux A, Berci G, Rose HB, Matloff JM, Forrester JS: Angioscopic visualization of blood vessel interior in animals and humans. Clin Cardiol 8: 65—70, 1985.
9. Moosdorf R, Scheld HH, Stertmann WA, Hehrlein FW: Koronare Endoskopie-Eine neue intraoperative Kontrollmethode nach Endarteriektomie der rechten Kranzarterie: Thorac Cardiovasc Surg 35 (Suppl I): 14—15, 1986 (Abstract).
10. Sherman CT, Litvack F, Grundfest W, Lee M, Hickey A, Chaux A, Kass R, Blanche C, Matloff J, Morgenstern L, Ganz W, Swan HJC, Forrester J: Coronary angioscopy in patients with unstable angina pectoris. N Engl J Med 315: 913—919, 1986.
11. Sherman CT, Litvack F, Grundfest W, Lee ME, Chaux A, Kass R, Swan HJC, Matloff J, Forrester JS: Fiberoptic coronary angioscopy identifies thrombus in all patients with unstable angina. Circulation 72 (Supp III): 112, 1985 (Abstract).
12. Spears JR, Marais HJ, Serur J, Paulin S, Grossman W: In vivo coronary angioscopy. Circulation 66 (Supp II): 366, 1982 (Abstract).
13. Spears JR, Marais HJ, Serur J, Pomerantzeff O, Geyer RP, Sipzener RS, Weintraub R, Thurer R, Paulin S, Gerstin R, Grossman W: In vivo coronary angioscopy. J Am Coll Cardiol 1(5): 1311—1314, 1983.
14. Sanborn TA, Rygaard JA, Westbrook BM, Lazar HL, McCormick JR, Roberts AJ: Intraoperative angioscopy of saphenous vein and coronary arteries. J Thorac Cardiovasc Surg 91: 339—343, 1986.

15. Dedichen H: Measurement of arterial blood flow during surgery. Acta Chir Scand 140: 363—369, 1974.
16. Denison AB, Spencer MP, Green HK: A square wave electromagnetic flowmeter for application to intact blood vessels. Circ Res 3: 39—46, 1955.
17. Terry HJ: The electromagnetic measurement of blood flow during arterial surgery. Bio-Med Eng 7: 466—473, 1972.
18. Kobinia G, Teiner G, Hagmüller GW, Krösl: Parameter bei der Beurteilung der intra-operativen Flowmessung. In: Hild R, Spaan G (eds): Therapiekontrolle in der Angiologie. Verlag Gerhard Witzstrock, Baden-Baden, Köln, New York, 1979, pp 260—264.
19. Sandmann W: Blutige une unblutige Flußmessung zur Qualitäts-kontrolle in der Arterien-chirurgie. In: Hild R, Spaan G (eds): Therapiekontrolle in der Angiologie. Verlag Gerhard Witzstrock, Baden-Baden, Köln, New York, 1979, pp 49—63.
20. Vollmar JF, Heyden B, Hamann H: Wertigkeit intraoperativer Kontrollverfahren aus chirurgischer Sicht. In: Hild R, Spaan G (eds): Therapiekontrolle in der Angiologie. Verlag Gerhard Witzstrock, Baden-Baden, Köln, New York, 1979, pp 92—95.
21. Engelman RM, Clements JM, Herrmann JB: Routine operative arteriography following vascular reconstruction. Surg Gynecol Obstet 128: 745—752, 1969.
22. Lange J, Maurer PC, Bonke S: Die intraoperative Angiographie — heute unentbehrlich in der Gefäßchirurgie. In: Hild R, Spaan G (eds): Therapiekontrolle in der Angiologie. Verlag Gerhard Witzstrock, Baden-Baden, Köln, New York, 1979, pp 292—924.
23. Likungu J, Grube E, Kirchhoff PG, Quade G, Schubert W: Intraoperative Darstellung der Koronararterien mit hochfrequentem Ultraschall vor und nach Revaskularisation. Herz/Kreisl 19: 199—202, 1987.
24. Vollmar J: Rekonstruktive Chirurgie der Arterien. Georg Thieme Verlag, Stuttgart, 1975, p 24.
25. Roberts AJ, Faro RS, Feldman RL, Conti CR, Knauf DG, Alexander JA, Pepine CJ: Comparison of early and long-term results with intraoperative transluminal balloon catheter dilatation and coronary artery bypass grafting. J Thorac Cardiovasc Surg 86: 435—440, 1983.
26. Vollmar J: Die Gefäßendoskopie. Ein neuer Weg der intraoperativen Gefäßdiagnostik. Endoscopy 4: 141—145, 1969.
27. Forrester JS, Litvack F, Grundfest W, Hickey A: A perspective of coronary disease seen through the arteries of living man. Circulation 75: 505—513, 1987.
28. Vallbracht C, Kress J, Schweitzer M, Wendt T, Schneider M, Kaltenbach M: Low speed rotational angioplasty — experimental results in postmortem human arteries. Abstract book Fifth Joint Meeting of the Working Groups of the European Society of Cardiology, September 5—10, Santiago, Spain, 1987.
29. Höfling B, Backa D, Stäblein A, Remberger K, Lauterjung L, Martin E: Erste Erfahrungen mit dem Atherektomie Katheter. Z Kardiol 76 (Suppl 1): 51, 1987 (Abstract).
30. Schwartz A, Aulich A, Lavkamp H: Percutaneous transluminal angioscopy: A new approach to intravascular interventional techniques. Laser 3: 30—32, 1987.
31. Moosdorf R, Kraushaar J, Glauber M, Kling D, Fitz J, Mulch J, Hehrlein FW: Experimental application of an Argonlaser for arterial desobliteration, heart valve decalcification and vascular anastomoses. Laser 3: 16—20, 1987.
32. Geschwind HJ: Treatment of cardiovascular disease by laser angioplasty. Laser 3: 6—15, 1987.
33. Abela GS, Normann S, Cohen D, Heldman RL, Geiser EA, Conti CR: Effects of carbon dioxide; Nd-YAG, and Argon laser radiation on coronary atheromatous plaques. Am J Cardiol 50: 1199—1205, 1982.
34. Crea F, Abela GS, Fenech A, Smith W, Pepine CJ, Conti CR: Translumial laser irradiation of coronary arteries in live dogs: an angiographic and morphologic study of acute effects. Am J Cardiol 57: 171—174, 1986.
35. Wollenek G, Laufer G, Haschkovitz H, Wolner E: Koronare Laser-Angioplastie. Herz 6: 351—356, 1985.

16. The angioscopic view of atherosclerotic cardiovascular disease

WARREN GRUNDFEST, F. LITVACK, J. SEGALOWITZ, D. GLICK, F. MOHR, A. HICKEY, and S. FORRESTER

SUMMARY. We have performed intraoperative coronary angioscopy on 134 patients. A total of 228 vessels (85 LAD, 46 Cx, 24 Diag., 26 RCA, 47 grafts) were examined. In 18 patients with stable angina, smooth atherosclerotic plaque was seen in 17. In 13 patients with accelerated angina, 11 showed plaque ulceration and 2 patients had no identifiable ulcerative lesions. In 17 patients with rest angina, 15 showed a combination of intraluminal thrombus or ulceration with subintimal hemorrhage, and in 2, only smooth plaque was observed. In 1 patient with rest angina secondary to a vein graft lesion, histological examination confirmed a ruptured plaque with superimposed thrombus. In 8 post-MI patients, all demonstrated ulcerated plaque, 4 of which had superimposed thrombus. In 9 patients after failed PTCA, a combination of flaps and thrombus, not always angiographically demonstrated, (2 of 9) were observed.

Angioscopy demonstrates a spectrum of coronary morphology from smooth plaque to ulceration and thrombosis. These morphologies correlate with clinical status from stable angina through unstable anginal syndromes including myocardial infarction to failed PTCA. Percutaneous application of this technology is feasible, and combined with these data suggests that alterations in therapy may be based on angioscopic observations.

Introduction

Our group has played an active role in developing the technology of angioscopy. Angioscopy allows the physician to inspect the intimal surface and observe luminal details of blood vessels at points distal from operative sites. As such, the physician is able to look at the effects of intraoperative and percutaneous therapy and assess the impact these interventions have had on the intimal surface of the arterial wall. This chapter presents an overview of endoscopic technology and the rapidly developing applications of this field to the diagnosis and treatment of atherosclerotic vascular disease.

Methodology

Early attempts at intravascular observation were hampered by the lack of

J. C. Reiber & P. W. Serruys (eds.), New Developments in Quantitative Coronary Arteriography,
261—270.

appropriate devices. Until recently, the fiberoptic imaging bundle could not be miniaturized, and the smallest endoscopes were not practical for intra-vascular use. Attempts at rigid endoscopy were hampered by the limited scope of application. In 1983, Spears [1] published a report outlining the use of a small prototype flexible endoscope to view the coronary ostium via a guide catheter. This report heralded a new era in fiberoptics: the development of miniaturized endoscopes. Our group at Cedars-Sinai then developed miniaturized devices for vascular endoscopy [2, 3]. Commercially available angioscopes range in size from 0.5 to 2.8 mm in outer diameter. To view larger diameter vessels (greater than 3 mm), we employ angioscopes that are 1.0 to 2.8 mm in diameter (Olympus, Rye, NY and American Edwards, Santa Ana, California). For smaller vessels, we have used angioscopes which are as small as 0.5 mm in diameter. This new technology pioneered by our colleague Dr. Tsvi Goldenberg (Advanced Interventional Systems, Costa Mesa, California) permits percutaneous insertion and imaging in coronary and distal tibial vessels. In these small endoscopes, an imaging bundle of 3,000–8,000 imaging fibers is surrounded by a concentric ring of illumination fibers. The optical system is then packaged in a plastic catheter. The stiffness of the imaging bundle and the catheter material determines the flexibility of the endoscope. At present, only the devices larger than 2.5 mm are steerable.

Illumination is delivered through a side port on the endoscope to a concentric ring of illumination fibers. We employ a 1,000 Watt xenon light source (Storz Corporation, Los Angeles, California), although in most situations, a 500 Watt source is acceptable.

The optical image presented at the proximal end of a miniaturized bundle is too small for useful direct visual observation. We therefore interface the endoscope to a video camera via a specially designed video-endoscope coupler. These couplers have varying degrees of magnification. Several coupler models are commercially available. But as yet, none are optimal for our use. A variety of video cameras are also available for endoscopy. When we want high quality permanent video records, we employ a low noise, high gain (Sharp XC801RP), three tube camera. This camera is cumbersome, and when we want adequate clinical information only, we use small 'chip' cameras weighing only a few ounces. Due to the lower resolution and contrast specifications, images obtained with these solid state cameras are not as clear as those obtained with the three tube professional cameras. However, the advantages of small size, low weight, and ease of use, of the chip cameras makes these devices generally preferable for angioscopic applications. Images are always viewed on a high resolution color monitor. The video tape recorder also significantly affects the resolution of the stored images. We employ a 3/4″ Sony tapedeck.

Current endoscopes tend to be fragile; imaging bundles or illumination fibers break easily. After 20 to 30 uses, the image quality degrades due to mechanical fracture of the fibers. The development of disposable low cost endoscopes is in progress, but they are not yet commercially available. We keep detailed records on the quality of the imaging bundles as they are delivered from the factory. All endoscopes are tested for minimum focus, spatial resolution, and flaws in the jacketing. Devices with minimum focal lengths greater than 5 mm are not applicable in intravascular imaging. The spatial resolution of currently available endoscopes exceeds 200 microns at 5 mm. Therefore, it is possible to obtain high resolution images with these devices.

The most common cause for poor images is the inability to remove blood from the imaging field. At present, no adequate commercial irrigation systems are available. We employ a variety of systems depending on the surgical site. In peripheral vascular applications, a pressurized crystaloid solution is delivered through either a concentric or coaxial irrigating catheter. This irrigating system usually consists of an 8 or 9″ introducer catheter with a side port, or a 16 or 18 gauge 5 inch long intravenous catheter.

In the coronary system, angioscopy is performed during bypass surgery. Crystaloid cardioplegia is infused, either through the aortic root or via an 18 or 20 gauge 2 inch intravenous catheter. We are starting to perform percutaneous coronary angioscopy using crystaloid irrigation at body temperature delivered via the guide catheter.

At surgery, the angioscope is inserted through an arteriotomy. Both the proximal and distal lumens are inspected. After completion of a distal graft anastomosis, the angioscope is inserted through the proximal limb of the graft to view the anastomosis.

In peripheral vascular bypass surgery, the angioscope can be inserted through a vein graft or synthetic graft as the operator desires. However, it is essential to have vascular control prior to angioscope insertion, because blood causes failure to obtain an image. When retrograde visualization is planned, a Fogarty balloon embolectomy catheter can be advanced proximally and the vessel irrigated prior to inspection. This works particularly well in the inspection of occluded limbs of aorto-bifemoral grafts. At present, all angioscopes lack distance markers which would be helpful in determining lesion locations. We guide these first-generation angioscopes by gentle manipulation of the vessel and rotation of the angioscope while it is being advanced. In many instances, better images are obtained on withdrawal of the angioscope than on insertion. To date, we have performed more than 130 coronary and 85 peripheral vascular angioscopies. We have obtained more than 250 angioscopic images. We have a 15% failure rate, primarily due to the inability to deliver sufficient volume of fluid to clear the imaging field.

Results of angioscopic investigation

Peripheral vascular

We have detected a variety of unsuspected technical errors which occur during vascular surgery. Of the 37 peripheral anastomoses angioscoped, five (13%) [5] were revised based on angioscopic images. Three of the revisions occurred in femoral popliteal bypass grafts, one in an axillary bypass graft, and one in the distal limb of an aorta bifemoral bypass graft. Revisions were for redundancy of graft material, intraluminal flaps or misplaced sutures that caused significant obstruction of flow. Figure 1 shows a typical example of a

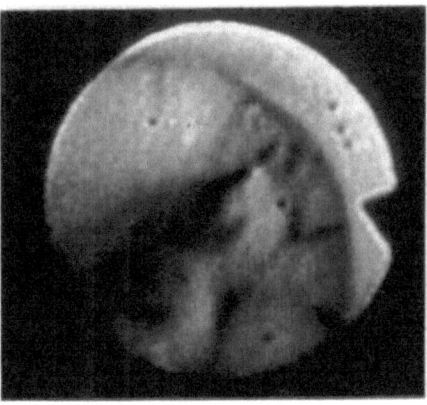

Figure 1. This angioscopic image shows the distal half of a distal anastamosis of a gortex supergeniculate femoral popliteal bypass graft. A large intimal flap stretching from the center of the field to the 6:30 position is seen obstructing the outflow track. Based on this angioscopic image, this anastamosis was revised.

large, filamentous flap obstructing the distal outflow in a femoral popliteal bypass graft. The novice angioscopist must learn that, to the inexperienced observer, a small flap can appear to be enormous if it is close to the distal tip of the angioscope. Whenever possible, lesions should be compared to the size of the distal or proximal orifice or adjacent suture material to estimate relative sizes. Of the 32 anastomoses which were felt to be technically successful by traditional surgical criteria, angioscopic inspection often revealed small intimal fragments which did not compromise flow. Figure 2 is an angioscopic photograph taken from an infrageniculate insitu femoral popliteal bypass graft. Several small flaps were seen angioscopically, the largest of which is in the center of this photograph. The lumen which occupies the upper quarter of the frame appears adequate, and this anastamosis was left in tact.

Although we have only anecdotal information about the prognostic value

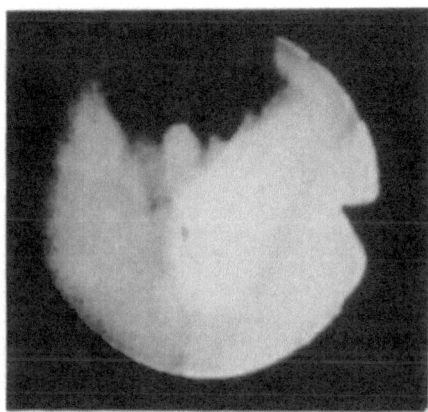

Figure 2. This angioscopic photograph was obtained after completion of an *in-situ* infrageniculate femoral popliteal bypass graft. While the distal lumen of the anastamosis was widely patent, small and probably insignificant flaps were seen. These flaps were left in place and did not appear to accumulate thrombus.

of angioscopy, it seems likely that the information we obtain is both unique and important. In three cases, we have performed angioscopic inspection. After completion, arteriography showed a normal anastomosis and outflow tract. Angioscopy showed obstructing vascular webs or thrombosis in all three. In two cases, no action was taken, and the vessels occluded 1—2 days post-operatively. In the third case, the thrombus was removed and an intimal flap was secured with an uneventful follow-up.

We have angioscoped 68 patients during femoral popliteal bypass surgery. Various techniques were used to create the bypass graft. Of the 17 *in-situ* procedures, 8 veins had intact valves at angioscopy, which led to repeat valve disruption. Angioscopy often revealed sclerotic vein segments in both *in-situ* and reverse saphenous vein grafts. Usually dilatation, or removal of overlying connective tissue was sufficient to achieve appropriate luminal diameter (< 3 mm). However, in 3 of 28 veins, angioscopic findings of localized sclerosis led to excision of the segment. In the 8 thrombectomies we have examined by angioscopy, 7 revealed residual thrombus, intimal flaps or disrupted plaque [4]. Figure 3 demonstrates the lumen of a dacron graft after an apparently successful attempt at embolectomy. On angioscopic inspection, a significant portion of the lumen was still occupied by thrombus and neointimal debris as seen in this figure. Repeat thrombectomy under angioscopic guidance resulted in a debris free lumen in all cases.

Coronary angioscopy

Angioscopy during coronary artery bypass surgery has revealed a smaller

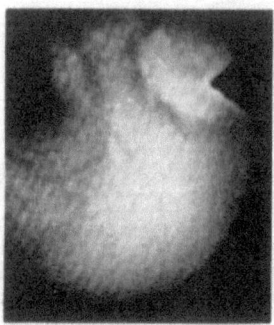

Figure 3. This figure was obtained from a 73 year old man undergoing embolectomy and thrombectomy of a vein graft. After multiple attempts, thrombectomy angioscopy was used to inspect the proximal portion of the vein. Upon inspection, this large flap seen between 3:00 and 5:00 was noted, as well as considerable residual thrombus. Under direct visualization, a Fogarty embolectomy balloon was passed, and after three additional tries, good results were achieved.

number of technical errors. In newly created anastomoses, three of 36 were found to have either misplaced sutures or intimal flaps. In three other cases, angioscopy led to revision of an old graft or placement of an additional graft.

Angioscopy has given us new insights into the nature of coronary ischemic syndromes. In patients with chronic stable angina, the intimal surface was typically smooth, yellow-white, and glistening without evidence of disruption, as illustrated in Fig. 4 [6]. In contrast, most patients with acute ischemic syndromes were observed to have intimal ulcerations and thrombus [7]. In patients with accelerated angina (defined as increasing frequency of angina

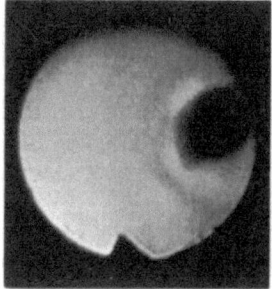

Figure 4. This figure shows the mid third of a left anterior descending coronary artery in a 71 year old patient with chronic stable angina. A lesion is seen encroaching on the lumen. The intimal surface is smooth yellow white and without intimal ulcerations.

without rest pain), we observed intimal ulcers and associated platelet aggregates. Figure 5 is an angioscopic view from a left anterior descending coronary artery from a patient with a two week history of accelerated angina. The posterior intimal surface in the center of the image is ulcerated and irregular with subintimal hemorrhage. In 18 patients with unstable angina at rest, the 'offending' artery (by ECG criteria) revealed thrombus and ulceration [8]. Figure 6 shows a typical obstructive thrombus taken from a patient with impending infarction. Of arteries observed post-infarction, some showed a variable combination of thrombus, ulceration, and intimal strands. Angioscopy provided information not seen at angiography. In most cases, the endothelial ulcer and the presence of partially occlusive thrombus was not detected by angiography. In 6 additional patients who had acute PTCA failure, intimal flaps and thrombus were seen in all, but were seen angiographically in only two [9].

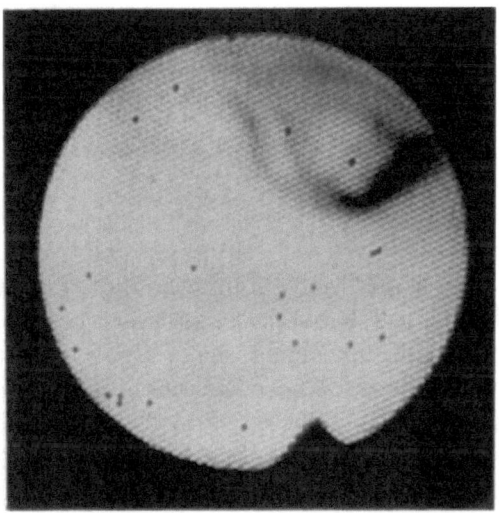

Figure 5. This figure shows the intimal surface of a patient with two weeks off accelerated angina. In the upper portion of the field, a discolored irregular surface can be seen. This is an ulcerated plaque with subintimal hemorrhage.

In peripheral vascular disease, correlation with the clinical syndromes are intrinsically less certain because syndromes are not as rigidly defined. In five patients with acute onset of leg pain at rest, we have observed ulcerative and thrombotic lesions in four [10]. Additionally, we have seen ulcerated and thrombotic lesions proximal to total obstructions in the superficial femoral artery. These observations suggest that endothelial ulceration often leads to thrombosis and/or distal embolization, i.e., that the ulcerative lesion with its subsequent sequela is the primary cause of acute vascular syndromes.

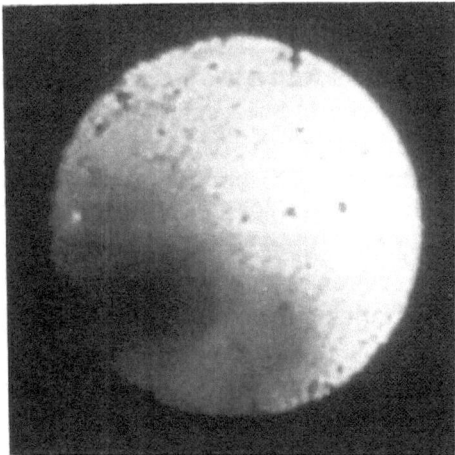

Figure 6. This angioscopic view taken from the LAD of a patient undergoing emergent bypass for acute recurrent ischemia shows the thrombotic nature of this coronary occlusion. The light of the angioscope can be seen reflecting off the thrombus in the left-hand side of the image from about 7:00 to 10:00. Despite vigorous irrigation, this thrombus could not be dislodged.

Complications of angioscopy

Initial designs of angioscopes were primitive. The early devices (some of which are still available) had sharp distal ends which could cause endothelial abrasion and relatively stiff, unyielding, shafts which made them difficult to manipulate in the vascular tree. A new generation of angioscopes has largely overcome these problems. Nevertheless, forceful manipulation, particularly when there is no image, is dangerous. One should also avoid a large angioscope in a small vessel, because forced dilatation can lead to intimal disruption over a long segment. In the peripheral vascular circulation, we usually employ no more than 200—300 cc of crystaloid solution per angioscopic inspection. In coronary applications, we have found that irrigation through the aortic root can lead to excessive infusion of cardioplegia, and therefore the preferred route of irrigant delivery is by coaxial catheter. We have had no complications from fluid overload. To date, using first-generation devices, we have observed four intimal flaps which may have resulted from angioscopy. In one case, a flap at a newly created distal anastamosis was thought to be secondary to vigorous angioscopic inspection. This anastomosis required revision. In the other three cases, small flaps were identified and thought to be secondary to the sharp nature of the angioscopic tip. In these three cases, no clinical sequela were observed.

Technical limitations

Present commercially available angioscopes lack intrinsic steering and irrigating systems. Another limitation is the time required to assemble the system. However, new prototype systems with improved instrumentation may overcome some limitations. Disposable angioscopes and angioscopes with *in-situ* valve cutters which can be operated under direct vision are currently under development. Construction of more flexible devices, with further miniaturization of the optics is also in progress, with the goals of developing a more user-friendly system, and enabling percutaneous coronary angioscopy.

Newer developments in angioplasty

Recently, several companies have begun development of angioscopes as small as 0.4 mm in diameter. These scopes are intended to be used through a guide wire or over a guide wire to allow visualization during percutaneous transluminal angioplasty. When fully developed these systems will allow for detection of flaps and or thrombus after PTCA which are otherwise not seen angiographically. In our experience, angioscopy is significantly more sensitive and specific in detecting thrombus and ulcers than is angiography. As percutaneous angioscopes develop and systems for angioscope delivery become perfected, we believe that percutaneous angioscopy may play a significant role in determining endpoints for balloon angioplasty. Angioscopy has the potential to be an effective tool in the hands of the cardiovascular physician to improve his understanding of both the pathophysiology of atherosclerotic vascular disease and the causes and extent of acute failure due to cardiovascular interventions. We believe that rapid progress towards percutaneous angioscopy will result in clinical systems that are available to the interventional cardiologist over the next two to three years.

Acknowledgements

The authors would like to express their appreciation for the Vascular Surgeons: Robert Foran, M.D., Lewis Cohen, M.D., Philip Levin, M.D., David Cossman, M.D., Richard Treiman, M.D., and Robert Carroll, M.D., and Cardiovascular Surgeons: Myles Lee, M.D., Aurelio Chaux, M.D., Jack Matloff, M.D., Carlos Blanche, M.D. and Robert Kass, M.D. who participated in this research and helped to collect much of the angioscopic data.
    The authors gratefully acknowledge the contributions of Tsvi Goldenberg,

Ph.D., James Laudenslager, Ph.D., Tom Pacala, Ph.D., and Thannasis Papaioannou, M.Sc. of the Cedars-Sinai Laser Research Center.

This work is supported in part by Imperial Grand Sweepstakes, the Grand Sweepstakes, and the Medallions Fund of Cedars-Sinai Medical Center. Their generous contributions are gratefully acknowledged.

This work is supported in part by the Specialized Centers of Research in Ischemic Heart Disease of the National Heart Lung and Blood Institute, award # HL-17651.

Drs. Grundfest and Litvack are recipients of NHLBI Clinical Investigator Awards, # 1K0HL-01522 and # K08HL-01381-01, respectively.

Parts of this chapter are reproduced with permission from NEJM, Journal of Vascular Surgery, Circulation, Journal of Thoracic and Cardiovascular Surgery, Journal of American College of Cardiology, and Hamovici's Vascular Surgery Third Edition.

References

1. Spears JR, Marais HJ, Serur J: In vivo coronary angioscopy. J Am Coll Cardiol 51: 1311—1314, 1983.
2. Litvack F, Grundfest WS, Lee ME, et al.: Angioscopic visualization of blood vessel interior in animals and humans. Clin Cardiol 8: 65—70, 1985.
3. Grundfest WS, Litvack F, Sherman CT: Delineation of peripheral and coronary detail by intraoperative angioscopy. Ann Surg 202: 394—400, 1984.
4. Glick D, Grundfest WS, Litvack F, et al.: Intraoperative decisions based on angioscopy. Manuscript in Preparation.
5. Grundfest WS, Litvack F, Hickey A, Doyle L, et al.: The current status of angioscopy and laser angioplasty. J Vas. Surg (5)4: 667—673, 1987.
6. Chaux A, Lee M, Blanche C, et al.: Intraoperative coronary angioscopy: technique and results in the initial 58 patients. J Thorac Cardiovas Surg 92: 972—976, 1986.
7. Forrester JS, Litvack F, Grundfest WS, Hickey A: New insights into the role of thrombus in the pathogenesis of acute and chronic coronary heart disease. Perspective Circ.
8. Grundfest WS, Litvack F, Sherman T, et al.: Definition of new pathophysiologic mechanisms and altered decisions: An outcome of intravascular angioscopy. J Am Coll Cardiol 2: 153a, 1986.
9. Hickey A, Litvack F, Grundfest WS, Sherman T, Lee M, Chaux A, et al.: In vivo angioscopy following balloon angioplasty. Circulation 74 (Supp. II): II—458, 1986.
10. Glick DG, Grundfest WS, Litvack F, Hickey A, Treiman, R, et al.: Intraoperative decisions based on angioscopy in peripheral vascular surgery. Society for Clinical Vasc. Surg. 15th Symp.: 44, 1987.

17. Percutaneously implantable endo-coronary prosthesis

JACQUES PUEL, F. JOFFRE, H. ROUSSEAU, A. COURTAULT, M. GALINIER, J. HADDAD, and J. P. BOUNHOURE

SUMMARY. A promising new approach to reduce post-dilatation restenosis is the use of self-expanding endocoronary scaffolding or wall stent device. So far we have implanted the stent in 25 coronary patients; in 24 of these patients this was done post-dilatation to prevent coronary restenosis, and in 1 case the stent was placed at a stenosis in a venous coronary artery bypass graft. There were 15 event-free implantations with excellent angiographic follow-up ranging from 3 to 12 months in 14 cases. Acute or early occlusion (before the tenth day post-implant) occurred in 10 cases, probably related to technical complications of the implantation in 2 cases, to inadequate heparinization in 3 cases, to previous transmural myocardial infarction distal to the stent in 3 cases, and to inadequate congruence between the stent and the native coronary artery in 2 cases. Thus, the risk of a thrombus is more acute in the first two weeks post-implant. However, we have noted that the rate of early occlusion is decreasing with our familiarization with the device, optimisation of the drug therapy and of the patient selection. Beyond this critical period, our preliminary results are encouraging and suggest that the intra-coronary stent might be a promising adjunct to transluminal·coronary angioplasty.

Introduction

"How do we stabilize the initially successful coronary angioplasty?" This is the main question after 10 years of experience. Indeed, the rate of restenosis during the first 6 months following transluminal coronary angioplasty is still as high as 30 to 40% and continues to compromise the overall results of this procedure [1]. According to recent pathological studies, restenosis has its genesis within the arterial wall and specifically within the cracks caused by the dilatation itself [2]. The concept of sealing these fissures has let to the development of the wall stent, a new form of a self-expanding scaffolding prosthesis, being a promising approach to the prevention of restenosis.

Extensive animal experiments (Fig. 1) showed good vessel tolerance, good patency of sidebranches and, in particular, an endothelialisation completely and homogeneously covering the stent filament after a few weeks [3—4]. Following these promising experimental studies and upon the approval by the hospital ethics committee, we performed the first implantation on March

J. C. Reiber & P. W. Serruys (eds.), New Developments in Quantitative Coronary Arteriography,
271—277.

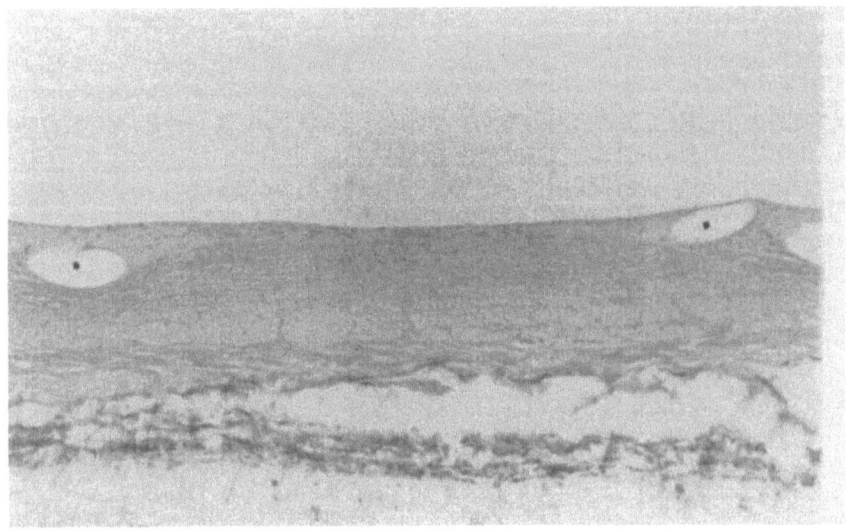

Figure 1. Longitudinal section of the stented coronary arterial wall 6 weeks after implantation. The stent is completely covered by a neointima. Asterisks indicate the spaces occupied by the stent filament.

28, 1986 in a patient, who had symptomatic restenosis 13 months after coronary angioplasty.

Description of the stent

The tubular stent is woven from a surgical grade stainless-steel alloy. The prosthesis consists of 16 wire filaments of 0.08 mm thickness. As a result, this prosthesis is pliable, self-expanding and geometrically stable. By longitudinal extension, it can be reduced in diameter and thus constrained on a small caliber catheter. The constraining doubled-over membrane is progressively rolled back and the device will return to its initial large diameter. When implanted, equilibrium is attained between the radial force of the stent and the elastic resistance of the vessel wall.

The outer diameter of the loaded catheter is 1.6 mm. Stents for vessel sizes up to 6 mm in diameter, can be mounted on this delivery system (Fig. 2).

Study population

Indications for the endoluminal stents were coronary restenosis after pre-

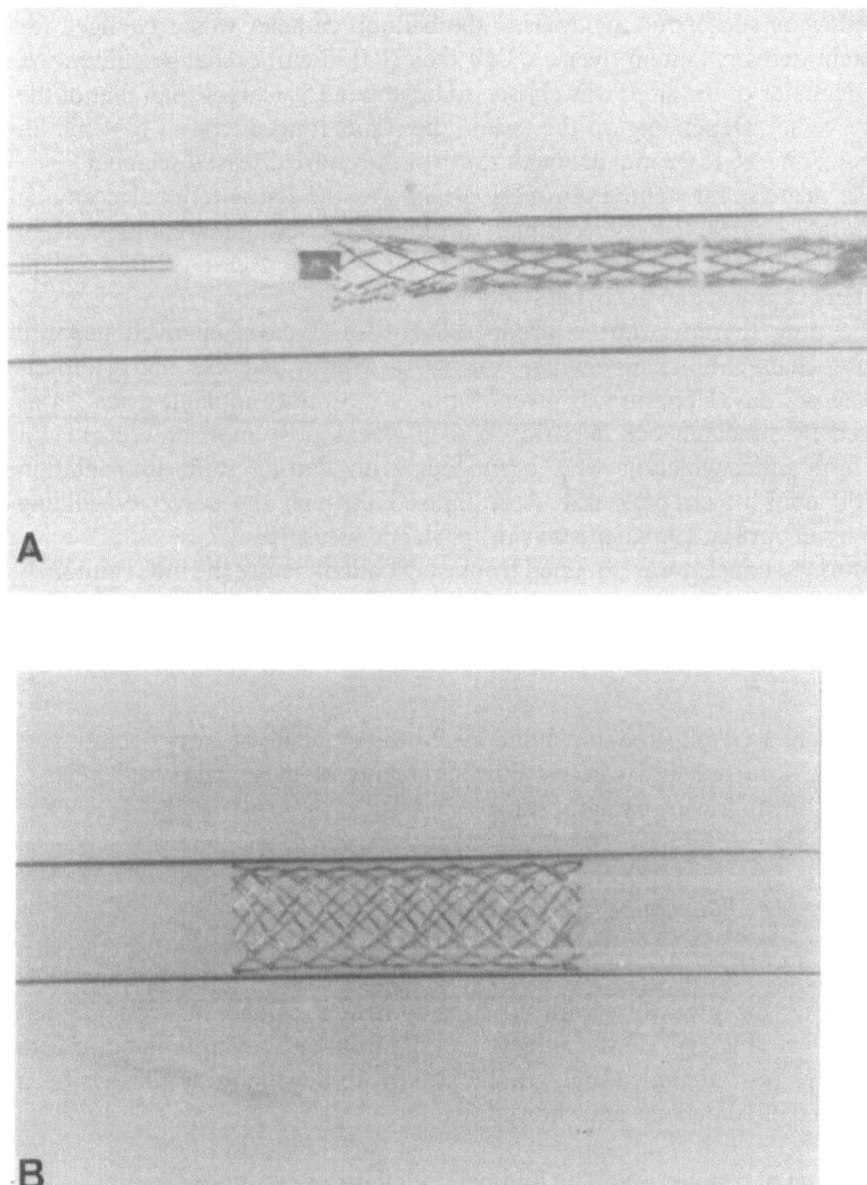

Figure 2. The self-expanding scaffolding prosthesis. (A) One-fourth of the stent open during deployment and (B) unconstrained.

vious dilatation (24 cases) and stenosis of aortocoronary-bypass graft (1 case). A total of twenty-five coronary stents were implanted in 24 patients following transluminal balloon angioplasty and in one patient without prior dilatation.

Following successful angioplasty, the balloon catheter was exchanged for the stent delivery system over a 0.014 inch (0.036 cm) exchange guide wire. The diameter of the stent was chosen to be about 15% larger than that of the native vessel. Depending on the lesion, the stents ranged from 3 to 4 mm in diameter and 15 to 23 mm in length to cover the entire diseased segment.

The dilated and stented coronary artery was the left anterior descending artery in 14 cases, the right coronary artery in 8 cases, the circumflex artery in 2 cases and a coronary artery bypass vein graft in 1 case (in this patient the stent was placed in the bypass graft itself).

The drug therapy, started preoperatively for 2 days, involved heparin, calcium-channel-blocking agents, 250 mg of aspirin and 225 mg of dipyridamole per day. Heparin was given during 9 days post-implant, when it was relayed by subcutaneous heparin up to 6 weeks post-implant. We did not use oral anticoagulation with acenocoumarol. During stent implantation 50,000 units of streptokinase were infused through the coronary guiding catheter in our last 13 patients as a prophylactic measure.

Informed consent was obtained from each patient before the intervention.

Results

There were 15 event-free implantations; however, acute or early occlusion of the stent occurred in 10 cases. Further details of these cases will be presented in the following paragraphs.

1. Event-free implantations (15 patients)

All patients recovered normally, underwent coronary angiography at 2 weeks after the procedure with no signs of restenosis and subsequently left the hospital (Fig. 3). These patients are all stress-test asymptomatic at 2 to 16 months post implant. Angiographic follow-up beyond 6 months has been performed in 10 patients and showed:

— No sign of restenosis and no luminal irregularities in 6 cases.
— Endoluminal stent smoothly embedded with no traces of serious luminal narrowing in 4 cases.
— Restenosis with a narrowing of more than 50%, across the proximal junction of the native vessel and the stent in 1 case.

2. Occlusion of the stent (10 patients)

Occlusion occurred acutely in 4 cases and early on before the tenth day

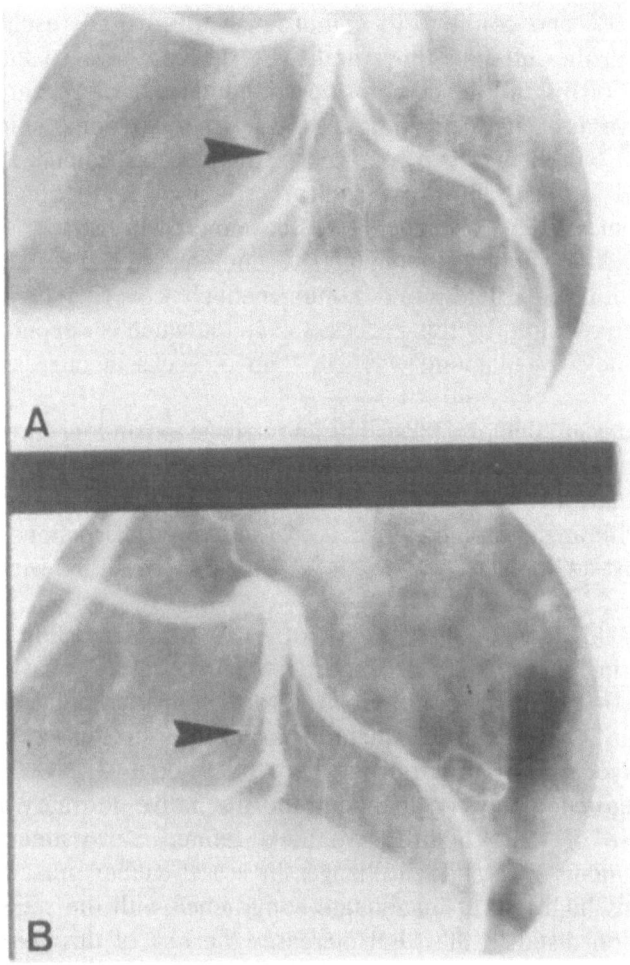

Figure 3. Left coronary artery before angioplasty (A) and 2 weeks after stent implantation (B).

post-implant in 6 cases. In 7 cases angioplasty and lytics were used. Of the 5 primary success cases, 3 reoccluded later. Two of these patients died; one patient (LAD stent), with previous right coronary artery and LAD vein bypass graft occlusions, was a very high risk case refused by the surgeons, and the other patient (LAD stent) died after elective LAD bypass graft following the stenting failure.

Discussion

The problem of restenosis following coronary angioplasty is presently one the main limitations of this promising procedure. The restenosis rates range from 30 to 40% and continue to compromise the overall results [1]. The operator's skill, the inflation times and drug therapy have so far failed to solve these problems and the need for new techniques that prevent restenosis is evident. Several designs including elastically self-expanding spirals of the memory metal type, have been reported in animal experiments [5—9]. The endo-prosthesis used in our first clinical serie was made of a new self-expanding stainless-steel (Medinvent SA, Lausanne, Switzerland).

All experimental studies in animals have demonstrated the occurrence of endothelialisation, completely and homogeneously covering the stent filament. The time required by this process [3, 7—9], which is dependent on the thickness of the wire filament, was less than 6 weeks in our experimental study.

Due to its design, this prosthesis has an intrinsic expanding force of about 2 atmospheres; only in a very limited number of cases this force would be sufficient to dilate a restenosis without prior balloon dilatation. For example, in one case with angiographic evidence of a narrowed dissection, developed 2 months post-angioplasty, we used the stent successfully without prior dilatation.

Our results in patients show a risk of early stent occlusion caused by thrombus during the first 10 days post-implant. Acute or early occlusion occurred in 10 patients, probably related to technical complications of the implantation in 2 cases, to inadequate heparinization in 3 cases, to previous transmural myocardial infarction distal to the stent in 3 cases and to in-adequate congruence between the stent and the native coronary artery in 2 cases. Because of these failures, we have refined our patient selection. Coronary segments with sudden changes in vessel caliber must be avoided because of this high risk of inadequate congruence with the stent. A transmural infarction distal to the stent increases the risk of thrombosis due to poor distal runoff. Indeed we have noted an occlusion in 3 out of 5 patients with an infarction distal to the location of the stent. However, we are now seeing a steady reduction in the number of acute occlusions, probably due to our familiarization with the device and optimisation of the patient selection. It also important to define an optimal drug therapy.

In 15 event-free implantations, our preliminary results revealed only 1 case of restenosis after angiographic follow-up ranging from 6 to 12 months. In this one patient with angiographic restenosis at 6 months post-implantation, the narrowed site is not in the middle of the stented segment, but on the junction between the proximal artery and the stent. This fact suggests that the stent did not cover the entire diseased segment; it incites us to implant longer prostheses.

Beyond this critical period, our preliminary results are encouraging and suggest that intracoronary stent might be a promising adjunct to transluminal coronary angioplasty. However, we do not know the long-term evolution;

therefore, further studies are needed to determine the benefits and the limitations. Only after these facts are known, this method may be used on a larger scale.

References

1. Leimgruber PP, Roubin GS, Hollman J, Cotsonis GA, Meier B, Douglas JS, King III SB, Gruentzig AR: Restenosis after successful coronary angioplasty in patients with single-vessel disease. Circulation 73: 710—717, 1986.
2. Austin GE, Ratliff NB, Hollman J, Tabei S, Phillips DF: Intimal proliferation of smooth muscle cells as an explanation for recurrent coronary artery stenosis after percutaneous transluminal coronary angioplasty. J Am Coll Cardiol 6: 369—375, 1985.
3. Sigwart U, Puel J, Mirkovitch V, Joffre F, Kappenberger L: Intravascular stents to prevent occlusion and restenosis after transluminal angioplasty. N Engl J Med 316: 701—706, 1987.
4. Puel J, Sigwart U, Joffre F, Rousseau H, Courtault A, Bounhoure JP: Percutaneously implantable endo-coronary prosthesis: Preliminary results in the treatment of post-dilation restenosis. J Am Coll Cardiol 9: 106A, 1987 (Abstract).
5. Dotter CT, Buschmann RW, McKinney MK, Rösch J: Transluminal expandable nitinol coil stent grafting: preliminary report. Radiology 147: 259—260, 1983.
6. Cragg A, Lund G, Rysavy J, Castaneda F, Castaneda-Zuniga W, Amplatz K: Nonsurgical placement of arterial endoprostheses: a new technique using nitinol wire. Radiology 147: 261—263, 1983.
7. Maass D, Zollikofer CL, Largiader F, Senning A: Radiological follow-up of transluminally inserted vascular endoprostheses: an experimental study using expanding spirals. Radiology 152: 659—663, 1984.
8. Palmaz JC, Sibbitt RR, Reuter SR, Tio FO, Rice WJ: Expandable intraluminal graft: a preliminary study. Radiology 156: 73—77, 1985.
9. Wright KC, Wallace S, Charnsangavej C, Carrasco CH, Gianturco C: Percutaneous endovascular stents: an experimental evaluation. Radiology 156: 69—72, 1985.

18. A coronary endoprosthesis to prevent restenosis and acute occlusion after percutaneous angioplasty: One and a half year of clinical experience

ULRICH SIGWART, S. GOLF, U. KAUFMANN, and
L. KAPPENBERGER

SUMMARY. The high incidence of chronic restenosis and acute occlusions seen after balloon dilatation of coronary arteries (PTCA) is a persisting problem. Despite improvements of equipment as well as drug treatment the restenosis rate is about 30% and the rate of acute occlusions is about 5% [1—3]. One way to overcome both these problems is to give mechanical support to the vessel wall using an endoprosthesis or stent. Such a device will also smooth the endothelial surface of the vessel which otherwise often is very rugged after the PTCA procedure, potentially preventing platelet aggregation and formation of thrombosis.

The endoprosthesis (stent)

A stent which consists of an elastic porous tube made from medical grade steel alloy was developed in cooperation with Medinvent SA, Lausanne. The tubular mesh form of the stent makes it highly flexible along its long axis and gives it a self-expanding capacity when released. Before deployment the stent is sandwiched in its restrained form between the shaft of the deploying catheter and a flexible double layered sheath. With the stent in correct position, retraction of the double layered sheath will free the stent and allow it to expand to its fully unrestrained elastic form [4]. A free stent and a stent halfway freed from its deploying catheter are shown in Fig. 1. The preceeding animal experiments and the first clinical experience with the stent have been reported elsewhere [4].

Patients. Follow-up. Drug treatment

Between April 1986 and mid October 1987, 64 stents have been implanted in 53 patients, their age ranging from 35 to 60 years (mean 55 years). Table 1 gives the location of the stents and the indication for stent implantation. Nine patients received two different stents in one or two procedures and two patients received three different stents in two and three different procedures.

J. C. Reiber & P. W. Serruys (eds.), New Developments in Quantitative Coronary Arteriography,
278—284.

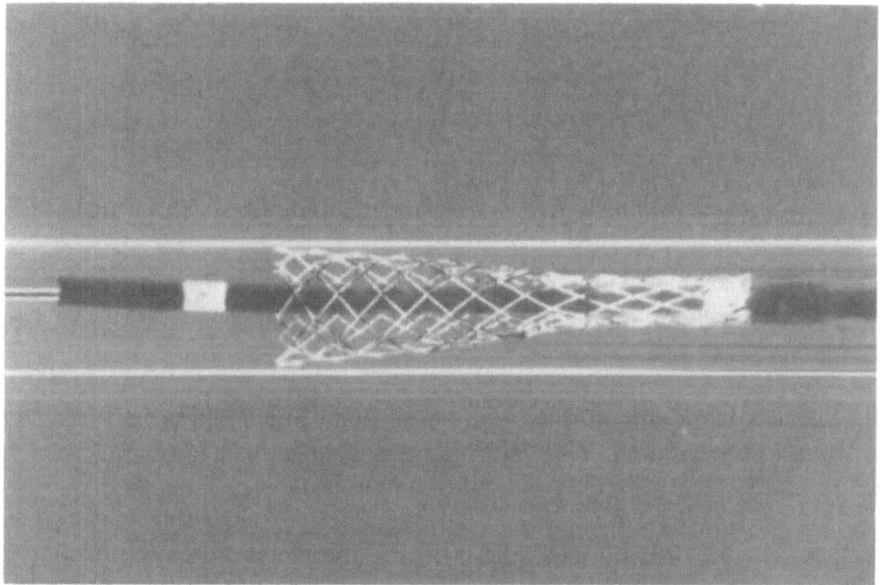

A

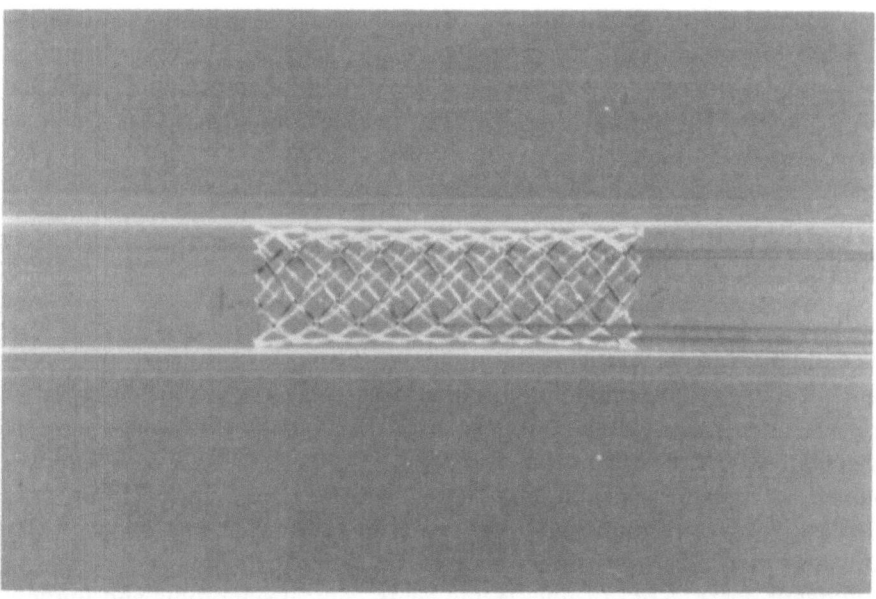

B

Figure 1. The endocoronary prosthesis or stent partly liberated from its deploying catheter (A); and in its free fully expanded form (B).

Table 1. 64 Coronary stents according to localization and indication.

	LAD	Cx	RCA	CABG	RIMA
Restenosis (elective)	22	5	9	19	1
Acute occlusion	3	0	5	0	0
Total	25	5	14	19	1

LAD = left anterior descending coronary artery; Cx = circumflex coronary artery; RCA = right coronary artery; CABG = coronary artery bypass graft; RIMA = right internal mammary artery.

All patients gave their informed consent to stent implantation according to the Helsinki Declaration. The indication for stent implantation was in each case posed by at least two cardiologists and one cardiovascular surgeon.

All patients have been clinically followed closely. Control angiography has been carried out the next morning after the implantation and then after 3 months, 6 months and one year. An exercise ECG has also been carried out after 6 weeks. One day before the implantation patients received antiplatelet drugs consisting of acetylsalicylic acid, dipyridamole and sulfinpyrazol. Immediately before implantation the patients received heparin intravenously. During deployment of the stents urokinase was given in a slow drip through the guiding catheter. After implantation heparin and then oral anticoagulants were continued for at least three months. A calcium antagonist (nifedipine) was also given.

Results

We have seen two cases of restenosis, both with stents in the left anterior descending artery (LAD). In one of these, the stenosis started in the left main coronary artery, extending into the stent in the LAD. Furthermore, we have seen four cases with a new stenosis of the stented vessel which were all located in different segments proximally to the stent. These cases are not counted as restenosis (Table 2). There have been one early closure and two late closures resulting in three cases of myocardial infarction (AMI). Altogether we have seen three deaths among the patients. In the case of early death post-CABG (Table 2), the acute clinical symptoms and findings strongly suggested occlusion of the stented vessel. During the emergency operation, the vessel was found open; however, the patient died from complications in the post-operative period. As stated previously, this patient probably had a serious attack of coronary spasm [4]. The case of late death post-CABG (Table 2) is the same patient recorded as having a serious new

Table 2. 64 Coronary stents in 53 patients: restenosis and complications.*

	No	%
Early closure (< 3 days)	1	1.7
Late closure	2	3.3
Restenosis	2	3.3
AMI	3	5
Early death (post-CABG)	1	1.7
Late death (post-CABG)	1	1.7
Late sudden death	1	1.7

CABG = coronary artery bypass graft.
* Some patients had more than one complication. The nine complications (not including restenosis) were altogether seen in 6 different patients.

stenosis of the left main coronary artery. This patient underwent a third elective bypass operation from which he did not recover due to post-operative complications. The case of late sudden death (Table 2) died at home without an autopsy being performed. Later it turned out that this patient had not taken his prescribed anti-coagulation therapy. The nine different complications (whereby restenosis is not counted as a true complication) summarized in Table 2 were seen in altogether six different patients. In the other patients no complications were seen except for a few cases of moderate bleeding and coronary spasms which could all be handled easily. Some intimal thickening within the stent has been seen in most patients. Except for the two patients with serious restenoses, these thickenings have never exceeded 20% of the overall luminal diameter. A typical example of successful coronary stenting is shown in Fig. 2.

Discussion

We have implanted 64 coronary endoprostheses (stents) in 53 patients and seen 9 serious complications among six patients, three of which were fatal. In the other 47 patients only a few minor and transient complications have been seen. There have been two cases of significant restenosis within or in close proximity of the stent. The number of restenoses is certainly lower than should be expected in view of the special selection of patients taken into consideration. Thus it is likely that the endoprosthesis is able to prevent restenosis after multiple angioplasties. The stent has also been successful in acute occlusions immediately following the PTCA procedure. The four cases with a new stenosis in the vessel proximally to the stent, were considered to be extensions of the underlying arteriosclerotic disease. Three of these were

A

B

C

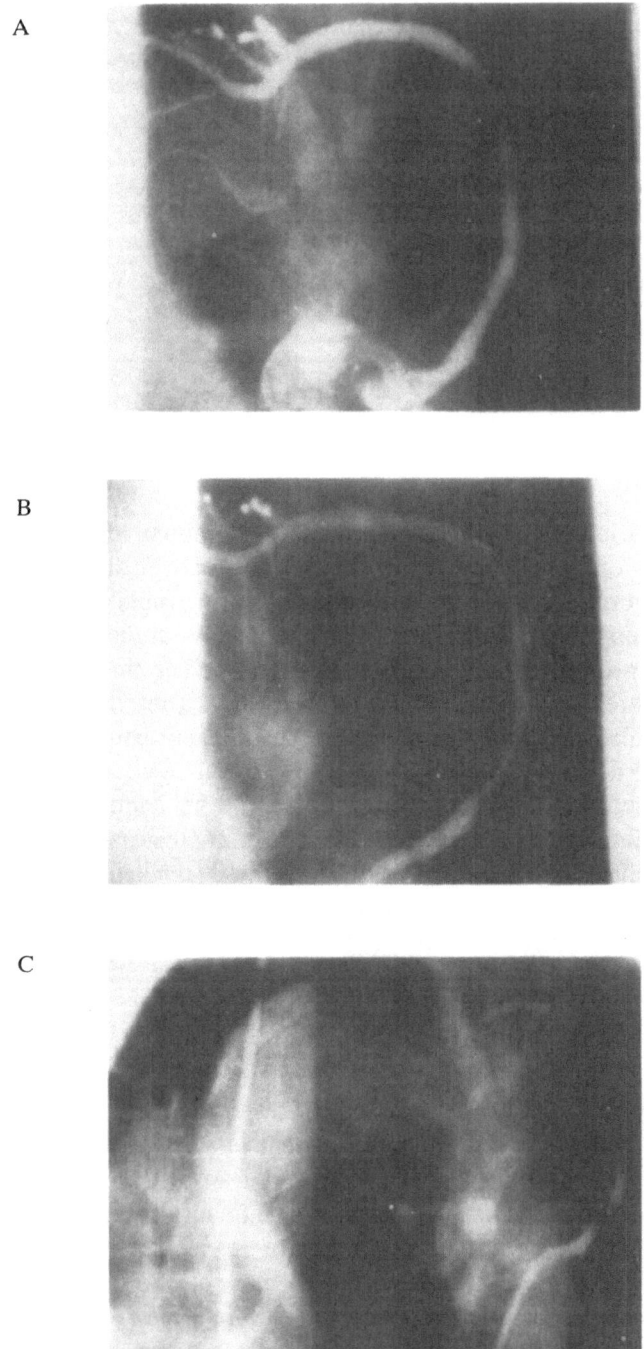

Figure 2. The right coronary artery with a very tight stenosis in its proximal part (A). After balloon dilatation the proximal part is still rugged and shows a residual stenosis (B), which has been smoothed away after stent implantation (C).

observed in bypass grafts, all of which were in bad general condition before the first stent implantation. It has been reported, however, that damage to the proximal part of the vessel wall by the instrumentation may provoke fibrous cellular hypoplesia and stenosis [5]. Although this mechanism is not very likely in these four cases, we cannot completely exclude it, since no histological examinations of the vessels could be undertaken for obvious reasons. On the other hand, the number of new stenoses seen in this patient group is close to that reported from follow-up after ordinary PTCA without stent implantation [6].

As for the safety of the stent and the implantation procedure, three fatal cases may seem to be a high toll and naturally are a matter of great concern. However, at least in two of these fatal cases, a direct relationship between the endoprosthesis and the fatal outcome is difficult to establish. The patient who died suddenly at home emphasizes the importance of drug treatment and a careful patient follow-up in the post implantation period.

The mechanism of the beneficial effect of the stent is largely unknown. Probably the most important factors are smoothing of the vessel wall, resistance to elastic recoil of the stenosis and improvement of blood flow pattern through the lesion [7—9]; pressure measurements have shown no residual pressure gradients after stenting. After endothelialization of the stent [4], the formed 'neo-intima' may also represent a barrier to further thrombosis and cell ingrowth.

Since no control groups were used, we think that all conclusions should be regarded with great caution. Taking into consideration that our patients presented multiple problems difficult to deal with, we think, however, that our results are encouraging. The rate of restenosis is certainly lower than what should be expected after yet another redilatation without stenting. The preliminary data suggest that the stent is also able to solve the problem of acute occlusion during the PTCA procedure. The complication rate is still high but steadily diminishing. During this time we have gained important experience and we feel confident to carry on with this treatment, keeping our minds highly alert to the long-term effects.

References

1. Holmes Jr DR, Vlietstra RE, Smith HC, Vetrovec GW, Kent KM, Cowley MJ, Faxon DP, Gruentzig AR, Kelsey SF, Detre KM, Van Raden MJ, Mock MB: Restenosis after percutaneous transluminal coronary angioplasty (PTCA): a report from the PTCA Registry of the National Heart, Lung and Blood Institute. Am J Cardiol 53: 77C—81C, 1984.
2. Leimgruber PP, Roubin GS, Hollman J, Cotsonis GA, Meier B, Douglas JS, King III SB, Gruentzig AR: Restenosis after successful coronary angioplasty in patients with single-vessel disease. Circulation 73: 710—717, 1986.
3. Sugrue DD, Vlietstra RE, Hammes LN, Holmes Jr DR: Repeat balloon coronary angioplasty for symptomatic restenoses: A note of caution. Eur Heart J 8: 697—701, 1987.

4. Sigwart U, Puel J, Mirkovitch V, Joffre F, Kappenberger L: Intravascular stents to prevent occlusion and restenosis after transluminal angioplasty. N Engl J Med. 316: 701—706, 1987.
5. Waller BF, Pinkerton CA, Foster LN: Morphologic evidence of accelerated left main coronary artery stenosis: a late complication of percutaneous transluminal balloon angioplasty of the proximal left anterior descending coronary artery. J Am Coll Cardiol 9: 1019—1023, 1987.
6. Joelson JM, Most AS, Williams DO: Angiographic findings when chest pain recurs after successful percutaneous transluminal coronary angioplasty. Am J Cardiol 60: 792—795, 1987.
7. Maass D, Demierre D, Deaton D, *et al.*: Transluminal implantation of self-adjusting expandable prostheses: Principles, techniques and results. Prog Artif Organs: 979—987, 1983.
8. Wright KC, Wallace S, Cgarnangavej C, Carrasco CH, Gianturco C: Percutaneous endovascular stents: An experimental evaluation. Radiology 156: 69—72, 1985.
9. Palmaz JC, Kopp DT, Hayashi H, Schatz RA, Hunter G, Tio FO, Garcia O, Alvarado R, Rees C, Thomas SC: Normal and stenotic renal arteries: experimental balloon-expandable intraluminal stenting. Radiology 164: 705—708, 1987.

Index of subjects